Mauro Di Pasquale, M.D.

Assistant Professor
University of Toronto
Toronto, Ontario, Canada

Amino Acids *and* Proteins *for the* Athlete

The Anabolic Edge

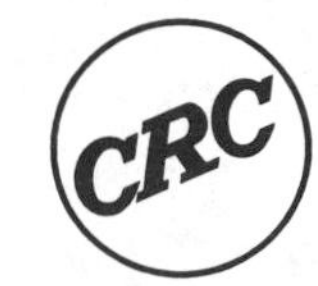

CRC Press
Boca Raton New York

Library of Congress Cataloging-in-Publication Data

Di Pasquale, Mauro G.
Amino acids and proteins for the athlete— the anabolic edge / Mauro Di Pasquale.
p. cm. -- (Nutrition in exercise and sport)
Includes bibliographical references and index.
ISBN 0-8493-8193-2
1. Proteins in human nutrition. 2. Amino acids in human nutrition.
3. Athletes--Nutrition. 4. Dietary supplements.
I. Title. II. Series.
QP551.D46 1997
612.3′98′088796--dc21 97-4307
CIP

International Standard Book Number 0-8493-8193-2
Library of Congress Card Number 97-4307
Printed in the United States of America 1 2 3 4 5 6 7 8 9 0
Printed on acid-free paper

NUTRITION in EXERCISE and SPORT

Editors, Ira Wolinsky and James F. Hickson, Jr.

Published Titles

Nutrients as Ergogenic Aids for Sports and Exercise
Luke R. Bucci

Nutrition in Exercise and Sport, 2nd Edition
Ira Wolinsky and James F. Hickson, Jr.

Exercise and Disease
Ronald R. Watson and Marianne Eisinger

Nutrition Applied to Injury Rehabilitation and Sports Medicine
Luke R. Bucci

Nutrition for the Recreational Athlete
Catherine G.R. Jackson

NUTRITION in EXERCISE and SPORT

Editor, Ira Wolinsky

Published Titles

Nutrition, Physical Activity, and Health in Early Life
Jana Parízková

Exercise and Immune Function
Laurie Hoffman-Goetz

Sports Nutrition: Minerals and Electrolytes
Constance Kies and Judy A. Driskell

Nutrition and the Female Athlete
Jaime S. Ruud

Body Fluid Balance: Exercise and Sport
Elsworth R. Buskirk and Susan M. Puhl

Handbook of Sports Nutrition: Vitamins and Trace Minerals
Ira Wolinsky and Judy A. Driskell

Sports Nutrition: Vitamins and Trace Elements
Ira Wolinsky and Judy A. Driskell

Forthcoming Titles

Nutrition Exercise and Sport, Third Edition
Ira Wolinsky and Judy A. Driskell

SERIES PREFACE

The CRC series, Nutrition in Exercise and Sport, provides a setting for in-depth exploration of the many and varied aspects of nutrition and exercise, including sports. The topic of exercise and sports nutrition has been a focus of research among scientists since the 1960s, and the healthful benefits of good nutrition and exercise have been appreciated. As our knowledge expands, it will be necessary to remember that there must be a range of diets and exercise regimes that will support excellent physical condition and performance. There is not a single diet-exercise treatment that can be the common denominator, or the single formula for health, or panacea for performance.

This series is dedicated to providing a stage upon which to explore these issues. Each volume provides a detailed and scholarly examination of some aspect of the topic.

Contributors from any bona fide area of nutrition and physical activity, including sports and the controversial, are welcome.

We welcome to the Series a timely and authoritative monograph on *Amino Acids and Proteins for the Athlete — The Anabolic Edge* by the very knowledgeable, energetic, and talented Mauro Di Pasquale, M.D.

Ira Wolinsky, Ph.D.
Series Editor

PREFACE

We need water and food to survive. Without water we can only survive 3 to 4 days. Without food, we can last a while longer. However, once our internal energy stores are exhausted, we perish. Our food contains, or at least should contain, the nutrients we need to live and grow.

While the carbohydrates, fats, and protein that make up our food are all important macronutrients, of the three, protein is the most important and versatile. Not only do proteins make up three quarters of body solids[1] (including structural and contractile proteins, enzymes, nucleoproteins, and proteins that transport oxygen) but protein and amino acids have potent biological effects on the body that involve all tissues in the body and extend to almost all metabolic processes.

Significant research has been conducted to determine the protein requirements of athletes and the effects of increasing both the amount and quality of dietary protein; the effects protein and amino acid supplements have on both athletic performance, primarily on muscle size and strength and energy metabolism; and the effects of specific amino acid supplements on metabolic and physiological responses to strength and endurance exercise.

There has recently been an increased interest in determining the ergogenic effect of specific amino acids. As we shall see, numerous studies have indicated that various amino acids are involved in the metabolic and physiological responses to both acute and chronic exercise. Because of a perceived need for protein, athletes have increased both their dietary protein consumption and the use of commercial protein and amino acid supplements.

In this book we will examine the available scientific and medical information in order to determine the physiological and pharmacological effects of protein and amino acids on lean body mass, body fat, strength, and endurance. Some of the information presented below will serve as a brief review of energy and protein metabolism in order to help the reader understand some of the more important information on just how proteins and amino acids can be used to increase lean body mass, and strength, lose body fat, and have a positive impact on athletic performance, health, disease, and longevity.

THE AUTHOR

Mauro G. Di Pasquale, M.D., M.R.O., M.F.S., is a licensed physician in Ontario, Canada specializing in Sports Medicine. He is an Assistant Professor at the University of Toronto researching and lecturing on athletic performance, nutritional supplements, and drug use in sports.

Dr. Di Pasquale holds an honors degree in Biological Science, majoring in Molecular Biochemistry (1968), and a medical degree (1971) both from the University of Toronto. He is certified as a Medical Review Officer (M.R.O.) by the Medical Review Officer Certification Council (MROCC), and as a Master of Fitness Sciences (M.F.S.) by the International Sports Sciences Association (ISSA).

Dr. Di Pasquale is the Drug Program Advisor to the World Wrestling Federation (WWF) and past Medical Director and Drug Program Advisor to the now defunct World Bodybuilding Federation (WBF). He is also the acting M.R.O. for the National Association for Stock Car Auto Racing (NASCAR).

He has been involved in international sports and drug testing for the past 30 years as an athlete, an administrator, and a physician. Dr. Di Pasquale was a world-class athlete for over 20 years, winning the world championships in powerlifting in 1976, and the World Games in the sport of Powerlifting in 1981. He was Canadian champion eight times, Pan American champion twice, and North American champion twice.

Dr. Di Pasquale was the chairman of the International Powerlifting Federation's Medical Committee for 8 years (1979–1987) and was on the committee for a total of 12 years. As chairman of the IPF Medical Committee, the Canadian Powerlifting Union Medical Committee, and the Canadian Amateur Federation of Bodybuilding Medical Committee, and as a consultant to various sporting federations he has had extensive exposure to athletic injuries and disabilities and drug use by athletes.

In the early 1980s Dr. Di Pasquale initiated and developed the IPF drug-testing protocols and procedures. At present, he is still actively involved with the IPF and the CPU (Canadian Powerlifting Union) as both a medical advisor and drug-testing officer.

Dr. Di Pasquale has written several books dealing with the use of drugs and nutritional supplements by athletes, including *Drug Use and Detection in Amateur Sports, Beyond Anabolic Steroids, Anabolic Steroid Side Effects, Fact Fiction and Treatment*, and *The Bodybuilding Supplement Review.* In the past 25 years he has written hundreds of articles on supplements, nutrition, drugs, and exercise for magazines and association journals, as well as numerous contributed chapters on anabolic steroids and drug testing to several fitness, weight, and sports medicine books.

At present, Dr. Di Pasquale has regular monthly columns and articles in several bodybuilding and powerlifting magazines, including *Muscle & Fitness, Men's Fitness, Flex; Iron Man, Muscle Mag International* and *Powerlifting U.S.A*. In the past few decades he has been on several Editorial Boards for various fitness and strength magazines and is presently on the Editorial Advisory Board of *Men's Fitness* and *Muscle and Fitness.*

He was the Editor-in chief of a quarterly international newsletter entitled *Drugs in Sports,* published in English, Spanish, and Italian. He is currently Editor-in-chief of a bimonthly newsletter entitled *The Anabolic Research Review.* Both newsletters contained information on the use of drugs and nutritional supplements by athletes.

Dr. Di Pasquale also acts as an international consultant and expert witness for athletes, amateur and professional sports bodies, and government agencies on legal matters relating to the use and abuse, and drug testing of anabolic steroids, growth hormone, and other ergogenic drugs and supplements.

CONTENTS

Chapter 3
Energy Metabolism 49

Chapter 4
Dietary Protein and Amino Acids 63

Chapter 5
Protein Foods vs. Protein and Amino Acid Supplements 89

Chapter 1

PROTEINS AND AMINO ACIDS

INTRODUCTION

The word protein comes from the Greek word "proteios" which means "of the first rank or importance". Protein is indeed important for life and is involved in every biological process within the body. The average human body is approximately 18% protein. Proteins are essential components of muscle, skin, cell membranes, blood, hormones, antibodies, enzymes, and genetic material and almost all other body tissues and components. They serve as structural components, biocatalysts (enzymes), antibodies, lubricants, messengers (hormones), and as carriers.

The contribution made by proteins to the energy value of most well-balanced diets is usually between 10 and 15% of the total and seldom exceeds 20%. In some athletes in power sports, and in bodybuilders who may be on very high-protein diets, the contribution can be as high as 50%, and in selective cases even more.

However, the energy contribution that proteins make in diets is usually secondary — their real importance lies in the fact that every cell in the body is partly composed of proteins which are subject to continuous wear and replacement. Carbohydrates and fats contain no nitrogen or sulfur, two essential elements in all proteins. Whereas the fat in the body can be derived from dietary carbohydrates and the carbohydrates from proteins, the proteins of the body are inevitably dependent for their formation and maintenance on the proteins in food. Proteins from food are digested and the resultant amino acids and peptides are absorbed and used to synthesize body proteins.

Proteins are large molecules with molecular weights ranging from 1000 to over 1,000,000 Da. In their native state some are soluble and some insoluble in water. Although there are a great variety of proteins that can be subdivided into various categories, they are all are made up of the same building blocks called amino acids.

Every species of animal has its characteristic proteins — the proteins of beef muscle, for instance, differ from those of pork muscle. It is the proteins that give each species its specific immunological characteristics and uniqueness.

Plants can synthesize all the amino acids they need from simple inorganic chemical compounds, but animals are unable to do this because they cannot synthesize the amino (NH_2) group. In order to obtain the amino acids necessary for building protein they must eat plants or other animals which have lived on plants.

The human body has a certain limited capability of converting one amino acid into another. This is achieved in the liver partly by the process of transamination, whereby an amino group is shifted from one molecule across to another under the influence of aminotransferase, the coenzyme of which is pyridoxal phosphate. However, the ability of the body to convert one amino acid into another is restricted. There are several amino acids which the body cannot make for itself and so must be obtained from the diet. These are termed essential amino acids.

Under normal circumstances, the adult human body can maintain nitrogenous equilibrium on a mixture of eight pure amino acids as its sole source of nitrogen. These eight are isoleucine, leucine, lysine, methionine, phenylalanine, threonine, tryptophan, and valine. Several amino acids, including arginine, histidine, and glutamine, are felt by some to be conditionally essential. That is, under certain conditions such as growth, these amino acids are not able to be synthesized in adequate amounts and thus need to be supplied in the diet.

Synthesis of the conditionally essential and nonessential amino acids depends mainly on the formation first of appropriate alpha-keto acids, the precursors of the respective amino acids. For instance, pyruvic acid, which is formed in large quantities during the glycolytic breakdown of glucose, is the keto acid precursor of the amino acid alanine. Then, by the process of transamination, an amino radical is transferred from certain amino acids to the alpha-keto acid while the keto oxygen is transferred to the donor of the amino radical. In the formation of alanine, for example, the amino radical is transferred to the pyruvic acid from one of several possible amino acid donors including asparagine, glutamine, glutamic acid, and aspartic acid.

Transamination is promoted by several enzymes among which are the aminotransferases, which are derivatives of pyridoxine (B_6), one of the B vitamins. Without this vitamin the nonessential amino acids are synthesized only poorly and, therefore, protein formation cannot proceed normally. The formation of protein can also be affected by other vitamins, minerals, and nutrients.

All proteins are made up of varying numbers of amino acids attached together in a specific sequence and having a specific architecture. The sequence of the amino acids differentiates one protein from another, and gives the protein special physiological and biological properties.

AMINO ACIDS

Amino acids are characterized by the presence of an amino (NH_2) group with basic properties (hence the term amino in amino acid) and a carboxyl (COOH) group with acidic properties (hence the term acid in amino acid), attached to the same carbon atom. The rest of the molecule varies with the particular amino acid. Since all amino acids contain both an acid and a base, they, unlike other biological material, are capable of both acid and base reactions in the body.

The structure of an amino acid may be represented by the formula:

$$\begin{array}{c} H \\ | \\ R - C - COOH \\ | \\ NH_2 \end{array}$$

where NH_2 is the amino group, COOH is the carboxyl group, and R represents the remainder of the molecule.

In the formation of protein, amino acids are linked together by the peptide linkage in which the basic (amino) group of one amino acid is linked to the carboxyl group of another, with the elimination of a molecule of water. Since all amino acids contain both NH_2 and COOH groups, long chains of amino acids may be formed. The resultant chain of amino acids therefore has an amino group at one end (the N-terminus) and a carboxyl group at the other end (the C-terminus). Amino acids with side chains possessing carboxyl groups are known as acidic amino acids; those with side chains possessing amino groups are known as basic amino acids; the remaining amino acids are termed neutral amino acids.

$$\mathrm{R{-}\underset{\displaystyle NH_2}{\overset{\displaystyle H}{C}}{-}COOH + NH_2{-}\underset{\displaystyle R}{\overset{\displaystyle H}{C}}{-}COOH}$$

$$= \mathrm{R{-}\underset{\displaystyle NH_2}{\overset{\displaystyle H}{C}}{-}CO\text{-}NH{-}\underset{\displaystyle R}{\overset{\displaystyle H}{C}}{-}COOH + H_2O}$$

These amino acid chains are called peptides or proteins. A chain of up to 100 amino acids is called a polypeptide. Two joined amino acids form a dipeptide, three form a tripeptide, and so on. A string of amino acids form a protein when more than 100 amino acids are joined together. The great variation in properties observed among proteins, whether it be the insulin secreted by the pancreas, the collagen found in connective tissues, or the hemoglobin of the blood, is largely due to the enormous number of ways in which these amino acids can be arranged.

However, there is more to a protein than the number of amino acids that make it up. A protein is a polypeptide chain (or a number of such chains) that has attained a unique, stable, three-dimensional shape (referred to as its native conformation), and is biologically active as a result. The shape of the protein is a result of interactions between various portions of the amino acids. If a protein is denatured by way of enzymes, heating, or by chemicals, changes occur in the shape of the protein. These changes, usually an uncoiling or unfolding of the protein structure, make the protein more vulnerable to degradation or digestion, destroying its biological effectiveness.

While the number of amino acids in various proteins can vary considerably (some proteins may contain hundreds of thousands of amino acids) there are only about 23 different amino acids that are used as building blocks for biological matter. Twenty or so of these amino acids are commonly found in animal protein and are the amino acids upon which we will concentrate in this book. The nature of the protein is determined by the types of amino acids in the protein, and also by the order in which they are joined.

All amino acids, save glycine, are asymmetrical and can assume different configurations in space, giving them the characteristic of chirality. Amino acids can, therefore, exist in two forms, designated D and L, both of which are found in nature. While both forms are found in nature and have biological effects, only the L form is found in proteins.

Protein and amino acids, like lipids and carbohydrates, are classified as macronutrients since they make up a large part of our diets. While there are recommended dietary protein intakes, there are no recommended dietary allowances set for individual amino acids.

Amino acids are involved in a number of important metabolic functions besides protein synthesis and the regulation of protein synthesis and catabolism. They can be precursors to neurotransmitters and also function as neurotransmitters. They are involved in energy production, ammonia and urea production, hormone synthesis, hormone activation and release, and in preventing oxidative damage through their antioxidant effects.

PROTEIN SYNTHESIS

In order to duplicate exact amino acid sequences, the body uses complex processes that allow copying of genetic information and translation of that information into the formation of specific proteins.

Nucleic acids are polymers of nucleotides. Ribonucleic acid (RNA) and deoxyribonucleic acid (DNA) are responsible for the storage, expression, and transmission of genetic information. The DNA of each individual creature is unique in the sequence of its nucleotide bases. It is this sequence which provides a set of instructions that ultimately directs each cell to synthesize a characteristic set of proteins.

Thus when a certain protein is needed, the cellular DNA provides a template of that protein that is carried to the ribosomes, the site of protein synthesis in the cell. Ribosomal RNA (rRNA) is an important constituent of the ribosomes and has a major functional role in many, and possibly all, ribosomal processes. The amino acid sequence of a polypeptide is specified by mRNA. The information is carried to the ribosome by a molecule of messenger RNA (mRNA). The mRNA transcribes, or copies, this genetic information from the DNA in a process appropriately called transcription.

In the process called translation, amino acids are assembled on ribosomes according to the sequence specified by the mRNA. As the ribosome travels along the mRNA chain and translates its code, the required amino acids (floating free in the cytoplasm) are brought to the ribosome by a specific transfer RNA (tRNA) molecule, of which there are at least one for each different amino acid. One by one, amino acids are linked together by peptide bonds until the sequence has been completed. A recognition process between the tRNA that is linked to the amino acid and the mRNA that is bound to the ribosome on which polypeptide synthesis takes place ensures that the correct amino acid is chosen for each successive amino acid addition. As well as information (specific order of amino acids), peptide bond formation in the cell requires energy to activate the incoming amino acid and link it to tRNA.

REGULATION OF PROTEIN SYNTHESIS

Following resistance training, the ribosomal machinery of skeletal muscle increases in activity and begins to decode mRNA molecules into protein more quickly.[2] This is likely in preparation for the replacement and hypertrophic adaptive response to exercise.

The amount of protein synthesis that takes place during and after exercise is dependent on several factors including a complete complement of precursor amino acids, specific acetylating enzymes, tRNA, and adequate ATP levels. While the relation of protein synthesis to the ambient concentrations of amino acids in the intracellular and extracellular pools has not been defined, it is possible to identify sets of intracellular amino acids that predict the level of protein synthesis, and to delineate combinations of plasma amino acids whose levels account for a significant portion of the variance in the intracellular predictor amino acids in normal human infants and adults.

In one study the intracellular concentrations of most amino acids were found to be higher than their concentrations in plasma, except for valine and citrulline, which were lower.[3] The "aminograms" in the two pools also were very different: 44% of the variance in protein synthesis was accounted for by the intracellular concentrations of leucine, glycine, alanine, and taurine in neonates, and 45% by a combination of threonine, valine, methionine, and histidine in adults. The intracellular concentrations of each of these predictor amino acids in adults were, in turn, related to different combinations of the plasma concentrations of threonine, phenylalanine, tryptophan, isoleucine, histidine, citrulline, ornithine, arginine, and glycine.

The increases in intracellular amino acid concentrations seen with exercise may reflect decreased protein synthesis, accelerated protein catabolism, an increase in amino acid transport into the cell, or combinations of these conditions. For example, an increase in protein synthesis would be expected to cause a decrease in amino acids, but this may be offset by an increase in intracellular availability due to increased transport. As well, altered intracellular amino acid levels may directly regulate exchange diffusion of intracellular for extracellular amino acid(s).

In order to have a net increase in protein synthesis so that there is an increase in the concentration of a protein in a cell, its rate of synthesis would have to increase or its breakdown decrease, or both. There are at least four ways in which the concentration of protein in a cell could be changed:

1. The rate of synthesis of the mRNA that codes for the particular protein(s) could be increased (known as transcriptional control).
2. The rate of synthesis of the polypeptide chain by the ribosomal-mRNA complex could be increased (known as translational control).
3. The rate of degradation of the mRNA could be decreased (also translational control).
4. The rate of degradation of the protein could be decreased.

The following table outlines some of the conditions or factors affecting protein synthesis. Many of these conditions and factors are interrelated.

TABLE 1 Some Conditions and Factors Affecting Protein Synthesis

Conditions or Factors	Effect on Rate of Protein Synthesis
Decreased protein intake	Decreased
Increased protein intake	Increased
Decreased energy intake	Decreased
Increased cellular hydration	Increased
Decreased cellular hydration	Decreased
Increased intake of leucine in presence of sufficiency of other amino acids	Increased
Increased intake of glutamine in presence of sufficiency of other amino acids	Increased
Lack of nervous stimulation	Decreased
Muscle stretch, or exercise	Increased
Overtraining	Decreased
Testosterone (and anabolic steroids)	Increased
Growth hormone	Increased
Insulin-like growth factor-1 (IGF-1)	Increased
Normal thyroxine levels	Increased
Excess thyroxine	Decreased
Catecholamines (including synthetic β-adrenergic agonist such as clenbuterol)	Increased
Glucocorticoids	Decreased
Physical trauma, infection	Decreased

CELLULAR HYDRATION AND PROTEIN SYNTHESIS

There are many factors that determine overall nitrogen balance as taking place in either a positive (anabolic) or negative (catabolic) direction, including stress, trauma, hormones, and nutritional substrate availability. One way in which these factors can directly trigger changes in protein turnover is by their effect on cellular hydration.[4] The state of intracellular hydration, or the amount of water inside cells, which is related to overall cell volume, is now thought to be one of the most important mechanisms in determining cellular protein synthesis and catabolism. It now appears that when a muscle cell's water content is high, anabolic or protein synthesis reactions are stimulated to occur. The converse is also true: when cells are dehydrated, protein synthesis decreases and catabolism increases.

It's important to understand that cellular hydration refers to an intracellular state and as such is different from extracellular hydration that is manifested either as water retention or volume depletion (extracellular dehydration) as measured by the degree of peripheral edema, overall blood volume, blood pressure, and serum concentrations of electrolytes.

While distinct, both intracellular and extracellular hydration have areas of overlap. Substances that promote extracellular water retention can likewise positively influence intracellular water retention. But this must not be misconstrued to mean that a general systemic water retention is in any way anabolic. In fact, one study showed that an increase in plasma volume induced by hypertonic fluids may come entirely at the expense of cell volume, not interstitial volume.[5] In this study, using isolated perfused cat calf muscle, the rapid increases in plasma osmolality caused by using NaCl or sucrose resulted in cellular dehydration.

The cell's intracellular hydration is largely determined by two factors:

1. The concentration and activity of various intracellular ions (sodium [Na^+], potassium [K^+], and chloride [Cl^-]), and
2. The concentration of certain substrates (particularly amino acids) within cells. These factors are chiefly independent of each other.

Each cell in the body has an electrical potential or gradient, based upon the intracellular and extracellular concentrations of the various ions mentioned above. These cells have a specific ion pump which keeps a relatively constant but different ion gradient outside and inside the cells by regulation of passage through the plasma membrane of the cell. These pump mechanisms require energy to maintain their operations, and this energy is derived from cellular metabolism of nutrients.

Many amino acids which are taken up in the cell for various bodily functions are actively transported from outside to inside by means of one of these pumps: the sodium ion-dependent pumps or transport systems are most common. These systems convert the energy of the electrochemical sodium gradient across the plasma membrane into osmotically active amino acid gradients with intracellular/extracellular concentration ratios of up to 30. Such gradients cause water to move into the cell and lead to cell swelling. For example, it has been shown that liver cells distend as much as 12% within 2 min under the influence of physiological concentrations of glutamine, and the increased cellular hydration is maintained as long as the amino acids are present.[6]

As the cell becomes more concentrated with substrate, free water diffuses through the cell's plasma membrane (osmosis) causing the cellular volume to enlarge. This signals the cell to take in more nutrients, thus stimulating protein synthesis and inhibiting further proteolysis. Also, as the cell expands there is more available space within it for the three-dimensional interaction of intracellular receptors and various substrates, hormones, and messenger molecules that carry signals for transcription of RNA, and later, DNA protein synthesis. It is the extent of the change in hydration (change in volume), rather than the mechanism underlying the change, that determines the extent of the proteolytic or protein-synthetic response of the cell.

Many factors such as hormones, adenosine, cytokines, serotonin, oxygen radicals, nutrient availability, amino acids, and metabolic flux can affect cellular hydration.[7,8] These factors either affect the efficiency of the machinery function (cellular pump mechanisms), the specific intracellular/extracellular ion gradients (through permeability changes in the cellular membrane), or the availability of substrate. Cell shrinkage is caused by the loss of Na^+ or K^+ concentration or the accumulation of Cl^-.

For example, hormones in both physiological and pharmacological concentrations modulate the activity of ion transport systems in the plasma membrane. Insulin, beta-adrenergic agonists, androgenic/anabolic steroids, and growth hormone increase cellular hydration by promoting the cellular accumulation of several ions or minerals (including potassium, sodium, and chloride secondary to the activation of the Na^+/H^+-antiporter, Na^+, K^+, $2Cl^-$ cotransport, and the Na^+/K^+ ATPase).[9] Glucagon, glucocorticoids, certain cytokines, and oxidative stress, on the other hand, cause cell shrinkage by opening Ba^{2+}-sensitive K^+ channels, which allows loss of K^+ from the cell.

Intracellular potassium plays a pivotal role in cellular hydration (and dehydration) by exerting a limiting effect on the other cell ions. In cellular hydration it controls the extent of cellular swelling, allowing just enough to promote the anabolic signal induced by swelling, but not enough to cause overhydration.

A recent study has shown that the nutritional state of an animal modifies the swelling potency of amino acids and hormones in liver and by this means affects proteolysis.[10] In livers from deprived of food rats for 24 h, the swelling responses to glycine, glutamine, and alanine were enhanced, whereas the insulin- and IGF-1-induced increases of cell volume were diminished. A stronger inhibition of proteolysis was observed in livers from food-deprived rats upon addition of the amino acids, whereas the insulin- and IGF-1-mediated inhibition of proteolysis was attenuated. This study also concluded that independent of the nutritional state, a close relationship between the cellular hydration state and the corresponding inhibition of proteolysis was observed, regardless of whether cell volume was modified by amino acids, hormones, hypoosmotic exposure, or bile acids.

It appears that any condition that results in stress or inflammation may lead to cell dehydration and consequent catabolism. Sepsis or infections, including viral replication and synthesis, that cause an increase in a substance called tumor necrosis factor also favor water loss from affected cells.[11,12] This may explain the catabolic effects typically seen in many viral diseases, including AIDS. Other factors leading to cell swelling or hydration include lactate, glycine oxidation, KIC (a leucine amino acid derivative), and urea synthesis from amino acids.[13]

Experimentally induced oxidative stress decreases cellular hydration by opening potassium (K^+) channels in the plasma membrane, possibly by oxidation of important thiol groups or by raising intracellular calcium (Ca^{2+}) concentration.[14] Thus it is possible that the oxidative stress that typically occurs during exercise may also promote cellular dehydration through the loss of cellular potassium.

CELLULAR HYDRATION AND AMINO ACIDS

The concentration uptake of some amino acids (i.e., those transported by sodium (Na^+)-dependent mechanisms into muscle and liver cells) can increase cellular hydration, thereby triggering a protein-anabolic signal. Such a case has been postulated for both glutamine and alanine.[15] In one recent study it was concluded that "it seems plausible to conclude that stimulation of K^+ inflow plays a major role in the mechanism of alanine-induced stimulation of protein synthesis through changes in cell volume."[16]

Cellular hydration also affects and is affected by cellular glycogen and amino acid content. Cell shrinkage stimulates glycogenolysis, proteolysis, and formation of organic osmolytes such as amino acids, methylamines, and polyols. Cell swelling stimulates formation of glycogen and proteins and cellular release of organic osmolytes. The effects of some hormones on protein synthesis may be partially mediated by their effects on glycogen. For example, while insulin promotes glycogen synthesis and increases cellular volume, glucagon works in an opposite direction through promoting liver glycogen breakdown and inducing cell shrinkage.

Several amino acids are known to stimulate glycogen synthesis via activation of glycogen synthase. The authors of one study also concluded that stimulation of glycogen synthesis by amino acids is due, at least in part, to an increase in hepatocyte volume resulting from amino acid uptake, and that hepatocyte swelling per se stimulates glycogen synthesis.[17]

The effects of both glutamine and alanine on cellular hydration and protein synthesis is discussed in more detail below.

ADAPTIVE RESPONSE TO EXERCISE

Exercise has profound effects on skeletal muscle. Skeletal muscle increases its contractile protein content resulting in muscular hypertrophy as it successfully adapts to increasing work loads. Studies have shown that certain stimuli produce muscle hypertrophy.

In a review on the effects of exercise on protein turnover in humans, Rennie et al. concluded the following:[18]

1. Exercise causes a substantial rise in amino acid catabolism.
2. Amino acids catabolized during exercise appear to become available through a fall in whole-body protein synthesis and a rise in whole-body protein breakdown.
3. After exercise, protein balance becomes positive through a rise in the rate of whole-body synthesis in excess of breakdown.
4. Studies of free 3-methylhistidine in muscle, plasma and urine samples suggest that exercise decreases the fractional rate of myofibrillar protein breakdown, in contrast with the apparent rise in whole-body breakdown.

In contrast to exercise, most of the increased proteolysis during fasting is due to the degradation of myofibrillar proteins (contractile proteins) in skeletal muscle.[19,20]

A number of studies have examined the influence of exercise on protein synthesis and protein degradation. In general, it seems that exercise suppresses protein synthesis and stimulates protein degradation in skeletal muscle proportional to the level of exertion. In one early study using rats, mild exercise decreased protein synthesis by 17%. More intense treadmill running reduced synthesis by 30% and an exhaustive 3-h run inhibited synthesis by 70%.[21]

Another study by the same author examined the effects of exhaustive running on protein degradation and found that exhaustive running stimulates protein degradation in skeletal muscle.[22] Other studies have also shown that exercise produces a catabolic condition. In one study looking at aerobic exercise in humans, 6 male subjects were exercised on a treadmill for 3.75 h at 50% $V0_2$max and the rates of protein synthesis and degradation were measured.[23] During exercise there was a 14% decrease in protein synthesis and a 54% increase in the rate of degradation.

This is one of the few studies to make measurements during recovery after exercise. The authors of this study found that, after exercise, protein synthesis increased above the initial resting levels while protein degradation decreased, returning eventually to preexercise levels. Any gains in the recovery phase therefore seem to be due to increases in protein synthesis rather than to decreases in protein catabolism.

In another study, multiple amino acid tracers were used to further elucidate the changes in protein synthesis and degradation which occur during prolonged aerobic exercise.[24,25] In these studies male subjects were exercised on a bicycle ergometer at 30% $V0_2$max for 105 min. The results of the study showed that while exercise inhibited protein synthesis, the degree of inhibition varied depending on the amino acid tracer used. For example, the authors found decreases in protein synthesis of 48% using labeled leucine and 17% using lysine. With the relatively light workloads used in these studies, there were no changes in protein degradation or increases in urea production.

Even though the acute effect of exercise on protein turnover is catabolic, the long-term effects are an overall increase in protein synthesis and lean body mass. Routine exercise produces maintenance or hypertrophy of muscle mass. There are few studies which have looked at the postexercise recovery of protein turnover. The above report and a later report by Devlin et al.[26] suggest that recovery occurs through stimulation of protein synthesis.

Preliminary studies reported in the second edition of *Nutrition in Exercise and Sport* provide additional support for this recovery pattern.[27] The authors found that after a 2-h bout of running on a motor-driven treadmill at 26/m protein synthesis in the gastrocnemius muscle was suppressed by 26 to 30% in fasted male rats. Recovery of protein synthesis occurred during the next 4 to 8 h even if the animals were withheld from eating. These data suggest that muscles have a very high capacity for recovery even during conditions of food restriction. However, as we shall see below, food intake and the use of certain nutritional supplements before and after exercise are important to the effects of exercise on muscle protein synthesis and on subsequent recovery.

Just what factors control protein synthesis during exercise remain largely unknown although there are some general trends and associations that have been recognized. For example, high-intensity, exhaustive bouts of exercise produce a transient catabolic effect on protein synthesis. This effect presumably is controlled at the translation level of protein synthesis. Transcription is depressed but RNA concentrations are unchanged during the relatively brief period of the exercise bout. At the level of translation, potential regulatory controls include (1) availability of substrates, (2) hormones, (3) energy states, and (4) initiation factors.[27]

EXERCISE-INDUCED AMINO ACID FLUX

The changes that occur in the BCAAs, alanine, and glutamine in the liver, plasma, and muscle during exercise suggest that individual amino acids may be limiting as substrates for protein synthesis and that they may be an important source of energy for various tissues and organs in the body. In general, decreases in protein synthesis and increases in protein degradation produce a net release of amino acids into the intracellular free pool which may or may not be reflected by increased plasma levels.

Exercise is accompanied by changes in anabolic and catabolic hormones. It would appear that the molecular mechanism for the action of these hormones on translation remains equivocal, but most evidence points to changes in the initiation phase of translation. We will examine the hormonal response to exercise in the next chapter.

The availability of energy may also be a limiting factor for muscle protein synthesis. Studies have found that decreases in protein synthesis that occur in proportion to the number of contractions induced by electrical stimulation were in proportion to the decline in the level of ATP in muscle cells.[28]

THE TIMING OF NUTRIENT AND PROTEIN INTAKE IN RELATION TO EXERCISE

Nutrient intake, protein intake, and the use of individual amino acids, and certain combinations of amino acids, in and around exercise, have specific physiological and pharmacological effects that can increase protein synthesis and the anabolic effects of exercise.

In one study, carbohydrate, protein, and carbohydrate-protein supplements were compared to determine their effects on muscle glycogen storage during recovery from prolonged exhaustive exercise and on protein synthesis.[28a] In this study, nine male subjects cycled for 2 h on three separate occasions to deplete their muscle glycogen stores. Immediately, and 2 h after each exercise bout, they ingested 112.0 g carbohydrate (CHO), 40.7 g of whey protein (PRO), or 112.0 g carbohydrate and 40.7 g protein (CHO-PRO). Blood samples were drawn before exercise, immediately after exercise, and throughout recovery. Muscle biopsies were taken from the vastus lateralis immediately and 4 h after exercise.

Interestingly enough (covered in more detail later in this book), during recovery the plasma glucose response of the CHO treatment was significantly greater than that of the

CHO-PRO treatment, but the plasma insulin response of the CHO-PRO treatment was significantly greater than that of the CHO treatment. Both the CHO and CHO-PRO treatments produced plasma-glucose and insulin responses that were greater than those produced by the PRO treatment. The results of the study suggest that post-exercise protein and carbohydrate supplementation increases muscle glycogen storage and enhances protein synthesis, likely secondary to the interaction of carbohydrate and protein on insulin secretion.

Thus, it would appear that the post-exercise intake of carbohydrates and protein is important in order to maximize protein synthesis. In an unpublished study, post-exercise net skeletal muscle protein balance, normally negative without nutrient supplementation, was increased by the provision of amino acids and glucose.[28b] The authors of the study state that earlier nutrient administration may be more effective to increase skeletal muscle-protein synthesis during recovery compared with a later administration. While the mechanisms for these effects are not entirely clear, increased insulin responsiveness earlier in the recovery period may be involved.

In another unpublished study, six normal, untrained men were studied during the intravenous infusion of a balanced amino acid mixture at rest and after a leg-resistance exercise routine, in order to test the influence of exercise on the regulation of muscle protein kinetics by hyperaminoacidemia.[28c] Leg muscle protein kinetics and transport of selected amino acids (alanine, phenylalanine, leucine, and lysine) were isotopically determined using a model based on arteriovenous blood samples and muscle biopsy.

The intravenous amino acid infusion resulted in comparable increases in arterial amino acid concentrations at rest and after exercise, whereas leg blood flow was greater after exercise than at rest. During hyperaminoacidemia, the increases in amino acid transport above basal were 30% to 100% greater after exercise than at rest. Increases in muscle protein synthesis were also greater after exercise than at rest.

Muscle protein breakdown was not significantly affected by hyperaminoacidemia either at rest or after exercise. The authors concluded that the stimulatory effect of exogenous amino acids on muscle protein synthesis is enhanced by prior exercise, perhaps in part due to enhanced blood flow. The results imply that protein intake immediately after exercise may be more anabolic than that ingested at some later time.

Another unpublished study looked at the effect of the timing of glucose supplementation upon fractional muscle protein synthetic rate (FSR), urinary urea excretion, and whole-body and myofibrillar protein degradation (WBPD and MPD, respectively) following resistance exercise.[28d] In this study, eight healthy males performed unilateral knee extensor exercises (8 sets /10 reps/85% 1RM). They received a carbohydrate (CHO) supplement (1g/kg) or placebo (PL) immediately (t=0 h) and 1 h (t=+1 h) post-exercise. The results of the study suggest that CHO supplementation (1g/kg) immediately and 1h following resistance exercise can decrease myofibrillar protein breakdown and urinary urea excretion, resulting in a more positive body protein balance.

Overall, the use of a balanced amino acid mixture along with glucose immediately after exercise and then again a short time later, would seem to optimize the immediate anabolic effects of exercise.

The use of the individual, and combinations of the amino acids both before, during, and after exercise also have significant effects on protein synthesis and the exercise and post-exercise hormonal milieu. These effects will be discussed further in Chapter 2 and under the individual amino acids.

Chapter 2

EXERCISE AND PROTEIN METABOLISM

INTRODUCTION

Exercise has been shown to have a profound influence on statural, hypertrophic, and reparative growth throughout the human life span in both men and women.[29,30] Exercise can facilitate statural growth and provides the necessary mechanical and metabolic stimuli (through the secretion of growth hormone and other anabolic hormones) that are necessary for hypertrophy of the musculoskeletal system and for reparative growth.

Exercise reverses the ultrastructural changes seen with immobilization (loss of myofilaments and shrinkage of muscle fibers),[31] and is such a potent anabolic stimulus that muscle hypertrophy can occur even under nutritionally unfavorable conditions or in the presence of wasting diseases such as AIDS[32] and malignancy.[33] It appears that increased tension development (either passive or active) is the critical event in initiating compensatory growth and that this process appears to be independent of growth hormone and insulin as well as testosterone and thyroid hormones.[34]

One recent study looked at the combined effects of exercise and energy restriction on muscle mass.[35] The findings of this study suggest that protein synthesis is stimulated by exercise even with energy-restricted diets and that energy intake and exercise have independent effects on the regulation of muscle mass and protein synthesis.

Another recent study looked at protein turnover rates of two human subjects during an unassisted crossing of Antarctica.[36] During the Austral summer of 1992-1993, two men walked 2300 km across Antarctica in 96 days, unassisted by other men, animals, or machines. During the journey they ate a high-energy diet of freeze-dried rations containing 56.7% fat, 35.5% carbohydrate, and 7.8% protein. Despite this high-energy intake, both men lost more than 20 kg in body weight due to extremely high energy expenditures. Studies of protein turnover using [^{15}N]glycine by the single-dose end-product method were made before, during, and after the journey, and these demonstrated considerable differences in the metabolic responses of the two men to the combined stresses of exercise, cold, and undernutrition. However, both men maintained high and relatively stable levels of protein synthesis during the expedition.

Thus even when one does not take in enough calories (usually intentionally while trying to lose weight) one can increase or at least maintain functioning muscle mass through exercise. Exercise, or more correctly, the right kind of exercise, is absolutely essential in producing muscle hypertrophy and for increasing lean body mass and strength. For example, in one study two groups of obese females were compared; one group exercised while the other group didn't.[37] Both groups were on a calorie-reduced diet that contained 80 g of protein. The weight-training group showed a significant hypertrophy in the muscles exercised although both groups lost the same weight.

Although muscle hypertrophy in certain muscles can occur under hypocaloric conditions, significant muscle hypertrophy cannot occur if there is an inadequate intake of protein. Dietary protein levels must be sufficiently high in order to provide the substrate needed for muscular hypertrophy. In general, in order to increase muscle mass increased exercise intensity must be accompanied by an increased dietary protein intake. When intensity of effort is high and the body is stimulated to adapt by increasing muscle mass, dietary protein intake must also be high.

As well, once a certain threshold of work intensity is crossed, dietary protein and certain protein and amino acid supplements become extremely important in augmenting the anabolic effects of exercise, not only by providing necessary substrates but by directly influencing proteins synthesis and catabolism and by influencing the hormonal milieu.

Acute bouts of exercise can induce measurable changes in protein, carbohydrate, and lipid metabolism. These changes are characterized by a change in protein catabolism and synthesis and an increased utilization of protein for gluconeogenesis and lipids for oxidative fuel.[38-41] Chronic daily exercise leads to adaptive processes that result in a net increase in total body as well as peripheral nitrogen stores.[42]

Exercise has profound effects on protein synthesis and degradation and on the endogenous anabolic and catabolic hormones, which in turn modulate the adaptation response to exercise.[43-54] In general, protein synthesis is suppressed during exercise while protein degradation appears to be increased; while in the recovery period during which hypertrophy occurs, protein synthesis is increased while protein degradation is suppressed in those muscles bearing the greatest load.[55-61]

While some studies show clear and consistent hormonal responses to exercise (as outlined below), others do not.[62-73] Some of the conflicting results may be the result of different exercise protocols. The kind of exercise stimulus, whether maximal, submaximal, acute, constant, etc., has an important effect on the hormonal response. For example, in one study that found an absence of a specific serum androgenic response with strength development the authors noted that the reason for this absence may be related to the fact that the constant exercise stimulus is not conducive to establishing clear-cut hormone-strength relationships.[74] As we shall see below, the effect of exercise on serum testosterone and growth hormone depends, among other things, on the intensity and duration of exercise. However, it has also been shown that levels of these two hormones vary in response to the fitness and expertise of the athlete.[75]

Both heavy resistance exercise and prolonged stressful exercise produce significant changes in serum levels of many potentially anabolic and catabolic hormones including testosterone, growth hormone, IGF-1, the catecholamines, insulin, and cortisol. The nature and extent of the hormonal responses can be quite different depending on many factors including the type and length of exercise, age, and training status.

Unless the exercise is prolonged or fatiguing, the general hormonal trend is an increase in growth hormone and cortisol and a decrease, or less commonly an increase, in testosterone during exercise. During the recovery period there is a fall in cortisol, a rise in GH, and a rise in testosterone. If there is a successful adaptive response to training, over several weeks the basal levels of testosterone and GH increase while those of cortisol decrease.

Overtraining, however, seems to have an adverse effect on serum hormone levels.[76] Although chronic overtraining appears to decrease the detrimental effects of stressful training on the endocrine system.[77] Age is definitely a factor although the authors of a recent study concluded that older individuals are capable of similar hormonal responses to submaximal exercise of identical durations and intensities as their young and middle-aged counterparts, and that chronic endurance training can enhance the hormonal response to exercise in all age groups.[78] In women, overtraining or endurance training may lead to hypothalamic-pituitary-ovarian axis suppression and exercise-induced amenorrhea.[79,80]

Hormonal responses may also differ during training and competition in the same sport. Thus in some sports there appear to be significant differences in plasma levels and urinary excretion of androgen hormones (testosterone, epitestosterone, androsterone, etiocholanolone, 11-hydroxy-androsterone, and 11-hydroxy-etiocholanolone) and plasma sex-hormone binding globulin (SHBG) after training and after competition. These differences may be due to the different stressors involved in competition in comparison to training. For example, in one study involving 16 professional racing cyclists, the urinary concentrations of androgen hormones decreased during the period of training and increased during competition, this being the reverse of what happened to SHBG plasma concentrations.[81]

Detraining has significant effects on hormonal parameters. A study which investigated the effects of 14 days of resistive exercise detraining on 12 power athletes found significant changes in serum hormones. Levels of plasma growth hormone, testosterone, and the testosterone to cortisol ratio increased, whereas plasma cortisol and creatine kinase enzyme levels decreased.[82] The authors remarked that changes in the hormonal milieu during detraining may be conducive to an enhanced anabolic process, but such changes may not materialize at the tissue level in the absence of the overload training stimulus.

THE HORMONES

The eight main hormones to consider when attempting to maximize the anabolic effects of exercise are:

- Testosterone (and in women especially, other androgens)
- Growth hormone (GH)
- Insulin-like growth factor-1 (IGF-1)
- Insulin
- Thyroid
- Cortisol
- Glucagon
- Catecholamines

Generally testosterone, GH, IGF-1, insulin, and physiological levels of thyroid are anabolic in nature, while the catecholamines, cortisol, glucagon, and high levels of thyroid hormone are catabolic. However, we must be careful in making absolute statements about the actions of specific hormones, since these actions are complex and interdependent. The hormones can act differently and sometimes contradictory depending on the metabolic environment and the presence of other hormones. When a number of influences coexist, the effect on any one hormone or group of hormones is difficult to predict.

The complex relationship among the gonadal and adrenal steroids — including the glucocorticoids, testosterone, and the hypothalamic-pituitary hormones — has yet to be fully elucidated. It is now known that many of the hypothalamic-releasing and pituitary-stimulating hormones cross react, stimulating more than just the supposed target glands. For example, there is some evidence to show that protirelin (TRH), besides stimulating thyrotropin (TSH) and thyroid secretion, also stimulates endogenous growth hormone, prolactin, and luteinizing hormone (LH), and therefore endogenous testosterone secretion.[83]

Although protein metabolism is felt to be a complicated balance between catabolic (glucocorticoids and thyroid hormones) and anabolic (insulin, growth hormone, and androgens) hormones,[84] this is not necessarily always the case. For example, at certain levels thyroid hormone can either be anabolic (physiological levels) or catabolic (higher levels) in its effect. Also some hormones have more than one mode of action. Insulin, for example, is a potent anticatabolic and anabolic hormone and is one of the most important factors controlling overall protein metabolism. As well, increasing serum insulin may cause a rise in endogenous androgens.[85] Thus we see a direct anabolic effect by the insulin and a possible indirect anabolic action by the increase in serum androgens.

A hormone can also regulate the secretion of other hormones and thereby produce a more complex spectrum of actions, an important instance being the stimulation by catecholamines of insulin and glucagon release. Therefore, when considering the physiological influence of alterations in certain circulating hormones, attention must be given to the impact these alterations have on other regulatory and counterregulatory hormones.

The metabolic roles of hormones that affect protein synthesis have been uncovered by a variety of studies including those on the catabolic effects of surgery, disease, and trauma, and the ways to counteract these effects. For example, several adjuvant therapies such as anabolic steroids,[86,87] pharmacologic doses of growth hormone,[88-90] insulin,[91] and amino acids that influence the hormones such as ornithine alpha-ketoglutarate,[92,93] branched-chain amino acids,[94,95] dipeptides,[96] and glutamine[97] have been instituted, supplementing postoperative nutrition to decrease protein catabolism and improve nitrogen retention.

Before we discuss the effects of dietary protein and protein and amino acid supplements on the anabolic and catabolic hormones, it's important to discuss the individual and collective roles of these hormones on protein metabolism.

GROWTH HORMONE

Growth hormone, a polypeptide (also known as GH, adenohypophyseal growth hormone, hypophyseal growth hormone, anterior pituitary growth hormone, phyone, pituitary growth hormone, somatotropic hormone, STH, and somatotropin) is one of the hormones produced by the anterior portion of the pituitary gland (situated at the base of the brain under the hypothalamus) under the regulation of the hypothalamic hormones, growth hormone releasing hormone (GHRH, somatoliberin), somatostatin, and galanin.[98-100] The anterior pituitary also secretes other hormones that have an effect on protein metabolism including LH, FSH, prolactin (PRL), adrenocorticotropic hormone (ACTH), and thyroid stimulating hormone (TSH).[101]

The metabolic effects of human growth hormone include promotion of protein conservation, stimulation of lipolysis, and fat oxidation. GH infusion increases lipolysis as evidenced by increases in glycerol and nonesterified fatty acid concentrations,[102] and also increases the incorporation of amino acids into protein.[103] In adults, the growth hormone/somatomedin C axis has been shown to be important in muscle homeostasis.[104,105] Therapeutic administration of growth hormone has been shown to reverse muscle loss associated with the aging process.[106]

GH administered to humans and animals results in nitrogen retention with an increase in protein synthesis and a decrease in protein catabolism. Quantitatively, the attenuation of losses of glutamine and alanine appear to dominate. This has led to the question of whether this anabolic agent should be used in connection with specific substrates, such as glutamine or glutamine precursors (such as alpha-ketogluterate) in therapeutic applications.[107]

While the presence of growth hormone is important for its physiological actions,[108] it is not merely a permissive effect since it appears that it is the total amount and pattern of GH secretion that are the determining factors of the growth rate.[109,110] In one study the effects of low and high GH on body composition, muscle protein metabolism, and serum lipids were studied in seven fit adults without GH deficiency.[111] The authors concluded that GH alters body composition and muscle protein metabolism, decreases stored and circulating lipids in fit adults with a pre-existing supranormal body composition, and that the magnitude of these effects were dose dependent.

In a study done to determine whether doubling the GH dose would enhance its anabolic effects and facilitate fat loss, the results showed that GH can induce significant anabolic responses even when caloric intake is decreased, and that the degree and duration of these anabolic responses are dependent on the GH dose given.[112]

While GH has been shown to increase protein synthesis if adequate caloric intake and dietary protein are provided,[113] the anticatabolic and anabolic effects of GH are evident even with calorie deprivation. In several studies it has been shown that increased levels of endogenous and exogenous GH result in nitrogen conservation despite restriction of dietary intake.[114,115]

GH has been found to be useful for decreasing the catabolic effects resulting from surgery and trauma,[116-129] conditions in which growth hormone levels are decreased.[130] In one study the protein kinetic response to exogenous GH in trauma patients fed parenterally was measured.[131] After 7 days of total parenteral nutrition (TPN) nitrogen balance was less negative, protein synthesis efficiency was higher, whole-body protein synthesis rate was higher, although still deficient (because of trauma), and IGF-1 and insulin levels were significantly elevated.

While GH is effective in most catabolic conditions, it is not in some instances. For example, GH has not been found to have significant anabolic or anticatabolic effects in the early stages of some acutely catabolic conditions including trauma. In one recent study the effect of GH on hormone and nitrogen metabolism in 14 patients with multiple injuries in the early phase of injury was evaluated.[132] In this study, administration of GH evoked a significant increase in plasma concentrations of GH, insulin-like growth factor-1 (IGF-1), and insulin-like growth factor binding-protein-3 (IGFBP-3). No significant differences were found for either daily or cumulative nitrogen balances in patients receiving GH and those receiving placebo. GH therapy did not affect skeletal muscle extracellular water, nor did it affect plasma or muscle concentrations of total free amino acids or glutamine.

As well, GH administration in exercising elderly men does not augment muscle fiber hypertrophy or tissue GH-IGF expression and suggests that deficits in the GH-IGF-1 axis with aging do not inhibit the skeletal muscle tissue response to training.[133]

Growth hormone (GH) and insulin-like growth factor-1 (IGF-1), especially the former, have immunoregulatory effects in addition to anabolic effects. The hormones may act to protect the host from lethal bacterial infection by promoting the maturation of myeloid cells, stimulating phagocyte migration, priming phagocytes for the production of superoxide anions and cytokines, and enhancing opsonic activity.[134]

Growth Hormone and Athletic Performance

Although GH is effective in certain catabolic states, the question still remains: does GH have an effect on protein synthesis and muscle hypertrophy secondary to exercise? It is felt by some that GH has a permissive effect on protein anabolism. But do increased levels of GH increase protein synthesis and have an anabolic effect?

Although the significance of GH release during exercise has yet to be fully elucidated, the overall actions of GH, including increasing growth, sparing glucose and utilizing fat as an energy source, affect the adaptive response to exercise. Prolonged intensive exercise causes elevated levels of GH and glucagon, and a reduced level of insulin in the blood. The GH response to exercise seems to depend on the severity of the exercise and on other factors such as emotional strain and the environmental temperature. It seems that the more adverse the conditions and the harsher the exercise, the more GH is produced.

Exercise is a potent stimulator of several hormones including GH.[135] However, of all the hormonal changes that take place with exercise, GH levels seem to be most affected especially after an acute bout of resistive exercise.[136] We know that the GH response to exercise is workload dependent, and that with increasing intensity GH secretion increases.[137] We also know that the GH response is greater with acute anaerobic exercise bouts involving large muscle masses and less with continuous aerobic activity.[138-140]

Almost all forms of exercise increase GH secretion, although there appears to be a higher increase in GH level after maximal exercise than after submaximal exercise.[141,142] Some studies, however, have not shown this relationship.[143] The results of one study suggest that the balance between oxygen demand and availability may be an important regulator of GH secretion during exercise.[144]

Several studies have documented the increased GH secretion that occurs during weight lifting, and during the subsequent recovery phase.[145] It appears that the secretion of GH varies according to the muscle group that is exercised, with smaller muscle groups leading to increased GH release. For example, in one study arm work elicited a greater serum GH response than leg work.[146]

As with insulin and glucagon, the availability of carbohydrates modulates the response of GH to exercise.[147] The administration of glucose excludes the response while during a carbohydrate-deficient state the response is exaggerated.

A recent study examined the effect of sprint and endurance training on GH secretion.[148] In this study 23 highly trained sprint (100 to 400 m) or endurance (1,500 to 10,000 m) athletes were tested for GH levels after a performance of a maximal 30-s sprint on a nonmotorized treadmill. There was a marked GH response for all athletes but the response was three times greater for the sprint-trained athletes than for the endurance-trained athletes. The sprint-trained athletes reached their peak GH values 20 to 30 min following exercise, whereas the endurance athletes reached a peak GH value 1 to 10 min postexercise; 1 h following exercise the GH level was still approximately 10 times baseline in the sprint-trained group.

The authors concluded that the GH response to the sprints was secondary to the metabolic responses (high blood lactate and plasma ammonia, low blood pH) and the power output generated during this type of exercise. The authors also speculated that long-term increase in GH in the sprint-trained group may result in an increase in protein synthesis and a decrease in protein catabolism, resulting in a retention or increase of skeletal muscle mass. The results of this study further corroborate the effect on high-intensity exercise on GH secretion, whether the stimulus for this increased secretion is lactic acid, serum pH, ATP depletion, low serum glucose, an oxygen deficit, or some other factors.

But while it is important to determine just what does affect GH secretion, the real question is whether the increased GH response results in an anabolic response or whether the increased GH secretion simply allows the more efficient use of stored body fat with no long-term effects on protein synthesis.

The increased secretion of GH during exercise may be physiologically important for one or all of the following: glucoregulatory, lipolytic, and anabolic actions. Its anabolic and glucoregulatory effects include the increase of protein synthesis in all cells (through an increased transcription of DNA leading to increased quantities of RNA), an increase in the metabolism of fatty acids, a decrease in glucose utilization throughout the body, and an increase in glucose formation (by the stimulation of hepatic gluconeogenesis).[149] GH increases the movement of amino acids from intracellular spaces into the cytoplasm and increases ribosomal protein synthesis.[150] As well, GH has significant anticatabolic effects.

Human growth hormone is a major lipolytic factor in the body that stimulates the release of fatty acids from adipose tissue into circulation and increases intracellular conversion of fatty acids into acetyl-CoA.[151] In one study the lipolytic effect of exogenous GH during caloric restriction, manifested by increases in glycerol concentrations and body fat loss, persisted well beyond its anabolic effects.[152] Thus, through the increased use of fatty acids for energy contributions, protein and glucose supplies are spared, permitting circulating levels of glucose to increase.

The anticatabolic effects of GH (decrease in the breakdown of cell protein) may be due to its effects on lipid metabolism. Growth hormone stimulates the release of fatty acids from adipose tissue into the circulation and increases the intracellular conversion of fatty acids into acetyl-CoA with subsequent utilization for this energy.[153] The increased supply of free fatty acids for energy metabolism has the effect of sparing protein and glucose stores.[154]

As well, lipogenesis is decreased by GH. Chronic administration of GH results in inhibition of glyceride synthesis and decreased body fat content.[155] The overall effect is an increase in fat metabolism, decreased body fat, and a decrease in protein catabolism. In one study administration of GH in a therapeutic dose for 2 weeks, despite apparently normal daytime levels of major metabolic hormones, induced significant increases in circulating lipid fuel substrates, increased energy expenditure, and lipid oxidation.[156]

Indirect promotion of growth can be seen in the enhanced action of other growth factors in the presence of GH. Kelley et al. observed that the presence of GH improves the anabolic action and tissue responsiveness to androgens.[157] In addition, Alen et al. demonstrated that androgens and anabolic steroids could increase the responsiveness of GH secretion during various secretion challenges.[158] The synergistic effects of GH and IGF-1 will be examined in detail below.

In addition to the better-recognized roles of growth hormone as mentioned above, growth hormone was recently proposed to play a major role in acid-base homeostasis.[159] Growth hormone accelerates renal acid secretion and thereby facilitates elimination of acid from the body fluids, a potentially important role during strenuous exercise when acidogenesis may limit performance.

Growth Hormone Synthesis and Secretion

Many psychological and physiological parameters affect growth hormone release. Among the many factors that increase growth hormone secretion are the various amino acids, especially arginine, L-dopa, L-tryptophan, tyrosine, and ornithine. The GH stimulating effects of the various amino acids are discussed in detail below. High-protein diets also seem to have an increased GH response, as against high-carbohydrate diets. In one study measuring the effect of isocaloric (500 kcal) protein and carbohydrate ingestion found that GH increased after both diets after an initial decline; the increase was greatest after protein intake and maximum was reached at 180 min.[160]

Endogenous control of growth hormone secretion has still not been fully elucidated although somatostatin and growth hormone-releasing hormone seem to be the ultimate mediators of most of the changes in growth hormone secretion, including the feedback effects from GH itself and IGF-1.[161-165] GH dysfunction is often associated with changes in one or both of these regulatory hormones.[166,167] For example:

- Arginine-induced GH release is mainly mediated by a decrease in somatostatinergic tone, while GH responses to insulin stress are probably mediated by both an increase in hypothalamic GHRH release and inhibition of somatostatin.[168,169]
- The mechanisms by which insulin-induced hypoglycemia, L-dopa, and arginine stimulate GH secretion are all different; a suppression of somatostatin release may be partially involved in the stimulatory mechanism of GH secretion by L-dopa; arginine suppresses somatostatin release from the hypothalamus to cause GH secretion.[170]
- Cholinergic pathways play an important role in the regulation of GH secretion mediated through their effects on somatostatin and GHRH.[171-173]
- The adrenergic system is involved in the neural control of GH secretion with both stimulatory and inhibitory influences mainly mediated via GHRH and/or somatostatin modulation.[174]
- The secretion of growth hormone and its plasma levels, as well as the response to GHRH is severely reduced in old people because of an increased somatostatin secretion by the hypothalamus.[175,176]
- Yohimbine, an alpha-2-antagonist, suppresses the pulsatile GH secretion either through the elimination of GHRH release or via enhanced somatostatin release.[177]
- In obesity, the basis for the derangements in GH secretion (an impairment of GH secretion elicited by all stimuli known to date) is associated with a state of chronic somatostatin hypersecretion.[178]
- The decrease in GH response after repeated stimulation with GHRH is partly caused by an elevation of somatostatin tonus.[179]
- Tamoxifen, a partial competitive antagonist to the estrogen receptor, is widely used clinically in the treatment of breast cancer. *In vitro* data show that tamoxifen suppresses serum IGF-1 levels by acting at the pituitary to inhibit GH release.[180] Another study has shown that the blunting of GH pulse amplitude by tamoxifen is mediated at least in part by increased release of endogenous somatostatin.[181]

INSULIN-LIKE GROWTH FACTOR-1 (IGF-1)

IGF-1 has been implicated in protein metabolism and in growth and growth processes of many tissues in animals.[182-186] IGF-1 has a structure similar to insulin,[187,188] and is thought to mediate most of the anabolic effects of growth hormone in the body.

The IGF peptides are bound tightly to plasma proteins (IGFBPs). Because of this binding their activity is extended to several hours as against the 20 to 30 min of the unbound forms. IGF-1 is produced in the liver, chondrocytes, kidney, muscle, pituitary, and gastrointestinal tract. The liver is the main source of circulating IGF-1.[189]

Levels of IGF-1 and IGFBP-3 (a GH-dependent protein that binds IGF-1) are tied in with GH secretion and increase when GH levels increase. Levels are also age dependent, with low levels in early childhood, a peak during adolescence, and a decline after age 50. As a consequence of protein binding, and thus controlled release, the concentration of IGF-1 remains relatively constant throughout the day, in contrast to the fluctuating levels of GH.

IGF-1 seems to have a split personality in that it exerts both GH and insulin-like actions on skeletal muscles[190] by increasing protein synthesis and decreasing protein breakdown. Both GH and IGF-1 seem to shift the metabolism to decreasing fat formation and increasing protein synthesis.

Since both GH and IGF-1 have been shown to have anabolic and anticatabolic effects under certain stressful and catabolic conditions, and since IGF-1 is an important mediator of the anabolic effects of GH, it has been suggested that IGF-1 may be used as a substitute for GH in catabolic states because IGF-1 is not felt to have certain side effects seen secondary to GH use.

IGF-1 and IGF-2 have been observed *in vitro* to increase glucose uptake and to possess antilipolytic activity in cell cultures,[191] but with a molar potency that is considerably less than that of insulin.[192,193] These findings have been reproduced *in vivo* during IGF-1 and -2 and insulin infusions in rats[194] and after the administration of IGF-1 and insulin bolus injections to human subjects.[195] Thus, when infused into humans IGF-1 produces a rapid lowering of blood glucose (hypoglycemia) but with much less potency comparable to insulin. High rates of infusion of IGF-1 induce hypoglycemia and decrease estimates of whole-body proteolysis, suggestive of a predominantly insulin-like effect.

IGF-2 is thought to be a less effective anabolic agent than IGF-1.[196,197] In one study the *in vivo* effects of 300-min infusions of recombinant IGF-1 and IGF-2 on glucose and protein metabolism were investigated in awake, fasted lambs.[198] The effects were compared with an insulin infusion that had the same hypoglycemic potential as the high-dose IGF-1 infusion. IGF-1 lowered blood glucose by increasing the rate of glucose clearance, in contrast to insulin which both increased clearance and reduced glucose production. Net protein loss was reduced, after infusion of low- and high-dose IGF-1 and insulin. IGF-2 infusion did not alter the rate of net protein loss. In contrast to insulin, high-dose IGF-1 infusion increased the rate of protein synthesis in skeletal and cardiac muscle and in hepatic tissue.

The authors of this study concluded that (1) protein metabolism is more sensitive than glucose metabolism to IGF-1 infusion, as protein loss was reduced by an IGF-1 infusion that did not alter glucose kinetics; (2) protein synthesis is increased by IGF-1 infusion but not by insulin infusion; and (3) IGF-2 is a less effective anabolic agent than IGF-1. The authors also speculated that the effects of IGF-1 on protein metabolism are not mediated by insulin receptors.

Unlike GH, IGF-1 by itself, even at levels associated with pharmacological levels of GH, does not seem to significantly affect protein metabolism,[199] but may play a role as a fat repartitioning agent.[200] However, if coinfused with total parenteral nutrition,[201] or if amino acids are added even to low-dose IGF-1 infusions, protein synthesis increases, but there may be little effect on protein catabolism (see below).

IGF-1 plays an important role in mediating the somatotrophic effects of growth hormone. GH induces the liver to synthesize IGF-1 and other somatomedins, and the GH/IGF axis plays an important role in growth regulation and improvements in muscle protein synthesis and whole-body nitrogen economy in humans.

IGF-1 not only exerts some insulin-like actions but is structurally similar to proinsulin (the immediate precursor to insulin). GH and insulin are in many ways interdependent. GH stimulates insulin release directly and also facilitates its release in response to various other factors. As well, GH-deficient individuals have impaired insulin release to glucose challenge. Because of the various actions and interactions, one might consider insulin, GH, and IGF-1 as part of the same family.

Investigations into the anabolic and anticatabolic effects of IGF-1, and any synergism shown with GH and insulin on protein metabolism, have yielded rather conflicting results. These studies, while showing the significant anabolic and anticatabolic effects of IGF-1, especially when acting synergistically with GH and/or insulin, are somewhat contradictory when delegating which actions are due to GH, IGF-1, and insulin. Although somewhat confusing, a review of the literature is presented below.

The purpose of one recent study was to examine the effects of a heavy-resistance exercise protocol known to dramatically elevate immunoreactive GH on circulating IGF-1 after the exercise stimulus.[202] Seven young men were asked to perform an eight-station heavy-resistance exercise protocol consisting of three sets of ten repetition maximum resistances with a 1-min rest between sets and exercises followed by a recovery day. In addition, a control day followed a nonexercise day to provide baseline data. According to the authors of the study, the subjects were required to have engaged in resistance training two to three times a week for the past year. The subjects were screened in this way to ensure that the participants were better able to tolerate the training performed.

Despite postexercise elevations in GH significantly above resting levels, there were no significant differences between pre- and postexercise total serum IGF-1 concentrations, and total serum IGF-1 concentrations did not increase the day after the exercise period. It is possible, explained the authors, that the amount of muscle damage sustained by the subjects during the training period does not require alterations in circulating IGF-1 and that local IGF-1 release may have been sufficient to provide for repair and/or adaptational processes.

Thus, these data demonstrate that a high-intensity bout of heavy-resistance exercise that increases circulating GH did not appear to affect IGF-1 concentrations over a 24-h recovery period in recreationally strength-trained and healthy young men. The conclusion was that IGF-1 concentrations following exercise may be independent of GH stimulatory mechanisms.

Another study examined the effects of infusing recombinant human growth hormone, insulin-like growth factor-1, the truncated IGF-1 analogue des(1-3)IGF-1, and insulin over a 7-day period in streptozotocin-induced diabetic rats. The authors concluded that IGF peptides stimulate muscle protein synthesis and improve nitrogen balance in diabetes without obviously influencing the abnormal carbohydrate metabolism. Moreover, des(1-3)IGF-1 is at least as potent as the full-length IGF-1.[203] Carcass fat increased substantially following insulin administration. This did not occur with the IGF peptides, suggesting that IGF predominantly stimulates the growth of lean tissue.

In another recent study the effects of giving either infusions of IGF-1 alone or combined with insulin and amino acids were examined.[204] The use of IGF-1 alone lowered insulin levels and produced no increases in muscle protein synthesis, while the use of IGF-1 combined with insulin and amino acids increased protein synthesis. Thus it appears that the protein-synthesizing effect of IGF-1 is limited and only becomes significant in the presence of adequate amounts of insulin and amino acids.

In this study, low-dose infusions of IGF-1 failed to increase muscle protein synthesis in rats because it either suppressed insulin secretion or lowered plasma amino acid levels. Adding amino acids not only prevented the fall in plasma amino acid levels, but also prevented the drop in insulin that occurs with IGF-1 alone.

This study also shows that insulin is an important modulator of IGF-1 action in regard to protein synthesis. Providing growth hormone with IGF-1 also prevents the decline in insulin commonly seen when IGF-1 is given alone. This may explain the apparent synergistic effect shown by some studies when growth hormone is combined with both IGF-1 and insulin.

In a series of studies[205-209] it was shown that:

- Although GH exerts some direct effects, some of its growth and anabolic effects are mediated by IGF-1.
- The muscle hypertrophic stimuli of work overload and passive stretch are associated with significantly increased muscle IGF-1 mRNA levels.
- GH significantly decreased body fat and increased the protein:fat ratio only in the animals with the restricted intake.
- Skeletal muscle weight was increased by GH regardless of food intake. Thus the anabolic effect of GH administered to hypophysectomized rats was independent of dietary intake.
- Muscle IGF-1 mRNA levels were also elevated by GH but unaffected by food intake. In contrast, serum IGF-1 levels were markedly reduced by undernutrition.
- GH increased IGF-1 mRNA concentration similarly in skeletal muscle in both rats with food available *ad libitum* and in pair-fed rats. Serum concentrations of insulin and IGF-1 were increased by GH in the rats with food available ad libitum but not in the pair-fed rats.

Decreased nutrition, therefore, modulated the action of GH but emphasized its nutrient partitioning effect, thus increasing the anabolic drive towards skeletal muscle growth; this appeared to be mediated by the local production of IGF-1 within the muscle. These data suggest that the anabolic action of GH on muscle can be mediated through the autocrine/paracrine action of the IGF-1 hormone. In contrast, insulin dramatically affected muscle protein synthesis rates but had no measurable effect upon muscle IGF-1 mRNA levels, which suggests that the anabolic action of this hormone is not mediated through the autocrine/paracrine action of IGF-1. These studies suggest that IGF-1 may mediate growth in muscle in response to variety of stimuli by autocrine/paracrine action or in response to certain stimuli, possibly by endocrine action.

It has been shown that IGFs stimulate protein synthesis and inhibit protein degradation at physiological concentrations.[210] Studies done on normal humans, comparing IGF-1 action to insulin action, suggest that insulin-like effects of IGF-1 in humans are mediated in part via IGF-1 receptors and in part via insulin receptors.[211] IGF-1 infusion has also been shown to directly increase protein synthesis in normal humans.[212]

In low doses it appears that the use of IGF-1 may be counterproductive in that not only is it not anabolic, but it inhibits insulin and GH secretion[213] and therefore decreases any anabolic effect from these hormones.

Although IGF-1 in high doses positively affects nitrogen balance, IGF-1 use alone may also be somewhat counterproductive since it induces hypoglycemia while simultaneously decreasing the production of GH and insulin. When GH and IGF-1 are administered simultaneously, however, nitrogen balance is remarkably improved.[214]

Only a few studies have looked at the effects of IGF-1 on protein synthesis in athletes. One recent study has shown that neither GH nor IGF-1 treatment results in increases in the rate of muscle protein synthesis or reduction in the rate of whole-body protein breakdown — metabolic alterations that would promote muscle protein anabolism in experienced weight lifters attempting to further increase muscle mass.[215]

In an even more recent study, however, larger doses of IGF-1 had significant anabolic effects in humans.[216] This study investigated whether recombinant human IGF-1 could serve as a protein-sparing nondiabetogenic agent. In this study 21 healthy volunteers were studied in 3 similar clinical models: IGF-1 alone, IGF-1 and prednisone, and prednisone alone. Prednisone, being a potent catabolic agent, was used to determine the anticatabolic effects of IGF-1. The authors of this study concluded that 100 μg/kg IGF-1 given twice daily (1) has GH-like effects on whole-body protein metabolism, (2) markedly diminishes the protein catabolic effect of glucocorticosteroids, and (3) is nondiabetogenic in prednisone-treated humans.

As a result of this and previous studies, the authors feel that IGF-1 offers promise in the treatment of protein catabolic states. IGF-1 may also be useful in treating various growth hormone-resistant and insulin-resistant disorders and perhaps as an adjunctive treatment in insulin (such as diabetes) and GH-deficient disorders.[217]

Overall, the majority of studies support the fact that IGF-1 has significant anabolic and anticatabolic effects, especially when acting with insulin and GH and when there is an adequate amount of certain amino acids. Thus increasing endogenous levels of IGF-1 could be useful for maximizing the effects of exercise on muscle mass and strength. Increasing amino acid intake and increasing endogenous levels of GH and insulin would increase the anabolic and anticatabolic effects of IGF-1. All of the anabolic and anticatabolic effects and the hormonal synergism can be mediated in part by the judicious use of protein and protein and amino acids supplements.

GH and IGF-1 Synergism

The use of GH as an anabolic agent is limited by its tendency to cause hyperglycemia and by its inability to reverse nitrogen wasting in some catabolic conditions. IGF-1 has a tendency to cause hypoglycemia. An hypothesis has been proposed that administration of GH with IGF-1 to patients after severe injury could be more effective than GH alone in promoting anabolic protein metabolism, resulting in synergistic nitrogen retention and improved wound healing and immunologic function.[218] A combination of GH and IGF-1 has been shown to be much more potent in improving nitrogen balance than either one alone, and also attenuates the hyperglycemia caused by GH alone and the hypoglycemia caused by IGF-1 alone.[219]

One study looked at the effects of giving both IGF-I and GH simultaneously to tube-fed rats.[220] The rats were catabolic, having been previously subjected to surgical stress. Results showed that weight gain on the combined hormone regime was doubled to that when given either hormone separately. IGF-I selectively increased visceral organ mass, while GH increased calf muscle mass. Both hormones increased carcass protein and water content while reducing fat. When IGF-I was given with GH, it reversed the elevated insulin level commonly observed when GH is taken alone.

In another study by the same author, the fractional rate of protein synthesis (Ks) in skeletal muscle, jejunal mucosa and muscularis, and liver were compared to investigate the differential effects of GH and IGF-1 on tissue protein synthesis in surgically stressed rats.[221] Body weight gain, nitrogen retention, and serum IGF-1 concentrations confirmed that GH plus IGF-1 additively increased anabolism. Serum insulin concentrations were significantly increased by GH and decreased by IGF-1. GH significantly increased Ks in skeletal muscle and jejunal muscularis; IGF-1 significantly increased Ks in jejunal mucosa and muscularis; and neither GH or IGF-1 altered Ks in liver. The authors concluded that GH and IGF-1 differentially increase tissue protein synthesis *in vivo.*

In another study, seven calorically restricted normal volunteers were treated with a combination of GH and IGF-1, and the effects on anabolism and carbohydrate metabolism were compared to treatment with IGF-1 alone.[222] The GH/IGF-1 combination caused significantly greater nitrogen retention compared to IGF-1 alone. GH/IGF-1 treatment resulted in substantial urinary potassium conservation, suggesting that most protein accretion occurred in muscle and connective tissue. GH attenuated the hypoglycemia induced by IGF-1 as indicated by fewer hypoglycemic episodes and higher capillary blood glucose concentrations on GH/IGF-1 compared to IGF-1 alone. These results suggest that the combination of GH and IGF-1 treatment is substantially more anabolic than either IGF-1 or GH alone. GH/IGF-1 treatment also attenuates the hypoglycemia caused by IGF-1 alone.

A recent report demonstrated in a group of calorically restricted (20 kcal/kg ideal body weight/day) normal volunteers that the combination of GH and IGF-1 treatment is substantially more anabolic than either GH or IGF-1 alone.[223]

Thus there are data that demonstrate that recombinant human IGF-1 has GH-like effects on protein metabolism, selectively stimulating whole-body protein synthesis. Additionally, recent studies suggest that the combination of recombinant human GH and IGF-1 might be more anabolic than either compound alone when administered to calorically deprived subjects.

While these studies examined the effects of GH and IGF-1 in surgically stressed or calorie-deprived subjects, a recent study using normally fed healthy individuals did not find a synergistic anabolic effect of GH and IGF-1.[224] In this study subjects receiving combination treatment had a significant increase in plasma IGF-1 concentrations. As expected, there was a significant decrease in leucine oxidation in subjects given combination therapy as well as a significant increase in leucine turnover; hence the nonoxidative leucine disposal, a measure of whole-body protein synthesis, was significantly increased. However, when the absolute changes in all three parameters of leucine kinetics were compared in the three treatment groups (GH alone, IGF-1 alone, and combined GH and IGF-1), there was no additive effect of combination treatment on whole-body protein anabolism.

The authors concluded that, contrary to the calorically deprived model, in normally fed individuals the coadministration of IGF-1 and GH at these doses is not more anabolic on whole-body protein than either compound given alone. This difference in observed effects in the fed and partly fasted state may be related to the difference in total insulin output and suggests a saturable capacity of the body to accumulate protein during normal substrate availability while the body is exposed to individual anabolic hormones. These data suggest a common pathway for GH and IGF-1 to enhance whole-body protein anabolism in the normally fed state.

It would appear from this study that the simultaneous use of GH and IGF-1, while synergistically effective in increasing protein synthesis in catabolic states, does not have the same effects in normally fed healthy individuals. However, this does not necessarily imply that this is the case in athletes. Both the catabolic effects of intense exercise and increasing amino acid availability by increasing the capacity of the body to accumulate protein and increasing substrate availability, may be mitigating factors in determining any synergistic effects of GH and IGF-1 in athletes.

Interestingly, in the natural state GH and IGF-1 are part of a feedback loop so that while IGF-1 levels may be dependent on GH, elevated IGF-1 levels inhibit GH release. Conversely a decrease in IGF-1, as induced by starvation, leads to a compensatory increase in GH release.

Thus it appears that in the natural state both peptides are not present together in elevated levels for any significant period of time. As shown above, amino acids increase the anabolic effects of both GH and IGF-1 so that protein and amino acid supplementation may allow an increased synergism between these two hormones. However, while certain amino acids have been shown to increase GH (and insulin) secretion, amino acids per se have not been shown to increase plasma IGF-1 levels,[225] although in one recent study protein intake was shown to increase fasted but not fed values of IGF-1.[226]

INSULIN

Insulin is produced in the pancreas and is made up of two amino acid chains connected together by a disulfide bridge. It is secreted in the blood where it is bound to carrier proteins and carried to muscle, liver, and other tissues. The main action of insulin is to regulate the glucose level in the blood. In order to do this insulin influences the metabolism of not only sugars or carbohydrates, but also fats and protein.

Nondiabetic people maintain their plasma glucose concentration within a narrow range at all times despite episodic and erratic food intake. During and after meals, insulin, along with other hormones such as glucagon, epinephrine, and growth hormone, regulates the amount of glucose in the blood so that it doesn't go "out of bounds" since both high and low serum glucose can cause problems.

When a meal is eaten, an immediate rise in insulin release occurs such that absorbed carbohydrate is rapidly transported into the liver, muscles, and other tissues. After meals, insulin levels drop as the amount of glucose in the blood decreases. Insulin helps ensure smooth control of plasma glucose throughout the day, regardless of how hectic and erratic our day is. Insulin exerts a permissive effect on nutrient storage processes including increasing the rate of amino acid uptake by muscle.[226-231]

Pancreatic beta cells increase their rate of insulin secretion within 30 s of exposure to increased glucose concentrations, and can shut down just as quickly. Insulin secretion follows a biphasic secretion pattern. An initial burst first occurs, thought to prime the pancreas for a later sustained secretion. While the first phase involves only stored insulin in the pancreas, the second, more sustained phase includes both stored and newly synthesized insulin. Type-II diabetes often features an absence of the initial insulin release phase.

Insulin acts as a nutrient storage hormone involving protein, fat, and carbohydrate synthesis and storage. It promotes processes that build up stores of these macronutrients and inhibits all processes that break down or release those same nutrients. Insulin promotes glucose and amino acid uptake and increases protein synthesis.[233] It would appear that insulin has anabolic properties on par with testosterone, GH, and IGF-1, although likely by different mechanisms,[232] and may be responsible for up to 30% of protein synthesis in skeletal muscle.

Studies have shown the dose-dependent suppressive effect of insulin on protein degradation[234-242] and the stimulatory effect of insulin and insulin/amino acid infusion on protein synthesis.[243-254] A recent study looked at the contribution of dietary amino acids and endogenous hyperinsulinemia to prandial protein anabolism.[255] The results of this study demonstrate that by increasing whole-body protein synthesis and decreasing proteolysis, dietary amino acids account for the largest part (approximately 90%) of postprandial protein anabolism.

In a review of the hormonal regulation of protein degradation in skeletal and cardiac muscle, the authors felt that insulin is probably the single most influential factor for regulating and maintaining positive nitrogen balance in heart and skeletal muscle.[256]

Insulin promotes protein synthesis by directly stimulating the uptake of amino acids by muscle cells as well of the uptake of those substrates (e.g., glucose) required to support the process.[257] One study looking at how insulin exerts its protein anabolic and/or anticatabolic effects in muscle tissue, used human Type I diabetic male patients as subjects, in both insulin-deprived and insulin-treated states.[258] Among the many other findings was that insulin augmented protein anabolism by decreasing leucine transamination to alpha-ketoisocaproate.

The issue has also been investigated using healthy volunteers with the aid of stable isotopic tracers of amino acids.[259] Calculations of muscle protein synthesis, breakdown, and amino acid transport were made. Insulin infusion into the femoral artery caused a decrease in tissue concentrations of free essential amino acids and an increase in the fractional synthesis rate of muscle protein. While insulin did not significantly modify the catabolic release of phenylalanine, leucine, and lysine, it did increase the rates of inward transport of leucine, lysine, and alanine in leg muscle tissue. The authors concluded that hyperinsulinemia, within the physiological range, promoted muscle protein anabolism primarily by stimulating protein synthesis independently of any effect on transmembrane transport.

Recent evidence shows that insulin may exert its protein anticatabolic effect through stimulating cell hydration.[260] Insulin stimulates cell transporter systems that result in a cellular accumulation of potassium, sodium, and chloride, leading to cell water retention. The resultant swelling, in turn, signals increased protein synthesis in the cell. Glucagon produces opposite effects (cell dehydration), and thus promotes protein catabolism.

Other studies have shown that insulin increases skeletal muscle protein synthesis and decreases skeletal muscle protein breakdown, especially if hypoacidemia is not present. It appears that adequate amino acids must be present to maximize insulin's effects on protein metabolism.[261] Interestingly, the use of certain amino acids may increase endogenous insulin as well as providing the needed amino acid substrates for protein synthesis.

In one recent study, the effects of insulin were measured *in vivo*.[262] *In vitro*, insulin has been shown to increase skeletal muscle (SM) protein synthesis and decrease SM protein breakdown. Whether these same effects are found *in vivo* in humans is less clear. The study of the effect of hyperinsulinemia (INS) on SM protein turnover (SMPT) is complicated by hypoaminoacidemia, which can obviate the true effect of insulin on SMPT. To prevent this, the authors studied the effect of INS on SMPT in the human forearm with amino acid (AA) infusion to ensure adequate substrate for full evaluation of insulin's effect. They found that protein balance became positive with INS + AA infusion.

Insulin can influence other anabolic hormones including GH,[263] IGF-1,[264,265] and testosterone[266] to further increase the overall anabolic effect. A study recently looked at the effects of insulin suppression after long-term diazoxide (an inhibitor of pancreatic insulin secretion) administration on testosterone and SHBG (sex hormone-binding globulin) blood concentrations in two groups of obese and healthy normal-weight men.[267] The results of this study demonstrated that insulin stimulates testosterone production while at the same time inhibiting SHBG in adult normal-weight healthy controls and obese individuals. The decrease in SHBG, without a parallel drop in total testosterone, increases the serum level of free testosterone, the active form of testosterone.

The authors of this study felt that insulin may increase testosterone levels through one or several mechanisms that include:

1. It may work synergistically with luteinizing hormone (LH), the pituitary hormone that dictates testicular testosterone production. It may do this by stimulating a testes enzyme called 11-beta-hydroxysteroid dehydrogenase which has been shown to relieve steroid-dependent inhibition of Leydig cell function and thus increase testosterone secretion.[267]
2. Insulin may suppress activity of a peripheral enzyme found in fat called aromatase. This enzyme converts testosterone into estrogen, thus decreasing plasma testosterone levels. By suppressing this enzyme, insulin raises free testosterone levels.

Although insulin increases both glycogen and fat storage, there is a clear-cut dissociation between the effects of insulin on protein, lipid, and glucose metabolism.[268] Thus while the effect of GH opposes the action of insulin on sugar uptake and fatty acid release, it complements the anabolic action of insulin on amino acid uptake.[269]

Thus insulin may have a synergistic protein-synthesizing effect with GH. Some believe that GH has a superior muscle protein-synthesizing effect compared to insulin, while insulin has a superior anticatabolic effect. Some studies, however, show that GH interferes with insulin's anticatabolic properties,[270] as do corticosteroids. The effects of glucocorticoid on basal muscle protein turnover are minimized by compensatory hyperinsulinemia, and glucocorticoids cause muscle resistance to insulin's antiproteolytic action.[271]

As well, insulin can suppress the stimulation by glucocorticoids of muscle protein catabolism.[272] In one study it was found that the administration of insulin and testosterone, and feeding a high-protein high-fat diet, minimized muscle protein wasting by counteracting insulin resistance caused by corticosterone, and masking the corticosterone receptor.[273]

Not only does insulin have potent anabolic effects either alone or in concert with other anabolic hormones, but insulin also increases the anabolic effect of certain amino acids. For example, the effect of glutamine on skeletal muscle includes the stimulation of protein synthesis which occurs in the absence or presence of insulin, the response being greater with insulin.[274]

Based on this capacity of insulin to stimulate testosterone production and inhibit SHBG production, it is possible that amino acids (with and without added carbohydrate) which stimulate insulin secretion, particularly after training, may result in an enhanced anabolic state.

Insulin, GH, and IGF-1 Synergism

As well as the GH/IGF-1 combination mentioned above, there are other studies supporting the synergistic effects on protein metabolism with combinations of other hormones. In one study, GH and insulin separately produced an increase in whole-body and skeletal muscle protein net balance. GH plus insulin was associated with a higher net balance of protein than was insulin alone.[275] There thus appears to be a synergistic improvement in whole-body and skeletal muscle protein kinetics when GH and insulin are used together. For example, together they reduce whole-body and skeletal muscle protein loss in cancer patients.[276] It has also been shown that insulin and IGF-1 have additive effects on protein metabolism.[277]

An increase in whole-body and skeletal muscle protein net balance was produced with separate administration of GH and insulin in postabsorptive normal volunteers, and a combination of GH and insulin was associated with a higher net balance of protein than either given separately.[278] Such a therapy of a combination of anabolic hormones or of specific nutrients would be expected to be of substantial value in limiting protein catabolism.

A recent study compared the metabolic and cardiovascular effects of recombinant human IGF-1 and insulin in six normal subjects.[279] Results showed that IGF-1 has a similar effect to insulin on glucose metabolism, except with a slower onset and longer duration of action. IGF-1 had no effect on free fatty acid levels in blood. IGF-1 also inhibits insulin secretion and increases cardiac output, heart rate, and stroke volume.

While other studies show that IGF-1 acutely reduces free fatty acid levels, this study showed no effect on fatty acids. This may have been due to the small number of study subjects (6). IGF-1 may directly inhibit insulin release at the level of the pancreatic beta-cells, where insulin is produced. In contrast to insulin, IGF-1 has a definite heart-stimulating action. Insulin only affects the heart in high doses, an effect thought to occur through a cross reaction with IGF-1 cell receptors in the heart.

This study underscores the fact that since IGF-1 can decrease blood glucose levels in a manner similar to that of insulin, large amounts taken under uncontrolled conditions may produce hypoglycemia as a common side effect.

THYROID HORMONES

The thyroid gland, located in the lower front part of the neck, secretes two iodinated amino acids, levothyroxine (T4, L-thyroxine, thyroxine) and liothyronine (T3, triiodothyronine), that are the active thyroid hormones. Triiodothyronine possesses five times the biological activity of L-thyroxine. The thyroid gland is the only source of endogenous T4. Normally, small amounts of T3 (about 15 to 20% of circulating T3) are secreted from the thyroid while the majority comes from the peripheral (mainly in the liver and kidneys) monodeiodination of T4.

Thyroid hormones are essential for the normal growth and development of many tissues and exert most of their effects by increasing the basal metabolic rate, controlling protein synthesis, and the enhancing the lipolytic response of fat cells to other hormones. Thyroxine increases the rate of metabolism of all cells, affects protein metabolism, and modulates energy production. The activity of the citric acid cycle (tricarboxylic acid cycle or Kreb's cycle) is diminished in the presence of high plasma levels of thyroid hormones and enhanced by the hypothyroid state.[280]

Under conditions of insufficient carbohydrates and fats thyroxine increases protein catabolism in order to provide substrates for gluconeogenesis.[281] On the other hand, under normal dietary conditions, including adequate protein intake, thyroxine, in concert with other hormones, can increase the rate of protein synthesis.

Thyroid hormone levels can be influenced by a number of factors. For example, too little or too much iodine in the diet can adversely affect thyroid hormone production. So can excess stress, lack of sleep, and the abuse of alcohol[282] or cocaine.[283]

In animals and humans hypothyroidism is associated with growth impairment, and hyperthyroidism with the development of a hypercatabolic state and skeletal muscle wasting.[284] Both states adversely affect muscle function. Thyrotoxicosis produces myopathy caused by net protein catabolism, accelerated basal metabolic rate, and impaired carbohydrate metabolism.[285]

Although T4 has some hormonal actions itself, it is primarily a prohormone, and most of the actions of thyroid hormones are mediated by T3. In the liver, and many other tissues including muscle, T3, within parenchymal cells, appears to be derived from (or to be in equilibrium with) T3 in plasma, whereas about 50% of intracellular T3 in the anterior pituitary and most T3 in brain is locally produced.[286] Thus, the actions of thyroid hormones in liver and muscle, as compared with the pituitary and the brain, might be expected to relate more closely to circulating levels of T3.

The amount of T3 formed varies considerably depending on the hormonal and nutrient environment. For example, T3 increases with overfeeding and with increased carbohydrate intake. Under some conditions such as fasting, a significant amount of T4 is converted peripherally (the thyroid gland is a minor source of both T3 and rT3) to reverse T3 (rT3) at the expense of T3 formation, resulting in lower serum levels of T3.[287-389]

Artifically increasing the levels of T3 results in protein catabolism. In one study with grossly obese subjects, T3 administration resulted in mostly body protein loss and only to a small extent the loss of body fat.[290]

rT3 is more biologically inactive and more calorigenically inactive than either T4 or T3, so diverting T4 metabolism/conversion into making rT3 instead of T3 can save the organism a significant expenditure of energy. Alterations in the metabolism of T4 to rT3 appear to be important in the adjustment of energy expenditure in various tissues during different metabolic and nutritional states.[291]

In acute nonthyroidal illness there are profound alterations in thyroid homeostasis. Most frequently, the "sick euthyroid syndrome" is produced in which the person does not experience clinical symptoms of hypothyroidism, but is physiologically hypothyroid and thus may experience a lowering effect on metabolism. This includes a reduction in serum T3 levels, low or normal T4, normal free T4 and elevated rT3, while TSH is normal.[292] The low serum T3 may be an adaptive mechanism of the body to lower the basic metabolic rate (BMR) and therefore conserve energy and minimize wasting.[293]

The increased conversion of T4 to rT3 and decreased T3 formation has been observed in severe systemic diseases, including starvation and fasting,[294-297] hepatic disease,[298] after surgery,[299] during treatment with corticosteroids,[300] and in high catecholamine states, such as burns.[301] In postoperative critically ill patients, Zaloga et al.[302] observed that although the serum thyroid-stimulating hormone (TSH) response to thyrotropin-releasing hormone (TRH) was normal after surgery, the maximal TRH-induced increase in serum TSH and the integrated serum TSH response to TRH were suppressed in the early postoperative period.

Starvation impairs T4 conversion to T3 and can increase rT3 formation both in humans and in animals.[303,304] When T3 is administered in physiologic amounts to fasting subjects, plasma T3 increases, T4 and rT3 are unchanged, thyroid-stimulating hormone (TSH) response to thyrotropin-releasing hormone (TRH) is diminished, and nitrogen excretion increases. This suggests that the low T3 levels during fasting spare muscle protein and that there is a lower set point for regulation of TSH secretion in fasting subjects.[305]

In humans, these changes in thyroid metabolism are more readily reversed by carbohydrate than by protein or fat.[306,307] The relative contributions of various tissues to T4 metabolism and where the effects of starvation and other influences of T4 conversion actually occur are not known, but the liver is undoubtedly a major site and has been most widely studied.

In an attempt to explain reverse T3 changes during protein-supplemented semistarvation, reverse T3 (rT3) and T3 changes have been evaluated in regard to bodyweight changes and changes of nutrient combustion.[308] The authors concluded that although no definite clue could be found for the rT3 increase during semistarvation, a combined effect of lipolysis and lean mass preservation is suggested.

Overfeeding results in an adaptive thermogenic response (a process whereby excess calories are converted to heat rather than stored as fat) that attenuates any resulting weight gain. Part of this adaptive response is related to an increase in thermogenesis manifested as an increase in the resting metabolic rate. Thyroid hormone, a well-known regulator of the biogenesis of mitochondria in many tissues, is also the major effector of the increased mitochondrial biogenesis in brown adipose tissue seen secondary to adaptive changes.[309]

Overeating leads to increased plasma levels of T3 and decreased levels of rT3 while a converse effect is seen in starvation, with decreased T3 and increased rT3 levels.[310] Starvation produces a rapid fall in the basal metabolic rate (BMR) of 20% or more, and impairs thermogenesis in parallel with the drop in thyroid hormone.

Besides the adverse physiological effects of large amounts of thyroid hormone (with associated neurological and cardiovascular complications), the significant muscle loss, and the suppression of the hypothalamic-pituitary-thyroid axis, there has recently been some evidence that both hyperthyroidism and thyroxine replacement therapy may be associated with subclinical liver damage.[311]

Thyroid Hormones and Protein Metabolism

The effects of low or high thyroid hormone levels on protein synthesis and skeletal muscle have been well documented. However, the studies looking at changes in thyroid levels during exercise are not consistent and give rise to some confusion.

Thyroxine and triiodothyronine stimulate both protein synthesis and degradation — depending on their levels and the presence and levels of other hormones and regulators. In physiological concentrations thyroid hormones stimulate the synthesis as well as the degradation of proteins, whereas in higher or supraphysiological doses protein catabolism (breakdown) predominates — as part of the overall hypermetabolism that occurs. Thus hypothyroidism suppresses muscle growth while hyperthyroidism increases protein catabolism.

The rate of protein degradation is significantly higher in hyperthyroid patients. In one study a significant positive correlation was found between serum T3 and rate of protein degradation in skeletal muscle.[312] This study demonstrated for the first time increased proteolysis in skeletal muscle tissue from patients with high serum T3 concentrations. Hyperthyroidism also increases the rate of glutamine release from skeletal muscle.[313]

Thus in hyperthyroidism or with the use of high doses of thyroid hormone, the net effect is muscle wasting (with an increase in the turnover of body protein) rather than hypertrophy. Prolonged use of large doses of thyroid may result in extensive muscular wasting. In contrast, an excess in thyroid hormone can produce cardiac muscle hypertrophy.[314]

One study investigated the responsiveness of protein metabolism to insulin as a mediator of the protein catabolic response to hyperthyroidism in humans.[315] Six healthy volunteers were studied in a postabsorptive state before and after oral intake of thyroid hormones. Insulin was infused for 140 min under euglycemic and eukalemic clamps. An appropriate amino acid infusion was used to blunt insulin-induced hypoaminoacidemia.

Hyperthyroidism induced a significant proteolysis and the oxidation and nonoxidative disposal of leucine. Insulin lowered proteolysis, and hyperthyroidism improved the ability of insulin to inhibit proteolysis. Insulin also moderately lowered protein synthesis in both control and hyperthyroid states. These changes in insulin action may provide a mechanism to save body protein during hyperthyroidism.

To study the role of thyroid hormones in exercise-induced muscle growth and protein synthesis, Katzeff et al. measured skeletal and cardiac muscle protein synthesis and MHC gene expression in hypothyroid rats allowed to exercise voluntarily.[316] The rats without exercise experience significant skeletal muscle atrophy while the exercise group did not. Exercise, therefore, seems to mediate the effects of hypothyroidism on skeletal muscle protein synthesis. Calorie-reduced diets, when combined with exercise, can result in an increase in protein synthesis which helps maintain lean body mass, aided by a decrease of T3 which protects the organism against energy deficit.[317]

The authors of one study investigating diurnal changes in whole-body protein turnover associated with the increasing fasting body nitrogen (N) losses and feeding gains with increasing protein intake in normal adults, found that thyroid hormones (free and total triiodothyronine) did not change in any state.[318] Resting metabolic rate in the fasted and fed state was not influenced by dietary protein intake, but was increased by feeding with no influence of dietary protein concentration.

A study investigated the relations between changes in plasma insulin and triiodothyronine (T3), and muscle growth and protein turnover in the rat in response to diets of varying protein concentrations.[319] The authors found that dietary energy had no identifiable influence on muscle growth. In contrast, increased dietary protein appeared to stimulate muscle growth directly by increasing muscle RNA content and inhibiting proteolysis, as well as increasing insulin and free T3 levels.

They also found that changes in rates of muscle growth were accompanied by parallel changes in rates of protein synthesis and degradation as well as parallel changes in concentrations of plasma insulin and free T3, to the extent that all these variables were highly correlated with each other. Insulin and free T3 stimulated each other as well as muscle protein turnover.

On the other hand, a study in rats found that high-protein diets decreased T3 levels. This study looked at the effects of a high-protein (30%, HP) and a medium-protein (15%, MP) diet in rats after 21 days of hindlimb unweighting.[320] With respect to pair-fed animals, a significant reduction in protein synthesis occurred (33%) in MP nonweight-bearing rats, whereas it was of lesser magnitude and not significant in HP rats. The authors concluded that because the circulating level of free triiodothyronine was reduced by 14% with the HP diet, this effect on protein synthesis may involve thyroid hormones.

It seems that with strenuous exercise, thyroid function decreases.[321] In some cases, one way to stop the decrease is to eat more;[322] another way appears to be by phosphate supplementation.[322a] However, some lowering of the T3 levels may be beneficial and lead to increased protein synthesis and a decreased energy deficit.

Thyroid Hormone and Other Hormones

Thyroid hormone may act synergistically or antagonize the anabolic effects of GH, IGF-1, insulin, and testosterone. The effect of thyroid hormone seems to vary in different species. For example, in both the rat and fish, thyroid hormone increases transcription of growth hormone mRNA in the pituitary and increases protein synthesis.[323]

In vitro studies on goat testicular cells have shown that T3 resulted in a dose-dependent increase in androgen release from testicular Leydig cells.[324] T3 also had additive stimulatory effects on LH-augmented androgen release from Leydig cells. In an *in vitro* study using sheep thyroid, thyroid cells were found to be a site for IGF action, binding, and production.[325] In this study IGF synthesis was enhanced consistently by recombinant growth hormone.

In humans, however, thyroid hormone seems to decrease GH effects possibly by reducing the bioavailability of IGF-1, and to antagonize the anabolic effects of testosterone and insulin. Thyroid hormones in excess, like glucocorticoids, increase the catabolism of fast glycolytic fibers, whereas androgens, catecholamines, and beta-agonists have been shown to be anabolic and produce an enlargement.[326] As well, thyroid hormone activity is reduced by androgens.[327] Decreases in thyroid hormone secretion and serum levels can occur secondary to the use of anabolic steroids.[328,329]

A recent study measured urea nitrogen synthesis rates and blood alanine levels concomitantly before, during, and after a 4-h constant intravenous infusion of alanine.[330] Eight normal male subjects were randomly studied four times: (1) after 10 days of subcutaneous saline injections, (2) after 10 days of subcutaneous growth hormone injections, (3) after 10 days of T3 administration, and (4) after 10 days given (2) + (3). The results of the study show GH decreased functional hepatic nitrogen clearance and that T3 has no effect on functional hepatic nitrogen clearance. However, given together with growth hormone, T3 abolishes the effect of growth hormone on functional hepatic nitrogen clearance. A possible mechanism is the known effect of thyroid hormones in reducing the bioavailability of IGF-1.

A decline in urea excretion is seen following long-term growth hormone administration, reflecting overall protein anabolism. Conversely, hyperthyroidism is characterized by increased urea synthesis and negative nitrogen metabolism. These seemingly opposite effects are presumed to reflect different actions on peripheral protein metabolism. The extent to which these hormonal systems have different direct effects on hepatic urea genesis has not been fully characterized.

In one study, therapy with growth hormone for 6 months to adult patients with growth hormone deficiency increased lean body mass, decreased fat mass, improved the sense of general well-being in most patients, increased bone turnover without a measurable increase in bone density, caused some minor changes in lipid and carbohydrate metabolism, and increased the metabolism of thyroxine to T3.[331] In the same study the authors felt that the mechanism by which thyroid hormone produces cardiac hypertrophy and myosin isoenzyme changes remains unclear but may involve IGF-1, another anabolic compound. In this study, levels of T4 and free T4 as well as rT3 decreased, while T3 increased during growth hormone treatment.

As well, it has been shown that physiological doses of insulin selectively attenuate the stimulatory effect of T3 on GH mRNA levels.[332] Thus insulin decreased the thyroid-increased GH synthesis. This suppressive effect of insulin occurs independently of protein synthesis and is presumably mediated both at a transcriptional and posttranscriptional level. Insulin has previously been shown to inhibit basal and stimulated rat GH (rGH) secretion as well as basal GH transcription in rat pituitary cells.

It appears that in humans, thyroid hormone changes are largely independent of changes in insulin and glucagon. The effect of isocaloric (500 kcal) protein and carbohydrate ingestion was studied in a crossover study in nine healthy humans. The physiological increase in insulin after carbohydrate ingestion, and the physiological increase in glucagon after protein ingestion was not associated with any changes in total T4, free T4, T3, free T3, or rT3.

TESTOSTERONE

The androgenic and anabolic actions of substances produced by the testes have been known for centuries. Two case reports by Sacchi[333] and Rowlands and Nicholson[334] comprise the early evidence of the influence of testicular androgens, specifically testosterone, on growth and musculoskeletal development. Kenyon and associates, in a series of studies extending from 1938 to 1944,[335-338] investigated and elucidated the metabolic effects of testosterone. They were the first to outline possible clinical uses for testosterone.

Stress has an adverse effect on serum testosterone levels. Decreased plasma testosterone levels have been observed after surgery[339,340] and myocardial infarction.[341] Woolfe et al.[342] observed that critically ill men and women have decreases in plasma concentrations of testosterone and estradiol, respectively. The latter explains the amenorrhea seen during such stressful situations. The exact cause is not clear but may be due to decreased or altered secretion of intrapituitary and suprapituitary substances (e.g., FSH and LH) and/or decreased response of the pituitary to gonadotropin-releasing hormone.[343]

Testosterone levels can increase or decrease with exercise. Some studies have shown that serum testosterone concentrations tend to increase if the resistance training session lasts for a relatively short period of time, say from 30 to 60 min,[344-349] and that repetitive, intense resistance training can reduce resting serum testosterone levels when the overall training stress is exceptionally high for too long a period.[350] For instance, it has been shown that 2 hours of resistance training twice a day can decrease resting testosterone concentrations.[351] This would be expected to lower the testosterone/cortisol (T/C) ratio, an indicator of changes in the anabolic-androgenic activity of the body,[352] in favor of a catabolic state.

Studies have found that women with low average testosterone:SHBG ratios (an index of the serum free testosterone concentration) did not increase their muscle mass to the same degree as those with higher ratios.[353] In women, the level of serum testosterone seems just as important for the development of muscle strength and hypertrophy during resistance training as in men.

Studies have shown that testosterone increases muscle protein synthesis and enhances strength, size, and athletic performance.[354] A recent study has definitively shown that supraphysiologic doses of testosterone significantly increases both muscle size and strength in normal men.[355] In this study 43 normal men were assigned to 4 different groups: placebo with no exercise, and testosterone with no exercise, placebo plus exercise, testosterone plus exercise. The men received injections of 600 mg of testosterone enanthate or placebo weekly for 10 weeks. The results of this study conclusively show that supraphysiologic doses of testosterone increase muscle mass and strength, both on its own and more so when combined with exercise.

Androgens such as testosterone (and their regulating hormones such as luteinizing hormone [LH]) and GH increase with short bursts of intense exercise as long as the bursts are not taken over too long a period of time so as to become exhausting. The level of testosterone, after a certain point in the exercise session, decreases with increased duration of intense exercise. Thus repetitive and prolonged heavy exercise can be counterproductive. Overtraining also results in chronically lowered serum levels of GH. We thus need to strike a balance between GH and testosterone increases both during and between exercise sessions.

In general, studies have shown a rise in testosterone levels and GH (both during and after the exercise) during short-term high-volume, high-strength-level exercises (such as weight-lifting, sprinting, etc.), while with strenuous prolonged exercises (such as marathon running and other endurance events, or with overtraining in high-strength-level exercise), the testosterone and GH levels are depressed while the cortisol levels are elevated.[356,357] Prolonged stressful exercise can lead to distinct hormonal adaptations that offset some of the changes involving the catecholamines, the hypothalamic-pituitary-testicular axis, and the hypothalamic-pituitary-adrenal axis.[358]

Acute resistance training has been shown to increase serum testosterone levels. A study by Falkel et al. measured the time course for skeletal muscle adaptations to heavy-resistance training in men and women.[359] The authors found that absolute and relative maximal dynamic strength was significantly increased after 4 weeks of training in both sexes. As well, there was an increase in the resting levels of serum testosterone after 4 weeks in men, and a decrease in cortisol after 6 weeks in men.

It has been shown that prolonged physical stress can decrease the serum levels of testosterone and increase serum levels of cortisol and dihydroepiandrosterone sulfate (DHEA-S).[360] In this study the circadian rhythm of hormones was abolished by the adverse conditions and physical stress.

Testosterone is felt to play a major role in the muscle hypertrophic response to exercise although its exact role has yet to be fully defined. As well, the implications of changes in total and free testosterone and in sex hormone-binding globulin (SHBG) have not been adequately investigated and there are many discrepancies in the literature. Although more studies are needed to define the role of testosterone in protein synthesis and the response to exercise, recent studies are providing us with some useful information.

A recent Italian study[361] tested the response of total testosterone, free testosterone (fT), SHBG, and non-SHBG-bound testosterone (NST) to the same exercise protocol in two different experiments on long-distance runners. The two experiments were carried out at the end of the general preparation of the second 4-month macrocycle of the annual training season. In each experiment, each athlete ran for 1 h at a predetermined speed, assessed during a previously performed field test. The first experiment was performed at 9:00 a.m.; the second at 3:00 p.m.

Total testosterone and SHBG decreased after the first experiment, but the value after the recovery period was significantly lower than the initial value only for SHBG. In the second experiment, both total testosterone and SHBG increased after exercise, but only total testosterone decreased significantly to the initial concentration after the rest period. In both experiments, NST and fT increased postexercise and decreased in the rest period to the initial values.

The authors referred to previous studies in which it has been shown that the decrease in SHBG keeps the biologically active fraction of testosterone at a fixed level. As the current study found that SHBG variations showed the same trend as total testosterone, and the values of the two parameters postexercise were positively correlated, the authors claimed that their results provide further support for these earlier findings. In addition, they concluded that their results are suggestive of a compensatory mechanism operating during exercise that maintains adequate concentrations of biologically active testosterone when total testosterone concentrations decrease.

Studies have also shown an increase of GH and IGF-1 with increasing levels of serum testosterone. In a recent study it was shown that there is an association between serum levels of free testosterone and SHBG on the one hand, and serum IGF-1 and IGFBP-1 on the other.[362] In this study serum levels of IGF-1 decreased both with increasing age and increasing sex hormone-binding globulin levels, but increased with increasing free testosterone.

As well as having anabolic effects, testosterone may also decrease muscle catabolism. This effect of testosterone can be seen in the decreased exercise-induced alanine levels seen with hypertestosteronemia.[363]

The anabolic and catabolic hormones influence each other and their combined effects can be synergistic or antagonistic depending on the hormones involved and on the overall environment. As we have seen, GH, IGF-1, testosterone, and insulin can act synergistically in increasing protein synthesis and decreasing protein catabolism, and without GH and IGF-1 testosterone has limited anabolic effects. However, the combined use of testosterone and IGF-1 results in a synergistic effect on protein metabolism.[364] As well, testosterone and anabolic steroids increase GH secretion[365,366] partly secondary to their aromatization to estradiol,[367] and also increase serum IGF-1 levels.[368]

CATABOLIC HORMONES

Testosterone, insulin, GH, and IGF-1 can generally be considered anabolic hormones as they increase protein synthesis or decrease protein degradation, or both. Corticosteroids (cortisol, cortisone, and other similar endogenous and exogenous glucocorticoid compounds), glucagon, and the catecholamines are the main catabolic hormones. Studies have shown that simultaneous physiologic elevations of the concentrations of the three hormones cortisol, glucagon, and epinephrine can accelerate net skeletal muscle proteolysis.[369]

The anabolic and catabolic hormones interact in complex and intricate ways and their serum levels often reflect the influences of their hormonal counterparts. An example is the interaction between insulin and cortisol. Glucocorticoids and insulin are major, antagonistic, long-term regulators of energy balance.[370] Studies have shown that insulin and corticosteroids interact to affect cellular metabolism in various ways depending on their respective serum levels. There are marked diurnal rhythms in function of the hypothalamic-pituitary-adrenal (HPA) axis under both basal and stress conditions. The HPA axis controls corticosteroid output from the adrenal and, in turn, forward elements of this axis are inhibited by feedback from circulating plasma corticosteroid levels.

A recent review proposed the hypothesis that normal diurnal rhythms in the HPA axis are highly regulated by activity in medial hypothalamic nuclei to effect an interaction between corticosteroids and insulin such that optimal metabolism results in response to changes in the fed or fasted state of the animal.[371] Corticosteroids interact with insulin on food intake and body composition, and corticosteroids also increase insulin secretion. Corticosteroids stimulate feeding at low doses but inhibit it at high doses; however, it is the high levels of insulin, induced by high levels of corticosteroids, that may inhibit feeding. Corticosteroids both synergize with and antagonize the effects of insulin. In the presence of elevated insulin stimulated by glucocorticoids and nutrition, stress causes less severe catabolic effects.

The metabolic responses to skeletal muscle stress and injury include accelerated net skeletal muscle protein breakdown associated with increased stress hormone and decreased insulin concentrations. In one study, temporary insulin suppression during physiologic increases in stress hormone concentrations amplified whole-body nitrogen loss and led to the development of accelerated net skeletal muscle protein breakdown.[372] Therefore, increasing or maintaining insulin levels and amino acid availability would likely decrease the catabolic response to exercise and other stressors.

Effect of the Catabolic Hormones on Skeletal Muscle Catabolism

The mobilization of amino acids from skeletal muscle is an adaptive response to stress. The liberated amino acids are oxidized and used as fuel, and they are taken up by the immune system, liver, and other visceral organs. The proteolysis of muscle under physical stress thus enables the body to shift protein resources from muscle to the more urgent needs of the immune system and visceral organs.

This shift is in large part mediated by circulating levels of cortisol, glucagon, epinephrine, and growth hormone. While there are other hormones and factors involved in this shift, there is less information on how these factors affect protein synthesis and degradation. For example, while increased local or circulating levels of interleukin 1 and tumor necrosis factor alpha (TNF-a) in patients with a systemic inflammatory process probably play a major role in sparing the visceral protein compartment at the expense of the skeletal muscle, it is not known if these two factors significantly affect protein metabolism under physical stress.

Increased plasma levels of the catabolic hormones glucagon, epinephrine, and cortisol secondary to trauma and sepsis affect the metabolic response to these stressors. Infusion of the three hormones causes significant negative nitrogen and potassium balances, glucose intolerance, hyperinsulinemia, insulin resistance, sodium retention, and peripheral leukocytosis.[373,374]

In a study set up to determine the part that these hormones have and whether they act synergistically, normal subjects were infused with hydrocortisone, glucagon, and epinephrine at levels that simulated the plasma levels seen after moderate injury.[375] The infusion produced increases in glucose production and decreases in glucose clearance. The effect was more pronounced when all three hormones were administered than when they were infused individually or in groups of two. The authors thus proposed that these hormones act synergistically.

In one study physiological elevations of plasma cortisol levels, as are encountered in stress and severe trauma, were produced in 6 normal subjects by infusing them with hydrocortisone for 64 h. Physiological hypercortisolemia produced increases in proteolysis, and in glutamine and alanine production (secondary to proteolysis and de novo synthesis).[376]

In another study, accelerated muscle protein breakdown was found after a mixture of the catabolic hormones were infused into normal rats.[377] The authors felt that although increased muscle proteolysis was mediated in part by catabolic hormones, reduced muscle protein synthesis and amino acid uptake are probably signaled by other substances or mechanisms. In yet another recent study set up to determine the acute *in vivo* response of human muscle protein to stress, arterial infusion of the catabolic hormones epinephrine, cortisol, and glucagon resulted in a net catabolism of human muscle protein by increasing the rate of protein breakdown in excess of an increased protein synthesis rate.[378]

However, the degree of nitrogen loss observed during the infusion of the counterregulatory hormones (glucagon, epinephrine, and cortisol) into normal subjects is less than that observed during injuries causing comparable increases in the counterregulatory hormones.[379] Studies have indicated that tumor necrosis factor (TNF) may be the principle catabolic monokine, with IL-1 potentiating skeletal muscle proteolysis.[380,381]

Increases or decreases in any or all of insulin, growth hormone, IGF-1, and testosterone may affect the individual or combined catabolic effects of cortisol, glucagon, and epinephrine. For example, the catabolic hormonal effects of cortisol, glucagon, and epinephrine may be significantly attenuated by a concurrent increase in serum insulin concentration, although how insulin may modify the catabolic hormonal effects remains to be fully elucidated. This modifying effect of insulin may itself be reduced if insulin concentration does not rise until after the catabolic hormonal effects have become established.

CATECHOLAMINES

Catecholamines exist in the circulation both as free catecholamines and as the sulfur conjugate that accounts for 60 to 90% of the total catecholamines.[382] The serum levels of the catecholamines norepinephrine[383] and epinephrine[384] have been observed to increase after a variety of stresses, including anxiety, hypotension,[385] hypothermia, hypercarbia, and accidental injury.[386]

Epinephrine is secreted by the adrenal medulla in response to sympathetic nervous system activation, while norepinephrine spills over into the plasma after release from the sympathetic nerve endings. The sympathetic nervous system, in turn, is controlled by the hypothalamus, the same area of the brain responsible for the excretion of releasing factors that initiate the secretion of other endocrine hormones. Plasma levels of epinephrine and norepinephrine do not necessarily increase concurrently.[387] In a study of major accidental injury, plasma epinephrine concentrations were increased for only a short period (about 48 h) while norepinephrine levels remained elevated for periods of up to 8 to 10 days.[388]

Plasma epinephrine concentrations reflect adrenomedullary secretion, whereas plasma norepinephrine concentrations are used as an index of sympathetic nervous system activity. It is important to realize that most of the norepinephrine released by sympathetic ganglia is removed from the synapse by re-uptake into the nerve ending.[389]

Epinephrine in physiologic doses results in glycogenolysis, increased hepatic gluconeogenesis with mobilization of gluconeogenic precursors from peripheral tissues, inhibition of insulin release, peripheral insulin resistance, and lipolysis.[390,391] Epinephrine is a potent stimulator of gluconeogenesis. This is demonstrated by the observation that during starvation there is no diminution in the ability of epinephrine to stimulate gluconeogenesis. This contrasts with glucagon's gluconeogenic ability, which is less in starved than fed subjects.[392]

Catecholamines are important in increasing glucose production rates during exercise. A recent study looked at defining the relative roles of catecholamine vs. glucagon/insulin responses in stimulating glucose production rates and found that the catecholamines are most important in the regulation of glucose production rates in intense exercise.[393]

Sympathoadrenal activation during physical and emotional stress results in release of epinephrine and norepinephrine into the circulation. Heavy exercise and trauma have been reported to result in a 10- to 20-fold elevation of plasma epinephrine concentrations above resting values.[394,395] Increased plasma catecholamine concentrations are associated with well-recognized changes in glucose,[396] fat,[397] and ketone body metabolism.[398,399]

Effects of Catecholamines on Protein Metabolism

The mediators of muscle breakdown may be many. Shaw et al. observed that alpha-adrenergic blockade reduces nitrogen losses.[400] Thus, adrenergic activity may be involved in catabolism. However, it seems that the catecholamines are not catabolic with regard to whole-body protein breakdown, although they do induce muscle protein proteolysis. For example, an epinephrine infusion will decrease proteolysis and thereby reduce circulating amino acid (except alanine) levels.[401,402]

There are only a small number of studies that have looked at the effects of catecholamines on protein metabolism in humans. Epinephrine administration results in decreased plasma concentrations of branched-chain amino acids in normal and diabetic subjects.[403] Epinephrine infusion into normal subjects has been shown to decrease whole-body proteolysis studied by tracer infusions of amino acids.[404] However, epinephrine infusion resulted in increased plasma insulin concentrations which may have confounded epinephrine's effects.

Epinephrine seems to have a split personality in that it has been shown to both increase and inhibit protein catabolism. For example, epinephrine has adrenergic effects, and beta-adrenergic stimulation has been reported to inhibit amino acid release from skeletal muscle.[405,406] As well, the results of some studies are consistent with an insulin-like effect of epinephrine.[407]

A more definitive study, however, has cleared up some of this confusion. This study looked at the effect of hyperepinephrinemia on leucine plasma flux, oxidation, and nonoxidative disappearance using 1-[^{13}C]leucine infusions.[408] The authors assessed the contribution of muscle proteins in epinephrine's effect on whole-body leucine kinetics by measuring net plasma leucine balance across the forearm and determining the role of beta-adrenergic receptors in mediating epinephrine's effect on leucine kinetics. They eliminated confounding effects of altered insulin and glucagon concentrations by administration of somatostatin with replacement infusions of the two pancreatic hormones.

Epinephrine was infused either alone or combined with propranolol (beta-blockade) into groups of six subjects fasted overnight; leucine flux, oxidation, and net plasma leucine forearm balance were determined during 180 min. All effects of epinephrine were independent of alternations in plasma insulin and glucagon concentrations since constant plasma insulin and glucagon concentrations were maintained in all studies by infusing somatostatin combined with insulin and glucagon replacements. During epinephrine infusion, net forearm leucine release increased threefold, suggesting that the 22% fall of total body leucine flux during epinephrine was the result of a considerably greater fall of leucine appearance from nonmuscle tissues such as splanchnic organs.

The results suggest that elevation of plasma epinephrine concentrations similar to those observed in severe stress results in redistribution of body proteins and exerts a whole body protein-sparing effect, but a catabolic effect on skeletal muscle tissue. Net forearm release of leucine increased during epinephrine, suggesting increased muscle proteolysis. The fall of total body leucine flux was therefore due to diminished proteolysis in nonmuscle tissues such as splanchnic organs. The effect of epinephrine on forearm blood flow agrees with a previous paper,[409] and largely explains the increase in net leucine forearm balance.

As well, epinephrine infusion resulted in a significant increase in plasma glucose concentrations. This effect was mediated via beta-adrenergic receptors. Hyperepinephrinemia also results in a significant increase in plasma FFA concentrations due to its lipolytic effect. This effect was also beta-receptor mediated.[410] Elevation of plasma FFA in dogs decreased leucine plasma flux, oxidation, and concentration.[411] The inhibitory effect of epinephrine on proteolysis is at least in part mediated through the increase in FFA.

Studies have demonstrated that epinephrine administration results in increased circulating plasma insulin concentrations in humans.[412] These may have decreased plasma leucine flux and amino acid concentrations.[413] To exclude the confounding effect of insulin these studies were performed using somatostatin with insulin and glucagon replacements to maintain constant plasma insulin and glucagon concentrations.

As well, the hypothesis that epinephrine reduces protein synthesis by virtue of its stimulatory effect on branched-chain amino acid oxidation[414] may be true in skeletal muscle but not in the splanchnic bed.

Thus, the present data suggest that acute hyperepinephrinemia results in redistribution of amino acids, with a catabolic effect on skeletal muscle. While muscles such as those of the forearm release amino acids, protein breakdown is inhibited in other tissues. Whether prolonged beta-adrenergic stimulation or blockade influence whole-body protein metabolism remains to be determined.

However, although increases in catecholamines can be generally considered catabolic, recent work has again pointed out the possible anabolic effects of these hormones. A recent study has shown that epinephrine directly inhibits proteolysis of skeletal muscle via the beta-adrenoceptor.[415] However, the decrease in proteolysis is likely more than offset by a decrease in protein synthesis, resulting in an overall catabolic response. Future studies will help define the role of the catecholamines in protein metabolism.

GLUCAGON

Glucagon, a hormone synthesized and secreted by the alpha-2 cells of the pancreatic islets of Langerhans, is not chemically or structurally related to insulin. Glucagon increases blood glucose concentration by stimulating hepatic glycogenolysis. Besides stimulating glycogenolysis and gluconeogenesis, glucagon stimulates hepatic ketogenesis.[416]

Some of the metabolic effects produced by glucagon in various tissues (e.g., liver, adipose tissue) are similar to those of epinephrine. Glucagon stimulates the formation of adenylate cyclase, which catalyzes the conversion of ATP to cAMP, particularly in the liver and in adipose tissue. Formation of cAMP initiates a series of intracellular reactions including activation of phosphorylase, which promote the degradation of glycogen to glucose. The increase in blood glucose concentration occurs within minutes. Endogenous secretion of glucagon is stimulated when blood glucose concentration is low or when serum insulin concentration is increased.

In general, the actions of glucagon are antagonistic to those of insulin; however, glucagon has been reported to stimulate insulin secretion in healthy individuals and in patients with Type II diabetes mellitus. Glucagon also has been reported to enhance peripheral utilization of glucose. The intensity of the hyperglycemic effect of glucagon depends on hepatic glycogen reserve and the presence of phosphorylases. The hyperglycemic effect of glucagon is increased and prolonged by concomitant administration of epinephrine. Glucagon produces extrahepatic effects that are independent of its hyperglycemic action. Glucagon has been shown to decrease plasma amino nitrogen concentration and decrease synthesis of protein and fat.

Despite the strong association between protein catabolic conditions and hyperglucagonemia, and enhanced glucagon secretion by amino acids, glucagon's effects on protein metabolism remain less clear than on glucose metabolism. Physiological hyperglucagonemia during insulin resistance is catabolic in the short term and indicates that glucagon may influence muscle protein metabolism acutely in humans.[417]

A study looking at the effects of physiological hyperglucagonemia on protein synthesis found that glucagon may reduce phenylalanine availability for protein synthesis.[418] A recent study concluded that glucagon is the pivotal hormone in amino acid disposal during an amino acid load and, by reducing the availability of amino acids, glucagon inhibits protein synthesis stimulated by amino acids.[419]

Glucagon and Insulin

Glucagon and insulin are both secreted by the pancreas, the former by alpha-cells and the latter by beta-cells. These endocrine secretions enter the portal vein so that the liver is exposed to high concentrations of these hormones. Glucagon increases hepatocyte cyclic AMP and promotes gluconeogenesis;[420] insulin has the opposite effect — it decreases intracellular cyclic AMP concentration and prevents gluconeogenesis. In addition, glucagon increases glycogenolysis, lipolysis, and hepatic ketogenesis in the liver during starvation and diabetic ketoacidosis. The receptor mechanism that increases cyclic AMP concentrations is not the same as used by adrenergic mediators.[421]

Stimulators of glucagon secretion include hypoglycemia, protein ingestion, amino acid infusion, endorphins, exercise, GH, epinephrine, and glucocorticoids.[422,423] Suppressors of glucagon secretion include the infusion and ingestion of glucose, somatostatin, and insulin.[424] Insulin is an anabolic hormone with a multitude of effects. In addition to its role in increasing glucose transport across the cell membranes of adipose tissue and muscle, it stimulates glycogen production, inhibits lipolysis in adipose tissue, inhibits hepatic ketogenesis, and increases the rate of amino acid transport and protein synthesis in muscle, adipose tissue, and liver.

The hormonal milieu of low insulin with elevated counterregulatory hormones, however they are brought about, is thought to be a stimulus to gluconeogenesis. The interaction of the counterregulatory hormones (glucagon, catecholamines, and cortisol) in the response to injury has been of great interest. It is likely that catecholamines and glucagon work synergistically because either infused alone into normal subjects only causes transient elevation in gluconeogenesis, whereas more prolonged gluconeogenesis is seen when they are infused together.[425]

Nevertheless, in both normal and high-protein diets, it is the glucagon to insulin ratio that is the major determinant of the degree of gluconeogenesis.[426] During starvation the ratio is increased (increased glucagon and decreased insulin levels) and gluconeogenesis is promoted, whereas the reverse is true in the fed state. After most types of major surgery[427] there is an increase in plasma glucagon, although some[428] have failed to observe an increase after abdominal hysterectomy. Like starvation, there is an increased glucagon:insulin ratio.

The amino acid composition of the diet influences the postprandial levels of plasma amino acids along with the hormones insulin and glucagon in humans fed single test meals identical in composition except for protein source.[429] Soy protein induces a low postprandial insulin/glucagon ratio in both hypercholesterolemic and normocholesterolemic subjects, while casein induces a high postprandial insulin/glucagon ratio.

Individual and groups of amino acids have varying effects on both insulin and glucagon.[430] In a recent study, the effects of intravenous infusion of 17 amino acids on the secretion of insulin, glucagon, and growth hormone, each at a dose of 3 mmol/kg over 30 min, were studied in 6 castrated male sheep.[431] Leucine was the most effective amino acid in stimulating insulin secretion but did not produce any increase in glucagon and GH secretion. Alanine, glycine, and serine induced a greater enhancement of both glucagon and insulin secretion than other amino acids. No amino acid was able to specifically stimulate glucagon secretion without also increasing insulin or GH secretion. With regard to insulin and glucagon secretion, amino acids could be divided into groups according to their R groups. Neutral straight-chain amino acids stimulated both insulin and glucagon secretion, with a greater secretory response to shorter C-chain amino acids. Branched-chain amino acids tended to enhance insulin and suppress glucagon secretion.

In another study the relationships between changes in the plasma levels of insulin and glucagon in response to the postprandial increments of circulating amino acids were studied under normal physiological conditions in healthy dogs.[432] Multiple correlation analyses indicated that only branched-chain AAs were significantly correlated with insulin increases and were devoid of a relationship to glucagon. Similarly, only ornithine, lysine, and glycine were significantly correlated with glucagon profiles and devoid of a relationship to insulin. The significance of individual glucagon-stimulating effects of alanine and arginine were masked by other amino acid interactions, as significant intercorrelation was found among all 13 amino acids.

CORTISOL

Cortisol is a vital hormone because it diverts glucose utilization from muscles to the brain, facilitates the action of catecholamines, and prevents the overreaction of the immune system to injury.[433] Cortisol has many actions including stimulating gluconeogenesis, increasing proteolysis[434] and alanine synthesis, sensitizing adipose tissue to the action of lipolytic hormones (GH and catecholamines), and anti-inflammatory action. In addition, it causes insulin resistance by decreasing the rate at which insulin activates the glucose uptake system, likely because of a postinsulin receptor block.[435,436]

Increased pituitary production of ACTH stimulates increased glucocorticoid production. Glucocorticoids have a negative feedback effect on ACTH production and can also stimulate the adrenomedullary secretion of catecholamines. The administration of 500 mg cortisol sodium succinate at the time of surgical incision attenuated the increase in plasma ACTH.[437] ACTH release is itself stimulated by corticotrophin releasing factor (CRF) and by catecholamines, vasopressin, and vasoactive intestinal peptide.[438]

Cortisol is increased in stress and is thought to be a major mediator of the response because adrenalectomized animals and patients with Addison's syndrome fare poorly when stressed. This was well demonstrated by the increased mortality rate observed following the use of etomidate to sedate critically ill patients.[439] It was subsequently discovered that etomidate blocks adrenal steroidogenesis, specifically by inhibiting 11-beta-hydroxylation and 17-alpha-hydroxylation.[440,441]

It appears that any type of stress monitored by the central nervous system is relayed to the hypothalamus, which responds by starting the stress hormone cascade beginning with CRF release. Such stresses can include trauma, anxiety, severe infections, hypoglycemia, surgery, and even intense exercise.

In a recent study looking at the effect of cortisol on energy expenditure and amino acid metabolism in humans,[442] the authors found that:

- Acute hypercortisolemia increased protein breakdown 5 to 20%, as measured by increases in leucine and phenylalanine appearance rates;
- Normalizing insulin during hypercortisolemia did not alter phenylalanine flux but enhanced the leucine appearance rate, the latter result indicating that insulin was affecting leucine metabolism during hypercortisolemia;
- The fraction of the leucine flux that was oxidized was not significantly increased with hypercortisolemia, but disposal by the nonoxidative route of leucine uptake for protein synthesis was increased;
- Hypercortisolemia increased cycling of amino acids by increasing protein breakdown and synthesis.

Cortisol can increase body fat levels especially when present in supraphysiological amounts such as is seen in Cushing's disease, where fat distribution increases in the face and abdominal area. As well, cortisol dramatically stimulates lipoprotein lipase, a fat-synthesizing enzyme.[443]

Cortisol, Amino Acids, and Other Hormones

Stress and increased cortisol levels have an adverse effect on serum testosterone levels. A primary anticatabolic effect of exogenous testosterone and the anabolic steroids lies in their interference with muscle cortisol metabolism.[444] As well, these compounds may prevent the growth-suppressing activity of cortisol.[445]

Growth hormone also inhibits the muscle catabolic actions of cortisol.[446] In addition, a recent study found that lowering the cortisol level in the blood enhances the response to growth hormone-releasing hormone in healthy adults.[447] High levels of cortisol blunt GH release during exercise and after taking GH releasers such as arginine. It does this by increasing the release of somatostatin, which blocks GH release in the brain.

Insulin-like growth factor-1 (IGF-1) can diminish the catabolic effects of cortisol without the side effects noted with GH therapy.[448] A recent study has shown that cortisol down-regulates the IGF-1 mRNA levels, indicating that some of the catabolic effects of glucocorticoids in humans is mediated via a reduced autocrine/paracrine expression of IGF-1.[449]

A recent study has shown that glutamine directly prevents the cortisol-induced destruction of muscle contractile proteins.[450] Animal studies have shown that a high-protein, high-fat diet coupled with the use of anabolic steroids will mitigate corticosterone-induced muscle breakdown.[451]

It has been shown that normal increases in cortisol results in stimulation of lipolysis, ketogenesis, and proteolysis, and that circadian variation in cortisol concentration is of physiologic significance in normal humans in that it helps to regulate both anabolic and catabolic events.[452] Even mild elevations in serum cortisol within the physiological range can increase the plasma glucose concentration and protein catabolism within a few hours in healthy individuals.[453,454]

Testosterone/Cortisol Ratio

It has been shown that stress or disease-induced increases in plasma cortisol and corticosterone, the use of long-term systemic (and to a lesser extent inhaled) corticosteroid therapy[455] results in diminished testosterone secretion from the testes. Glucocorticoids suppress testicular steroidogenesis (and adrenal steroidogenesis) in two ways: by inhibiting the anterior pituitary secretion of LH, perhaps secondary to alteration of hypothalamic GnRH secretion,[456] and by directly inhibiting testicular function. The end result is catabolic, with a breakdown of muscle and tendon tissue — counterproductive for athletic performance.

It appears that the level of 11-beta-hydroxysteroid dehydrogenase (11-beta-OHSD) in Leydig cells dictates the level of intracellular glucocorticoid available to the glucocorticoid receptor and thus the potency of corticosteroid as an inhibitor of testosterone secretion.[457] Thus, lowered enzyme activity increases glucocorticoid-dependent inhibition of testosterone production.

One study examined the part played by the glucocorticoids in the ACTH inhibitory effect on plasma testosterone levels in men.[458] Plasma androstenedione, testosterone, cortisol, and LH were measured in 8 normal men, before and after the following tests: ACTH stimulation (2 mg metyrapone, i.m. administration 500 mg/every 4 h/6 times) and dexamethasone suppression (8 mg/d/3 d). In addition, androstenedione and testosterone were evaluated under human chorionic gonadotrophin (5000 IU HCG/d/3 d) before and after dexamethasone suppression (8 mg/d/6 d).

In all patients, ACTH decreased plasma testosterone. In contrast, after metyrapone the mean plasma testosterone was increased. This increase, though not statistically significant, was observed in all patients but one. Both tests resulted in a significant increase of plasma androstenedione. Dexamethasone suppressed both testosterone and androstenedione levels. None of the three tests had a significant effect on the LH concentration. HCG injection increased the mean plasma testosterone. Dexamethasone significantly depressed the testosterone response to HCG. These data are consistent with the following conclusions:

1. The decrease of plasma testosterone levels observed in men after ACTH administration is not observed after metyrapone-induced ACTH increase. This confirms that it is related to cortisol levels rather than to ACTH itself.
2. Glucocorticoids act directly on testicular biosynthesis since they do not induce any change in LH secretion and since dexamethasone reduces testosterone response to HCG.

Testosterone/Cortisol Ratio and Exercise

Cortisol (which induces the breakdown of cellular proteins) increases with increased duration of intense exercise.

In athletes that are training effectively, basal testosterone levels rise as do cortisol levels. Although exercise increases cortisol, well-conditioned athletes show less cortisol secretion during exercise compared to their out-of-shape peers.[459] In overtrained athletes, however, cortisol levels rise more and testosterone levels decline. Thus, one measure of overtraining is the testosterone/cortisol ratio. An elevated cortisol in relation to testosterone suggests overtraining, although a recent study has shown that this may not necessarily be true with some athletes. The results of this study indicate that in endurance trained cyclists, decreased testosterone levels, increased cortisol levels and a decreased testosterone: cortisol ratio does not automatically lead to a decrease in performance or a state of overtraining.[459a]

As well as their direct catabolic effects, cortisol and adrenocorticotrophin hormone (ACTH) have been shown to inhibit luteinizing hormone and testosterone secretion through an effect on both the hypothalamic-pituitary axis (decreasing the secretion of LH and GnRH) and directly on the testes.[460-466] The end result is catabolic, with a breakdown of muscle and tendon tissue — counterproductive for strength-related athletic performance, and for increasing lean body mass.

Endogenous androgens and synthetic anabolic steroids are powerful anabolic compounds partly because of their antiglucocorticoid effects. From the literature it can be seen that these compounds may act as an antiglucocorticoid in at least two ways: by competing with the glucocorticoid receptors and thus blocking their uptake, and by suppressing adrenal glucocorticoid production both directly and by suppressing ACTH. In the rat there is some evidence that anabolic steroids can act via muscle glucocorticoid receptors, thereby antagonizing the catabolic activity of endogenous glucocorticoids, rather than via muscle androgen receptors.[467]

Interestingly, at least some of the protein anabolic effects of anabolic-androgenic steroids on skeletal muscle have been suggested to be due to the inhibition of protein catabolism in this tissue.[468] As noted above, anabolic-androgenic steroids have been hypothesized to enhance muscle hypertrophy via an antagonism of catabolic activity induced by endogenous glucocorticoids, such as cortisol. Thus, anabolic-androgenic steroids may reduce the activity of proteolytic enzyme pathways in skeletal muscle that are dependent on the presence of glucocorticoids for activation.

Endogenous hormones are essential for physiological reactions and adaptations during physical work and influence the recovery phase after exercise by modulating anabolic and catabolic processes. Testosterone and cortisol play significant roles in the metabolism of protein. Both are competitive agonists at the receptor level of muscular cells. The testosterone/cortisol ratio can be used as an indication of the anabolic/catabolic balance and for monitoring fitness, overtraining, and overstrain in strenuous and ultraendurance exercise.[469,470] Decreases in the testosterone/cortisol (and insulin/glucagon ratios — see above) seen during prolonged exercise are consistent with reduced muscle protein synthesis. This ratio decreases in relation to the intensity and duration of physical exercise (the depression in protein synthesis is proportional to the duration and intensity of exercise) as well as during periods of intense training or repetitive competition, and can be reversed by regenerative measures.

It seems likely that the testosterone/cortisol ratio indicates not only the actual physiological strain in training, but also overtraining, especially if other factors are considered. These other factors could include the absolute values of both hormones and the hormonal response to a standardized exhaustive exercise test performed with an intensity of 10% above the individual anaerobic threshold.[471] This response is typically a decreased maximum rise of pituitary hormones (corticotrophin, growth hormone), catecholamines, cortisol, and insulin.

Myofibrillar proteolysis appears to proceed by a pathway in which glucocorticoids (e.g., cortisol or hydrocortisone and to a much lesser degree corticosterone) are essential for the activation.[472] Thus, conditions which may tend to elevate the cortisol concentration, such as overtraining or undernutrition, could lead to an enhanced rate of myofibrillar proteolysis and consequently to muscle atrophy. In support of this view, it has been shown that the response in skeletal muscle to undernutrition is predominantly a decrease in mass, whereas the response in visceral tissues is mainly a reduction in the rate of metabolic activity.[473]

An imbalance between the overall strain experienced during exercise training and the athlete's tolerance of such effort may induce an overreaching or overtraining syndrome. This failure to adapt to training load results in long-term hormonal and biochemical changes that are counterproductive. Overtraining syndrome is characterized by diminished sport-specific physical performance, accelerated fatiguability, and subjective symptoms of stress. Overtraining results in chronically decreased levels of testosterone and growth hormone (GH) and increased levels of cortisol.

It has been shown that, in muscle energy restriction, protein deficiency and corticosterone treatment induces parallel inhibitions of growth and protein synthesis, mediated by similar graded reductions in ribosomal capacity and activity.[474]

Exercise affects hormonal levels both during and after exercise, including during sleep.[475] In one study it was found that long-duration exercise (LDE) of moderate intensity, but not LDE of low intensity, during the daytime changes the typical temporal patterns of hormone release during subsequent nocturnal sleep. During the no-exercise nights, the typical secretory patterns were present with peak concentrations of GH and nadir concentrations of cortisol during the first half of sleep, but increased cortisol levels and minimum GH levels during the second part of sleep. Testosterone concentrations increased during the second half of sleep. LDE of moderate intensity reduced rapid-eye-movement sleep.

Levels of testosterone decreased with increasing intensity of daytime exercise. Moderate, but not low-intensity LDE decreased GH levels in the first half and increased GH levels in the second half of sleep. Also, LDE of moderate intensity but not LDE of low intensity increased cortisol levels during the first half and decreased cortisol secretion during the second half of sleep. Results suggest that nocturnal profiles of GH and cortisol concentrations may serve to indicate the disturbance of normal anabolic functions of sleep due to daytime exercise.

Although cortisol and GH often rise simultaneously as testosterone decreases, there are ways of exercising to minimize cortisol and maximize GH and testosterone.[476-478]

THE EFFECT OF DIETARY NUTRIENTS ON TESTOSTERONE AND THE TESTOSTERONE-CORTISOL RATIO

As we have seen, changing certain training variables such as exercise intensity, duration, and type of exercise can affect the levels of the various anabolic and catabolic hormones. Not as much is known, however, about the effects of dietary nutrients and nutritional supplements on exercise-induced hormonal changes.

A number of studies have shown that both testosterone and cortisol levels can be influenced by dietary manipulation. For example one study has shown that a high-protein, high-fat diet may reduce corticosterone-induced muscle proteolysis.[478a] As well, a recent study measured the effects of dietary fat and fiber on plasma and urine androgens and estrogens in men. The study had a crossover design and included 43 healthy men aged 19 to 56 years.[478b] Men were initially randomly assigned to either a low-fat, high-fiber or high-fat, low-fiber diet for 10 weeks and after a 2-week washout period crossed over to the other diet. The energy content of diets was varied to maintain constant body weight, but averaged approximately 13.3 MJ (3170 kcal)/day on both diets. The low-fat diet provided 18.8% of energy from fat with a ratio of polyunsaturated to saturated fat (P:S) of 1.3, whereas the high-fat diet provided 41.0% of energy from fat with a P:S of 0.6.

Mean plasma concentrations of total- and sex-hormone-binding-globulin (SHBG)-bound testosterone were 13% and 15% higher, respectively, on the high-fat, low-fiber diet and the difference from the low-fat, high-fiber diet was significant for the SHBG-bound fraction. Men's daily urinary excretion of testosterone also was 13% higher with the high-fat, low-fiber diet than with the low-fat, high-fiber diet. Conversely, their urinary excretion of estradiol and estrone and their 2-hydroxy metabolites were 12 to 28% lower with the high-fat, low-fiber diet.

The beneficial effects of dietary fat on serum testosterone was also seen in another earlier study.[478c] This study found that in men a decrease in dietary fat content and an increase in the degree of unsaturation of fatty acids reduces the serum concentrations of androstenedione, testosterone and free testosterone. During the low fat period a significant negative correlation between serum prolactin and androgens was observed. The study also found that with the exception of a small but non-significant decrease in serum estradiol-17 beta, the other hormone parameters were practically unaffected by the dietary manipulation.

Other studies have also shown that dietary changes, including both the amount and composition of the various macronutrients, can significantly affects serum testosterone and cortisol.[478d-f] Results of these studies show that diet can alter endogenous levels of sex hormones and cortisol in both men and women.

A recent study investigated the influence of dietary nutrients on basal and exercise-induced concentrations of testosterone (T) and cortisol (C).[478g] In this study, 12 men performed a bench press exercise protocol (5 sets to failure using a 10-repetitions maximum load) and a jump squat protocol (5 sets of 10 repetitions using 30% of each subject's 1-repetition maximum squat) with 2 min of rest between all sets. A blood sample was obtained at preexercise and 5 min postexercise for determination of serum T and C. Subjects also completed detailed dietary food records for a total of 17 days.

As expected there was a significant increase in postexercise T compared with preexercise values for both the bench press (7.4%) and jump squat (15=2E1%) protocols; C was not significantly different from preexercise concentrations. Interestingly the authors found a significant correlations between preexercise T and percent energy protein, percent energy fat, saturated fatty acids, monounsaturated fatty acids, the polyunsaturated fat-to-saturated fat, and the protein-to-carbohydrate ratio. There were no significant correlations observed between any nutritional variables and preexercise C or the absolute increase in T and C after exercise.

While these data confirm that high-intensity resistance exercise results in elevated postexercise T concentrations, they also show that dietary nutrients are capable of modulating resting concentrations of T and increasing resting testosterone cortisol ratios.

Further discussions on the effects of individual amino acids on endogenous hormonal levels and subsequently on the anabolic effects of exercise can be found under the individual amino acids.

ANABOLIC AND ANTICATABOLIC EFFECTS OF AMINO ACIDS

There are several studies that document the hormonal changes secondary to dietary protein and amino acid intake. Increased blood amino acid levels, secondary to a high protein meal, have been shown to cause insulin and growth hormone levels to rise.[574] Increasing these hormones as well as increasing amino acid levels, but at the same time decreasing muscle catabolism, leads to an enhanced anabolic response. As well, studies have shown that the hormone response to exercise is modified by branched-chain amino acid (BCAA) ingestion.[575]

A recent study looked at the effects of active amino acids and dipeptides as anabolic agents on surgically induced wound healing in lower extremity skeletal muscles in diabetic and normal rats.[576] Their data suggest that amino acids, primarily methionine, and dipeptides methionine-glutamine and tryptophan-isoleucine have a profound anabolic effect on muscle wound healing and on protein synthesis. They found that the amino acid and two dipeptides could override or block the increase in glucocorticoid levels found in diabetic patients.

Another study on rats demonstrated that dietary protein appeared to stimulate muscle growth directly by increasing muscle RNA content and inhibiting proteolysis, as well as increasing insulin and free T3 levels.[577] This apparent direct influence of dietary protein on muscle has also been found in humans. RNA turnover is also regulated by amino acids either directly,[578-581] or via cellular hydration[582] (see above).

Studies have shown that the anabolic effects of intense training are enhanced by a diet high in protein (it is well known that a high-protein diet is essential for the anabolic effects of anabolic steroids[583]). When intensity of effort is maximal and stimulates an adaptive response, protein needs increase in order to provide increased muscle mass. As well, in a recent study it has been shown that protein taken after training may increase both insulin and growth hormone levels, and thus have anabolic effects.[584] The authors of this study examined the effect of carbohydrate and/or protein supplements on the hormonal state of the body after weight-training exercise.

Nine experienced male weight lifters were given water (Control) or an isocaloric carbohydrate (CHO; 1.5 g/kg body wt), protein (PRO; 1.38 g/kg body wt), or carbohydrate-protein (CHO/PRO; 1.06 g carbohydrate/kg body wt and 0.41 g protein/kg) supplement immediately and 2 h after a standardized weight-training workout. CHO/PRO stimulated higher insulin concentrations than PRO and Control. CHO/PRO led to an increase in growth hormone 6 h postexercise that was greater than PRO and Control.

The results of this study (and another study mentioned above[28a]) suggest that nutritive supplements after weight-training exercise can produce a hormonal environment during recovery that may be favorable to muscle growth secondary to insulin and growth hormone elevations.

Increased amino acid availability has been shown to directly influence protein synthesis, especially within a few hours after physical exercise. The rate of protein synthesis, protein catabolism, and amino acid transport is normally increased after exercise and depends on amino acid availability.[585] If there is an increase in the availability of amino acids during this postexercise time interval or window then the catabolic processes are more than offset by the increased anabolic processes, resulting in an overall increase in cellular contractile protein. Thus it is vital to increase the absorption of amino acids as quickly as possible after exercise.

Major operative trauma has been shown to result in increases in arterial levels of glucagon, cortisol, and norepinephrine, a relative lack of insulin, increased muscle proteolysis, increased efflux of amino acids (taurine, serine, glycine, valine, methionine, isoleucine, leucine, phenylalanine, lysine, arginine, and total amino acid nitrogen) and lactate from muscle, and negative nitrogen balance.[586]

A recent study has shown that the signs of muscle protein catabolism elicited by administration of stress hormones can be attenuated by simultaneous administration of a conventional amino acid solution, although the solution used did not contain glutamine.[587] In this study healthy male volunteers were administered a stress-hormone infusion including epinephrine, cortisol, and glucagon either alone or combined with a balanced glutamine-free amino acid solution over a period of 6 h. After 6 h of the stress-hormone infusion, a decrease was observed in skeletal muscle protein synthesis as measured by the size distribution and concentration of ribosomes.[588]

The decrease was prevented by an infusion of the balanced amino acid solution. Following the triple-hormone infusion, a decrease was noted in the content of the total free amino acids in both muscle and plasma. After including amino acids in the infusion solution, the significant decrease in muscle glutamine caused by the triple hormones was not seen. Plasma cortisol, insulin, and glucose increased in response to the triple-hormone infusion alone or in combination with amino acids.

There has been much interest recently in the metabolism of the individual amino acids, especially glutamine. Glutamine is the most abundant amino acid in blood. Its levels in muscle and blood decrease markedly following injury and sepsis, and it is consumed rapidly by replicating cells such as fibroblasts, lymphocytes, and intestinal endothelial cells. Glutamine and alanine transport two thirds of the circulating amino acid nitrogen, and in the postabsorptive and injured state comprise more than 50% of the amino acids released by muscle.[589]

In the stressed state, the glutamine released by muscle is taken up by the intestinal tract where some is converted to alanine, which is then converted by the liver to glucose. It is likely that a good portion of the alanine converted by hepatic gluconeogenesis is supplied by the intestine. Glutamine is also metabolized to ammonia by the gut. The ammonia is then transported by the portal vein directly to the liver for disposal via the urea cycle. In the stressed state it appears that glutamine can replace glucose as a fuel.[589] Similar observations have been made during glucocorticoid administration.[590] It is possible that the use of glutamine may decrease protein catabolism in the intestine and in skeletal muscle under certain conditions.

Further discussions on the effects of amino acids on endogenous hormonal levels and subsequently on the anabolic effects of exercise can be found under the individual amino acids.

OTHER FACTORS AFFECTING PROTEIN SYNTHESIS

Recent investigation has demonstrated that the response to stress is mediated by complex interactions between the nervous, endocrine, immune, and hematopoietic systems. Thus, besides the anabolic and catabolic hormones we've been discussing there are many other factors and variables that are likely involved in protein metabolism. Not only is the neuroendocrine system operative, but monokines and lymphokines such as interleukin-1 (IL-1), interleukin-6 (IL-6), and tumor necrosis factor (TNF) also play important roles. However, their roles in the response to physical stress have not yet been adequately defined. We do know, however, that these processes can significantly affect protein metabolism.

Injury (surgical, traumatic, and burn) and sepsis result in accelerated protein breakdown.[479] This is manifest by increased urinary nitrogen loss, increased peripheral release of amino acids, and inhibited muscle amino acid uptake observed in sepsis. The amino acids originate from both injured tissue and uninjured skeletal muscle and are transported to the liver for conversion to glucose (gluconeogenesis) and protein synthesis.

The negative nitrogen balance observed in such patients represents the net result of breakdown and synthesis; with breakdown increased and synthesis either increased or diminished.[480] Jahoor et al. observed in burned children that the amount of protein breakdown was consistently elevated to the same degree during the acute and convalescent phases, whereas synthesis increased in the latter phase and caused a positive nitrogen balance.[481] Different muscle groups respond differently to injury and sepsis, with some undergoing more proteolysis than others.[482] Amino acid uptake by the liver is enhanced with resultant increased gluconeogenesis. Also, hepatic protein synthesis of selected proteins (acute phase reactants) increases while others decrease (such as transferrin, albumin, retinols, and prealbumin).

The acute phase reactants include fibrinogen, complement, C-reactive protein, haptoglobin, alpha-1 acid glycoprotein, alpha-1 antitrypsin, alpha-1 antichymotrypsin, ceruloplasmin, ferritin, and serum amyloid A.[483] The degree of acute phase response is proportional to the level of tissue injury. Stimulators of the acute phase reactants include cytokines, such as IL-1, TNF, IL-6, ciliary neurotrophic factor (CNTF), a member of the (IL-6) superfamily, and gamma-IFN,[484-488] neuroendocrine mediators (specifically glucocorticoids), and possibly toxic products such as bacterial lipopolysaccharides. It has been observed that after IL-1 stimulation the total amount of protein synthesized does not increase, but rather synthesis of the acute phase proteins is favored. Another study has found that in response to exercise there is a stimulation of the synthesis of some acute phase proteins, which may be a mechanism whereby nitrogen resulting from muscle protein breakdown is spared.[489]

A recent study has shown that TNF has significant short-term and long term effects on protein synthesis.[490] Earlier work demonstrated that a single subcutaneous dose of 50 μg of TNF significantly increased skeletal muscle protein synthesis and breakdown in the tumor-bearing rat.[1] Some of the earlier work demonstrated that TNF can reduce food intake, weight gain, and enhance muscle catabolism.[491,492] In this recent study a 50-μg subcutaneous dose of TNF was shown to acutely alter amino acid transport with an early catabolic and later anabolic effect.

As we can see, the various factors that regulate protein metabolism are complex and interrelated. For example, stimulation of the immune system results in a series of metabolic changes that are antagonistic toward growth. Monokines, including IL-1, IL-6, and TNF, appear to mediate homeorhetic response, which alters the partitioning of dietary nutrients away from growth and skeletal muscle accretion in favor of metabolic processes which support the immune response and disease resistance. These alterations include decreased skeletal muscle accretion due to increased rates of protein degradation and decreased protein synthesis, use of dietary amino acids for gluconeogenesis and as an energy source instead of for muscle protein accretion, and the release of hormones such as insulin, glucagon, and corticosterone.[493]

EICOSANOIDS AND MUSCLE PROTEIN SYNTHESIS

Eicosanoids are physiologically active metabolites of the essential fatty acids with important effects on the immune,[494-500] cardiovascular,[501-506] reproductive[507-513] and central nervous system[514-516] and include leukotrienes, lipoxins, prostaglandins, and the thromboxanes.[517] The essential fatty acids, linoleic and alpha-linolenic acid, are converted to other fatty acids including eicosapentaenoic acid (EPA), docosahexaenoic acid (DHA), dihomo-gamma-linolenic acid (DGLA), and arachidonic acid, from which the eicosanoids are synthesized. Synthesis of eicosanoids is initiated by signal transduction cascades which result in the hydrolysis of free arachidonic acid from membrane phospholipids.[518]

Since eicosanoids act locally in and around the tissues in which they are produced, they are not hormones but autacoids, although they have hormone-like effects and influence hormonal function.[519] Virtually all cells in the body can form some of the eicosanoids, but tissues differ in enzyme profile and consequently in the products they form. They also differ in their ability to be affected by specific eicosanoids. Eicosanoids are not stored to any degree and must be synthesized in response to immediate need. They are rapidly synthesized, released, and degraded.

The eicosanoids are both stimulated by and stimulate the production of other autocrine and paracrine messengers[520,521] and hormones (such as insulin, glucagon, growth hormone, insulin-like growth factor-1, cortisol, and the sex hormones)[522-532] and are partly responsible for the effects of, and work synergistically with, other hormones and growth factors.[533,534] For example, studies have indicated that TNF may be the principal catabolic monokine, with IL-1 potentiating skeletal muscle proteolysis.[535] Reports indicate that *in vitro* proteolysis could be blocked by cyclooxygenase inhibitors, leading to the possibility that catabolism is mediated by prostaglandins, specifically E2.[536]

In gastrectomy patients the administration of indomethacin postoperatively resulted in reduced fever, attenuated cortisol and catecholamine increase, and reduced protein loss.[537] It is unclear whether just the reduction of fever (central cyclooxygenase inhibition) or another action of the indomethacin, e.g., peripheral cyclooxygenase inhibition, is operative. On the other hand, other *in vivo* studies in burned and septic rats indicate that indomethacin is unable to block proteolysis.[538,539] This implies that prostaglandins may not be the mediators of proteolysis.

Eicosanoids and cytokines released from one cell activate their receptors on neighboring cells, interact with each other, and affect each other's production, release, and degradation.[540,541] The cytokines interleukin-1 and tumor necrosis factor enhance arachidonic acid release, probably by inducing the synthesis of phospholipase A2 and possibly other enzymes involved in the metabolism of phospholipids.[542] In turn, arachidonic acid itself may act as a second messenger, synergizing with other agents, as well as serving as the precursor for prostaglandins and various other bioactive eicosanoids.

Like all eicosanoids, prostaglandins are autocrine and paracrine in behavior, and influence the metabolism and growth of the same and neighboring cells in which they are synthesized.[543,544] Prostaglandins are known regulators of protein turnover in skeletal muscle, with PGE2 and PGF2α stimulating protein degradation and protein synthesis rates, respectively.[545-549] In one study, when rat skeletal or cardiac muscles were incubated with arachidonate, rates of protein breakdown rose and protein balance became more negative.[550] Aspirin or indomethacin, which prevented synthesis of PGE2, markedly reduced this effect.

PGF2α directly stimulates protein synthesis in skeletal muscle, but does not affect protein degradation,[551] whereas PGE2 enhances rates of protein degradation without affecting protein synthesis.[552] Prostaglandins regulate the muscle hypertrophic response to insulin and tension/stretch.[553] PGF2α appears to be involved in the stimulation of protein synthesis by insulin in muscle from fasted animals and to mediate stretch-induced increases in protein synthesis in muscle.[554] The repletion of muscle protein after disuse atrophy is also a PGF2α-dependent event.[555]

Prostaglandins have also been reported to be involved in the catabolic effect of the synthetic glucocorticoid dexamethasone. The main effect of glucocorticoids on prostaglandin metabolism is to lower the availability of free arachidonic acid.[556] Prostaglandin synthesis in skeletal muscle has been shown to increase during high-intensity exercise in both humans[557] and animals.[558]

These findings suggest that cyclooxygenase inhibitors may be useful in the treatment of patients showing excessive protein breakdown.

Although controversial data exist in the literature, there are a number of studies that implicate arachidonic acid and prostaglandins in steroidogenesis, specifically in testosterone production and on leuteinizing hormone. In one study the effects of single and repeated administration of $PGF_{2\alpha}$ on the secretion of testosterone and the effect of $PGF_{2\alpha}$ on the action of human chorionic gonadotropin (hCG) were investigated in adult male rats.[559] The results of the study indicate that repeated stimulation by $PGF_{2\alpha}$ directly inhibits testosterone production in the rat testis without mediation by LH.

In another study in rats, arachidonic acid metabolites were found to be intratesticular factors which can regulate LH-stimulated testicular steroidogenesis.[560] In this study the use of inhibitors of prostaglandin production led to a decrease in the LH-stimulated increase in secretion of testosterone. The use of vitamin E (antioxidant and inhibitor of lipoxygenase) enhanced LH-stimulated androgen production.

In a recent study, arachidonic acid induced a dose-related increase of testosterone formation and, at the highest dose, stimulated the production of prostaglandin E_2 (PGE_2), leukotrienes B4 (LTB4), and C4 (LTC4) by purified rat Leydig cells.[561] In this study, the contemporary addition of the prostaglandin synthesis blocker, indomethacin, and arachidonic acid further increased testosterone formation and decreased PGE_2 levels. The findings of this study suggest that: (1) exogenous AA stimulates T secretion; (2) conversion of AA to cycloxygenated and lipoxygenated metabolites is not required for its steroidogenic effect; and (3) cycloxygenated and lipoxygenated compounds play a diverse modulatory role in testicular steroidogenesis.

In a recent study aspirin was found to inhibit the stimulatory activity of naloxone on LH release, suggesting that the inhibitory tone of opioids on GnRH secretion may be caused by the block of hypothalamic prostaglandin biosynthesis with consequent inhibition of

PGE2-induced GnRH secretion.[562] Together, these results suggest that the arachadonic acid effects on testosterone production are mediated by metabolite(s) of the cyclooxygenase pathway.

Other major metabolites of arachidonic acid such as the prostacyclins and thromboxanes also have effects on protein metabolism and cellular growth.[563] For example, the vasoconstrictor eicosanoid, thromboxane, has a direct stimulatory effect on extracellular matrix protein production. In one study two different thromboxane analogues resulted in increased production of components of the extracellular matrix, including fibronectin and the basement membrane proteins laminin and type IV collagen.[564] These results suggest a potential role for thromboxane as a mediator of the sclerotic and fibrotic responses to injury.

In another study the effects of the thromboxane A2 mimetic, U-46619, on the biosynthesis of human mesangial cell proteins was evaluated.[565] Cellular tubulin and collagen type IV, but not actin, were markedly stimulated by U-46619.

While it would be advantageous to be able to direct eicosanoid production so that "good eicosanoids" would be produced deferentially to bad eicosanoids, it is difficult to do so because of the complexity of eicosanoid production, action, and metabolism. Unfortunately, we do not, as yet, know a lot about the dietary influences that affect the known eicosanoids and thus can make only limited use of any knowledge we do have.

For example, prostaglandins can be both good and bad. Unfortunately it is difficult to stimulate the good ones and not the bad ones. If we decrease the formation of prostaglandins from arachidonic acid we inhibit the formation of both good and bad prostaglandins. Of more relevance for dieters, it is not possible to differentially stimulate the production of PGI_2 that has a lipolytic action from PGE_2 which has an antilipolytic action. Both prostaglandins belong to the series 2 prostaglandins and are formed from arachidonic acid.

At present some treatment strategies using the essential fatty acids have tentatively been formulated to try and take advantage of the good eicosanoids. For example, Omega-3 fatty acids found in fish oils can decrease production of some arachidonate metabolites and increase levels of certain prostaglandins. Feeding of these fatty acids has been used as a therapeutic strategy to diminish platelet aggregation by decreasing TXA2 and increasing TXA3 synthesis by platelets.

Omega-3, like LNA and eicosapentaenoic and docosahexaenoic acid (known as EPA and DHA, respectively), are critical to anyone concerned with dieting. They increase fatty acid oxidation (burning of fat) and basal metabolic rates and lower cholesterol. Omega-3 fatty acids also provide an anabolic effect by increasing the binding of IGF-1 to skeletal muscle and improving insulin sensitivity, even on diets high in fat which have a tendency to decrease insulin sensitivity.[566] As well, fish oils may also have important implications for women prone to osteoporosis since they appear to decrease calcium excretion.[567]

Omega-3s also stimulate prostaglandin production.[568] Prostaglandins are eicosanoids that regulate activity in body cells on a moment-to-moment basis and are involved in critical functions like blood pressure regulation, insulin sensitivity, and immune system and anti-inflammatory responses. They're also involved in literally hundreds of other functions, many of which have yet to be fully identified in research. If one has a problem producing prostaglandins or experiences an imbalance between the different kinds of prostaglandins, overall health can be significantly affected.

The series 3 prostaglandins are formed from EPA. As well, EPA reduces the production of the bad prostaglandins from arachidonic acid. EPA deficiency can lead to high blood pressure, hormonal dysfunction, impaired immune function, coagulation problems, inflammatory changes, dry itchy skin, peripheral edema, and many other conditions.

A number of nonsteroidal anti-inflammatory agents, including salicylates, indomethacin, diclofenac, mefenamic acid, piroxicam, sulindac, phenylbutazone, and ibuprofen, have been found to variably influence the formation of prostaglandins[569-573] and thus to influence protein synthesis and catabolism. For example, indomethacin, a cyclooxygenase inhibitor, blocks the conversion of arachidonic acid, via the cyclooxygenase pathway, into prostaglandins, endoperoxides, and thromboxanes. Aspirin also functions in this way.

As we have seen, recent discoveries have demonstrated that hormones and growth factors exert their effects in part through eicosanoids. Thus there are significant implications in the manipulation of these compounds for exercise-induced muscle hypertrophy and for athletic performance. The future will demonstrate these compounds to be critical not only in intracellular (molecular) events, but also in the effects they produce that are far from the source of origin. Once more studies are done and more information is available, we should be able to change our diet and supplements to manipulate these compounds and maximize their anabolic potential.

Chapter 3

ENERGY METABOLISM

INTRODUCTION

The human body, through metabolic and hormonal controls, has evolved to meet its continuous metabolic needs even though eating, and thus provision of essential nutrients, is intermittent.

In the postabsorptive period (after a meal has been completely digested and the resulting nutrients absorbed into the body — usually 6 to 12 h after a meal, during which the transition from the postprandial to the fasting state occurs), and even under fasting conditions (as long as the fasting state is not extensive), the body tends to keep a constant energy output by utilizing dietary sources when available and at other times by mobilizing internal substrates (glycogen, cellular and body fat, cellular protein) that can be used as energy sources.

Postabsorptive energy sources include circulating glucose, fatty acids and triglycerides, liver and muscle glycogen, muscle triglycerides, the branched-chain amino acids (used by skeletal muscle), and the amino acids alanine and glutamine (released from skeletal muscle and used for gluconeogenesis in the case of glutamine directly as fuel by the immune system and gastrointestinal tract).[592,593] In a normal 70-kg human these postabsorptive energy sources provide up to 1200 kcal (800 calories from carbohydrate sources). These sources are exhausted in less than 24 h if no other food is consumed.

In an individual that is dieting to lose weight, or in an athlete that is limiting both caloric and fat intake in order to maximize lean body mass and minimize body fat, these sources may amount to less than 500 kcal since liver and muscle glycogen levels as well as circulating triglycerides and fatty acids are often limited, and, in the case of the athlete, would easily be exhausted during a training session. In cases where the available energy is used up while training, other energy sources are called upon to supply the energy needed both during and after training until nutrients are able to be absorbed from a posttraining meal.

Fatty acids and ketones formed by the catabolism of body fat (triglycerides) can be used by most tissues in the body. However, in the short term certain tissues such as the brain can only use glucose for energy. Thus glucose or substances that can be converted to glucose are vital to survival. The lack of glucose in the short term results in the formation of glucose through gluconeogenesis, a process by which glucose is formed from other substrates, mainly lactate, pyruvate, glycerol, and amino acids.[594-596] Amino acids, a major substrate for glucose production, comes from skeletal muscle, leading to a loss of both contractile and noncontractile protein.

Short-term extreme adaptations to energy needs beyond the immediate available energy are varied. Certain tissues, such as the heart, kidney, and skeletal muscle, change their primary fuel substrate from glucose to fatty acids and ketone bodies rather readily. Others, like the brain, take longer and only use glucose (from gluconeogenesis) and ketones as energy sources.[597]

Although fatty acids cannot be directly converted to glucose, the energy produced from the oxidation of FFA can be used to fuel the conversion of certain other substrates into glucose (gluconeogenesis being an energy-requiring process), thus sparing somewhat the use of structural and contractile protein for glucose formation. For example, lactate and pyruvate are formed from anaerobic glycolysis and released systemically. In the liver they are converted to glucose, which is then released for other tissues to use. This shuttle is called the Cori cycle.[598,599] As well, the energy garnered through fatty acid oxidation is used for transforming glycerol into glucose.

With ongoing energy deprivation or low carbohydrate intake other adaptations appear. The brain, which ordinarily obtains energy only by glucose oxidation, acquires the ability to use keto acids for its fuel requirements, and this further contributes to protein conservation.

GLYCOGENOLYSIS AND GLUCONEOGENESIS

As we have seen, certain processes such as glycogenolysis, gluconeogenesis, increasing fatty acid oxidation, utilization of ketones, proteolysis, and others insure that the body has a continuous supply of available energy and substrates for its metabolic needs.

The rise in blood glucose and the subsequent rise in insulin that occur after a meal promote glycogen storage in liver and muscle and fat deposition in adipose tissue, skeletal muscle, and liver. After a meal both glucose and insulin levels fall and liver glycogen through the process of glycogenolysis becomes the primary source of available glucose.

Maintenance of plasma glucose concentrations within a narrow range despite wide fluctuations in the demand (e.g., vigorous exercise) and supply (e.g., large carbohydrate meals) of glucose results from coordination of factors that regulate glucose release into and removal from the circulation.[600]

Lactate, pyruvate, glycerol, and certain amino acids are used by the liver and kidney to form glucose. Under normal conditions, amino acids, especially alanine and glutamine, serve as major substrates for gluconeogenesis (see below under the individual amino acids).[601]

In one study the contribution under various nutritional regimens of several amino acids and lactate to gluconeogenesis was estimated by measuring the glucose formation from ^{14}C-labeled substrates.[602] Isolated rat hepatocytes were incubated for 60 min in a Krebs-Ringer bicarbonate buffer, pH 7.4, containing lactate, pyruvate, and all the amino acids at concentrations similar to their physiological levels found in rat plasma, with one precursor labeled in each flask. In all conditions, lactate was the major glucose precursor, providing over 60% of the glucose formed. Glutamine and alanine were the major amino acid precursors of glucose, contributing 9.8 and 10.6% of the glucose formed, respectively, in hepatocytes isolated from starved rats. Serine, glycine, and threonine also contributed to gluconeogenesis in the starved liver cells at 2.6, 2.1, and 3.8%, respectively, of the glucose formed.

In this study it was shown that the availability of dietary carbohydrates varies the gluconeogenic response. The rate of glucose formation from the isolated hepatocytes of the starved rats and those fed either high protein or high fat was higher than from rats fed a nonpurified diet.

The low insulin and the high glucagon output that characterizes the postabsorptive phase and fasting (the lower the glucose level the lower the insulin and higher the glucagon output) stimulates both glycogenolysis and gluconeogenesis. Initially, approximately 70 to 75% of the hepatic glucose output is derived from glycogenolysis and the remainder from gluconeogenesis.

Starvation is associated initially with an increased release of the gluconeogenic amino acids from muscles and an increase in gluconeogenesis.[603] In one study looking at amino acid balance across forearm muscles in postabsorptive (overnight fasted) subjects, fasting significantly reduced basal insulin and increased glucagon, and increased muscle release of the principal glycogenic amino acids (alanine, glutamine, glycine, threonine, serine, methionine, tyrosine, and lysine).[604] In this study alanine release increased 59.4%. The increase in release for all amino acids averaged 69.4% and was statistically significant for threonine, serine, glycine, alanine, alpha-aminobutyrate, methionine, tyrosine, and lysine. In the same study 7 subjects were also fasted for 60 h. In these subjects there was a reduction of amino acid release as the fasting continued.

Since these changes reproduce those observed after a few days of total fasting, it has been suggested that it is the carbohydrate restriction itself, and the subsequent decrease in insulin and increase in glucagon, which is responsible for the metabolic and hormonal adaptations of brief fasting.[605] A reduction in the release of substrate amino acids from skeletal muscle largely explains the decrease in gluconeogenesis characterizing prolonged starvation.

A similar response, an initial increase in gluconeogenesis followed in time by a decrease, is seen in trauma such as burn injury[606] and in prolonged exercise.[607]

During prolonged mild exercise that increases the hepatic glucose output twofold, the relative contribution of gluconeogenesis to the overall hepatic output increases from 25 to 45%, indicating a threefold rise in the absolute rate of gluconeogenesis. After 12 to 13 h of fasting, hepatic gluconeogenesis replaces glycogenolysis as the main source of glucose.[608]

HORMONAL CONTROL OF GLUCONEOGENESIS

Among the hormones responsible for a rise in gluconeogenesis one must take into account adrenaline, glucagon, glucocorticoids, growth hormone, and insulin. These hormones can act either directly on the gluconeogenic enzymes or on the mobilization of precursors necessary for gluconeogenesis (the three-carbon precursors, including lactate, alanine, and glycerol). On a moment-to-moment basis, however, these processes are controlled mainly by the glucocorticoids, insulin, and glucagon, whose secretions are reciprocally influenced by the plasma glucose concentration. The glucocorticoids increase the activity of the glucose-alanine cycle. Insulin decreases the supply of gluconeogenic substrates and inhibits the glucose-alanine cycle. Thus, the exercise-induced hypoinsulinemia is a promoting factor in gluconeogenesis. In the resting postabsorptive state, release of glucose from the liver (usually equally via glycogenolysis and gluconeogenesis) is the key regulated process.

Glycogenolysis depends on the relative activities of glycogen synthase and phosphorylase, the latter being the more important. The activities of fructose-1,6-diphosphatase, phosphoenolpyruvate carboxylkinase, and pyruvate dehydrogenase, whose main precursors are lactate, alanine, and glutamine, regulate gluconeogenesis.

In the immediate postprandial state, due to the availability of substrates coming from the GI tract, suppression of liver glucose output and stimulation of skeletal muscle glucose uptake are the most important factors. Glucose disposal by insulin-sensitive tissues is regulated initially at the transport step and then mainly by glycogen synthase, phosphofructokinase, and pyruvate dehydrogenase. Hormonally induced changes in intracellular fructose 2,6-bisphosphate concentrations play a key role in muscle glycolytic flux and in both glycolytic and gluconeogenic flux in the liver.

Under stressful conditions (e.g., hypoglycemia, trauma, vigorous exercise), increased secretion of other hormones such as adrenaline, cortisol, and growth hormone, and increased activity of the sympathetic nervous system, come into play. Their actions to increase hepatic glucose output and to suppress tissue glucose uptake are partly mediated by increases in tissue fatty acid oxidation.

In diabetes, the most common disorder of glucose homeostasis, fasting hyperglycemia, results primarily from excessive release of glucose by the liver due to increased gluconeogenesis; postprandial hyperglycemia results from both impaired suppression of hepatic glucose release and impaired skeletal muscle glucose uptake. These abnormalities are usually due to the combination of impaired insulin secretion and tissue resistance to insulin.

As noted above, under normal conditions the amount of readily available energy coming from carbohydrate sources is only about 800 kcal — and includes the 120 g or so of glycogen from the body's skeletal muscle, 70 g of glycogen in the liver and 10 g of glucose in the blood. Adipose tissue, on the other hand, provides an almost limitless supply of available energy: about 100,000 calories from the average person's 15 kg of fat.

Free fatty acids from adipose tissue and intramuscular stores, and muscle glycogen provide energy both at rest and during low-intensity exercise. At these levels, substrate availability does not limit activity since there is so much potential energy available from body fat. FFA mobilization from adipose tissue (catecholamines stimulate adipose lipase which breaks each triglyceride molecule down to form one glycerol and three fatty acid molecules) starts with any kind of activity. FFA is metabolized in muscle cells to acetyl-CoA that subsequently enters the citric acid cycle, forming ATP as it is oxidatively metabolized.

While FFA mobilization may lag at first, it soon results in high FFA blood levels of up to six times the normal level. These levels of FFA are so high that it can't all be utilized by muscle. Perhaps one of the reasons for the overproduction of FFA is to release glycerol, a substrate for gluconeogenesis.

USE OF AA FOR ENERGY — CATABOLIC EFFECTS OF EXERCISE

Typical responses to acute exercise are suppressed protein synthesis and elevated protein degradation. Comparison of these responses in muscle containing various types of fibers indicated that the rate of protein synthesis was suppressed and the rate of protein degradation was elevated mainly in muscles less active during exercise. Thus, the less active muscles, but not those that fulfill the main task during exercise performance, are used as a reservoir for mobilization of protein resources. The exercise-induced catabolism is not extended to contractile proteins. During exercise the catabolic response is extended to the smooth muscle of the gastrointestinal tract, lymphoid tissue, liver, and kidney.

Both the antianabolic and catabolic effects have to be considered as tools for mobilization of protein resources during a stressful situation. As a result, an increased pool of available free amino acids is created. Due to the suppressed protein synthesis, the free amino acids pool is used for supplying the necessary protein synthesis by "building materials" only to a minor extent. The amino acids are mainly used for additional energy supply to contracting muscles.

There are at least three pathways connecting free amino acids with energy processes. One of these consists in the oxidation of branched-chain amino acids. The main site of this pathway is the contracting muscle. An increased oxidation of leucine during exercise was established in human as well as in animal studies. The metabolism of several amino acids leads to the formation of metabolites of the citric cycle, which also has a beneficial effect on muscle metabolism by increasing the capacity of the citric cycle for oxidizing the acetyl-CoA units generated from pyruvate and free fatty acids.

AMINO ACID METABOLISM IN MUSCLE

There are three principal sources of amino acids for energy metabolism: dietary protein, plasma and tissue free amino acid pools, and endogenous tissue protein.

All three sources are in equilibrium. Dietary protein is a relatively minor source of amino acids during normal exercise since ingesting a large protein meal prior to exercise is rarely done. The plasma pool of free amino acids is much smaller than the free amino acid pool of human skeletal muscle largely because skeletal muscle makes up about 40% of body weight and contains about 75% of the whole-body free amino acids.

The free amino acid pools, however, are much smaller than the amount of amino acids available from endogenous protein breakdown. It has been estimated that the intramuscular amino acid pool contains less that 1% of the metabolically active amino acids. It has also been estimated that the amount of leucine oxidized during a prolonged exercise bout is approximately 25 times greater than the free leucine concentration in muscle, liver, and plasma. Therefore, the free amino acid pool is only a minor source of amino acids during exercise, whereas the most important source is endogenous protein breakdown.

PATHWAYS OF AMINO ACID METABOLISM IN MUSCLE

Many of the amino acids can be oxidized by skeletal muscle, including alanine, arginine, aspartate, cysteine, glutamate, glycine, phenylalanine, threonine, tyrosine, and the three BCAAs. Not all of these amino acids, however, have the same metabolic potential in muscle and it appears that the BCAAs are the dominant amino acids oxidized by skeletal muscle. The catabolism of amino acids involves the removal of the alpha-amino group by transamination or oxidative deamination, followed by conversion of the carbon skeleton to metabolites that are common to the pathways of carbohydrate and fat metabolism. It should be noted that the avenues available for amino acid catabolism and conversion are extensive, and the final products, their fates, and the pathways available to them are all quite complex.

SKELETAL MUSCLE CATABOLISM

Significant gaps remain in our knowledge of the pathways of amino acid catabolism in humans. Sufficient information, however, does exist to allow a broad picture of the overall process of amino acid oxidation to be developed along with approximate quantitative assessments of the role played by liver, muscle, kidney, and small intestine. For example, one study found that amino acids are the major fuel of liver, i.e., their oxidative conversion to glucose accounts for about one half of the daily oxygen consumption of the liver, and no other fuel contributes nearly so importantly.[609]

The daily supply of amino acids provided in the diet cannot be totally oxidized to CO_2 in the liver because such a process would provide far more ATP than the liver could utilize and not enough ATP would be generated in other tissues. Instead, most amino acids are oxidatively converted to glucose. This results in an overall ATP production during amino acid oxidation very nearly equal to the ATP required to convert amino acid carbon to glucose.

ATP is thus produced in the muscle cells both by anaerobic glycolysis and oxidation of amino acids, while ATP is used up in liver cells to produce glucose from the carbon skeletons. Thus the glucose-alanine cycle in an indirect way transfers ATP from the liver to the peripheral tissues.

It is commonly thought that only ATP, PC, and glycolysis (the conversion of glucose into pyruvic acid) provide cellular energy under anaerobic conditions. Such is not the case, however, since several studies have shown that amino acid catabolism also provides a source of anaerobic energy production.[610]

In a study on anoxic heart muscle, glutamate and aspartate catabolized at a higher rate as compared with oxygenation.[611] The data obtained from this study suggest that the constant influx of intermediates into the cycle from amino acids is supported by coupled transamination of glutamate and aspartate. This leads to the formation of ATP and GTP in the citric acid or tricarboxylic acid cycle during blocking of aerobic energy production. Succinate, a component of the citric acid cycle, is thought to result from amino acid catabolism.

Another study on cat heart papillary muscle found that supplying hypoxic, contracting muscles with aspartate resulted in maintenance of muscular function to some extent and led to augmented release of succinate and lactate.[612] The data from this study indicate that anaerobic succinate formation is correlated to the energy-requiring processes of the myocardium. Maintenance of myocardial function by the supply of amino acids may be related to their conversion into succinate. In some studies it has been shown that glutamate may be used as an anaerobic fuel in the human heart through conversion to succinate coupled with GTP formation.[613]

Since amino acids can be used as fuel in both aerobic and anaerobic states, muscle catabolism occurs under both conditions to provide the needed substrates. The use of parenteral or enteral amino acid mixtures and combinations of specific amino acids can attenuate this catabolic and counterproductive response to exercise.

OXIDATION OF AMINO ACIDS

Once the needed proteins are synthesized and the amino acid pools replenished, additional amino acids are degraded and used for energy or stored mainly as fat and to a lesser extent as glycogen. The primary site for degradation of most amino acids is the liver. The liver is unique because of its capacity to degrade amino acids and to synthesize urea for elimination of the amino nitrogen.

The first step in the degradation of amino acids begins with deamination — the removal of the alpha-amino group from the amino acid to produce an oxoacid, which may be a simple metabolic intermediate itself (e.g., pyruvate) or be converted to a simple metabolic intermediate via a specific metabolic pathway. The intermediates are either oxidized via the citric acid cycle or converted to glucose via gluconeogenesis. For instance, deaminated alanine is pyruvic acid. This can be converted into glucose or glycogen. Or it can be converted into acetyl-CoA, which can then be polymerized into fatty acids. Also, two molecules of acetyl-CoA can condense to form acetoacetic acid, which is one of the ketone bodies.

Deamination occurs mainly by transamination, the transfer of the amino group to some other acceptor compound. Deamination generally occurs by the following transamination pathway:

alpha-ketoglutaric acid + amino acid
$\rightarrow$ glutamic acid + alpha-keto acid

glutamic acid + NAD^+ + H_2O
$\rightarrow$ NADH + H^+ + NH_3 + alpha-Ketoglutaric acid

Note from this schema that the amino group from the amino acid is transferred to alpha-ketoglutaric acid, which then becomes glutamic acid. The glutamic acid can then transfer the amino group to still other substances or can release it in the form of ammonia (NH_3). In the process of losing the amino group the glutamic acid once again becomes alpha-ketoglutaric acid, so that the cycle can be repeated again and again.

To initiate this process, the excess amino acids in the cells, especially in the liver, induce the activation of large quantities of aminotransferases, the enzymes responsible for initiating most deaminations. Hepatic tissue contains high concentrations of the degradative enzymes, including the aminotransferases (with the exception of the branched-chain aminotransferase) which remove the alpha-amino groups during the first step in amino acid degradation. Branched-chain aminotransferase results in the release of branched chain amino acids (BCAA) into circulation and is exclusively a mitochondrial enzyme in skeletal muscles.[614]

For example, degradation of the BCAAs is initiated by the reversible transamination of the BCAA to the alpha-keto acid with transfer of the alpha-amino group to alpha-ketoglutarate, forming glutamate. This step appears to be nearly at equilibrium with little physiological control. The second and rate-limiting step is decarboxylation of the branched-chain keto acids by branched-chain keto acid dehydrogenase (BCKAD). BCKAD activity is highly regulated by phosphorylation and dephosphorylation to the inactive and active forms, respectively. This step is stimulated by increases in the concentration of the leucine keto acid, alpha-ketoisocaproate (KIC).

During periods of increased energy needs, such as starvation, trauma, and exercise, increased levels of BCAAs stimulate BCKAD and the BCAAs are degraded to produce energy in skeletal muscle. During absorption periods when muscles are using glucose as a primary fuel, muscle transaminates the BCAA and releases the keto acids into circulation for complete oxidation by the liver or kidney. In the liver these intermediates, formed either in the liver or from other tissues, are either oxidized via the citric acid cycle or converted to glucose via gluconeogenesis. A deaminated amino acid can enter the citric acid cycle at different levels including acetyl-CoA, pyruvate, oxaloacetate, alpha-ketoglutarate, succinyl-CoA, or fumarate.[615] Both isoleucine and valine form succinyl-CoA, whereas leucine forms acetyl-CoA. Of these, only the carbons of acetyl-CoA from leucine can be oxidized directly in the citric acid cycle; the other intermediates must first be converted to pyruvate via phosphoenolpyruvate before their carbons are available for oxidation in the citric acid cycle as acetyl-CoA.

Within skeletal muscle, BCAA degradation involves transfer of the alpha-amino group to ketogluterate to form glutamate. Glutamate serves as an important intermediate in nitrogen metabolism. While glutamate is formed *de novo* in skeletal muscle, there is no net release. Once the amino group is transferred to glutamate there are three primary fates. The amino group can be transferred either to pyruvate in synthesis of alanine or onto oxaloacetate for the synthesis of aspartate, or the glutamate can release the amino group in the form of ammonia and reform ketogluterate, at the same time releasing two hydrogen atoms which are oxidized to form ATP. Alanine is released from muscle into circulation and is ultimately removed by the liver for gluconeogenesis. Aspartate is an important component of the purine nucleotide cycle, which is central to maintaining the pool of ATP in muscle. The purine nucleotide cycle serves to regenerate IMP and also produces fumarate and free ammonia (NH_3). The ammonia can be combined with glutamate via glutamine synthetase to form glutamine (glutamate + ammonia + ATP $\rightarrow$ glutamine + ADP).[616] Glutamine is ultimately released from muscle, with the majority of glutamine being used by the gut and the immune system as a primary energy source.

Together, alanine and glutamine represent 60 to 80% of the amino acids released from skeletal muscle while they account for only 18% of the amino acids in muscle protein. During exercise, glutamine synthesis and glutamine levels in muscle decline due to inhibition of glutamine synthetase.

The net effect of oxidation of amino acids to glucose in the liver is to make nearly two thirds of the total energy available from the oxidation of amino acids available to peripheral tissues, without necessitating that peripheral tissues synthesize the complex array of enzymes needed to support direct amino acid oxidation.

As a balanced mixture of amino acids is oxidized in the liver, nearly all carbon from glucogenic amino acids flows into the mitochondrial aspartate pool and is actively transported out of the mitochondria via the aspartate-glutamate antiport linked to proton entry. In the cytoplasm the aspartate is converted to fumarate utilizing urea cycle enzymes; the fumarate flows via oxaloacetate to phosphoenolpyruvate and on to glucose.

Thus, carbon flow through the urea cycle is normally interlinked with gluconeogenic carbon flow because these metabolic pathways share a common step. Liver mitochondria experience a severe nonvolatile acid load during amino acid oxidation. It is suggested that this acid load is alleviated mainly by the respiratory chain proton pump in a form of uncoupled respiration.

Besides providing substrates for energy production, the use of certain amino acids increases the utilization of other substrates such as free fatty acids (FFA).

ALANINE AND GLUTAMINE

Intense exercise has dramatic effects on amino acid metabolism. After an exhausting load, a significant rise and concurrent drop of serum isoleucine, threonine, ornithine, leucine, serine, glycine, asparagine, and glutamine occurs, with a rise in serum alanine.[617] The rise of alanine suggests the existence of a glucose-alanine cycle (see below). The drop of branched amino acids is probably due to their enhanced entry into muscles. The drop of glutamine reflects increased use by the gut and immune system, even though the release of glutamine by muscle cells increases secondary to proteolysis.

Similarly, under stress, glucose consumption increases and the efflux of lactate, alanine, glutamine, and total amino acid nitrogen (i.e., net muscle protein catabolism) increases.

In a series of studies, Brown et al. have shown that catabolic hormones alone fail to reproduce the stress-induced efflux of amino acids.[618] In this study the net balance of amino acids was determined in 5 healthy volunteers prior to and following a 2-h infusion of the catabolic hormones epinephrine, cortisol, and glucagon into the femoral artery. This hormonal simulation of stress in normal volunteers increased glutamine efflux from the leg to an extent similar to that of burn patients.

Alanine efflux, however, was not affected by the hormonal infusion. Because alanine efflux constituted a major proportion of the total peripheral amino acid catabolism in the burn patients, there was significantly less total amino acid nitrogen loss from the healthy volunteers receiving the stress hormones. Thus catabolic hormones alone fail to reproduce the stress-induced pattern and quantity of amino acid efflux from human skeletal muscle. This discrepancy is largely due to an unresponsiveness of alanine to hormonally induced muscle protein catabolism.

In states of stress alanine becomes increasingly important to sustain increases in gluconeogenesis. Alanine, via deamination to pyruvate, is a principal precursor for hepatic gluconeogenesis and is normally produced secondary to insulin resistance — important since insulin is known to inhibit muscle protein breakdown, especially in severely stressed states.

In another study Brown et al. have shown that alanine efflux may depend on pyruvate availability during stress, and the rate of glycolysis within peripheral tissues may be a major factor in regulating the quantity of alanine efflux.[619]

Several studies have hypothesized that alanine decreases plasma ketone body levels by increasing availability of oxaloacetate, thus allowing acetyl groups to enter the citric acid cycle and releasing coenzyme A (CoA). The significant elevation in plasma free carnitine concentration found after alanine ingestion is consistent with the hypothesis that alanine increases the oxidation of acetyl-CoA by providing oxaloacetate for the citric acid cycle.[620]

Glutamine also becomes increasingly important during stress, both due to its role as a major precursor for ammoniagenesis by the kidney and its avid consumption by visceral organs, fibroblasts, and lymphoid tissue.[621]

The authors of this study suggest that "any attempt to minimize muscle protein catabolism should be accompanied by amino acid supplementation, especially of glutamine and alanine." Thus the provision of exogenous alanine may decrease insulin resistance, and the provision of exogenous alanine and glutamine may decrease the need to obtain these amino acids from endogenous protein and therefore decrease muscle protein breakdown.

INTERORGAN EXCHANGE OF AMINO ACIDS

Many of the alterations in the hormonal ensemble during exercise favor (or even constitute the main cause of) protein and amino acid mobilization. As a result of exercise, there is an interorgan exchange of amino acids, particularly the BCAAs, alanine, and glutamine. The main features of this interorgan exchange include:

- The movement of the branched-chain amino acids (leucine, valine, and isoleucine) from the splanchnic bed (liver and gut) to skeletal muscles.
- The movement of alanine from muscle to the liver.
- The movement of glutamine from muscle to the gut.

The interorgan exchange of these amino acids has several functions including:

- Maintaining amino acid precursors for protein synthesis.
- Assisting in the elimination of nitrogen wastes.
- Providing substrates for gluconeogenesis.
- Providing glutamine for gut and immune system function.
- Maintaining the purine nucleotide cycle.

Early studies by Felig et al. provided evidence about amino acid movement among tissues.[622] By examining arterial-venous differences in substrate concentrations across tissues, they observed that skeletal muscle had a net uptake of BCAAs with a subsequent release of alanine greater than the amount present in muscle protein. The released alanine was removed by the splanchnic bed. On the basis of these observations, they proposed the existence of a glucose-alanine cycle for maintenance of blood glucose and the shuttling of nitrogen and gluconeogenic substrate from muscle to liver.

Another study by Ahlborg et al. using 6 untrained adult males examined the arterial-venous differences across the splanchnic bed and across the leg during 4 h of cycling at 30% of $V0_2$max.[623] They observed decreases in plasma glucose and insulin, and increases in glucagon and free fatty acids. Plasma glucose declined from a preexercise level of 90 mg/dl but stabilized at 60 mg/dl as release of glucose by the liver continued throughout the exercise period. Glucose remained an important fuel throughout exercise, but there was a significant increase in use of free fatty acids.

There was also a significant increase in amino acid flux, including a fourfold increase in the release of branched-chain amino acids from the splanchnic area and a corresponding increase in the uptake by exercising muscles. In return, muscles released alanine, which was removed by the liver for gluconeogenesis. This study demonstrated a change in amino acid flux during exercise, with movement of branched-chain amino acids from visceral tissues to skeletal muscles and the return of alanine as a precursor for hepatic synthesis of glucose.

Lemon and Mullin further established the relationship of amino acid metabolism to glucose homeostasis.[624] In this study they demonstrated a dramatic increase in sweat urea nitrogen in men previously depleted of glycogen stores and exercised for 1 h at 61% $V0_2$max, but no change in urinary urea nitrogen. The authors found that amino acid catabolism provided 10.4% of total energy for the exercise in carbohydrate-depleted individuals while in the carbohydrate-loaded group protein provided 4.4% of the energy needs. These results suggest that production of nitrogen wastes during exercise is related to carbohydrate status and that sweating may be an important mechanism for elimination of nitrogen wastes. Other studies also support the relationship of increased amino acid degradation with maintenance of hepatic glucose production.[625,626]

Exercise and periods of food restriction or fasting share many similarities in amino acid metabolism. In both there is a net release of amino acids from protein due to suppression of protein synthesis, and an increase in protein breakdown. This change in protein turnover results in an increase in tissue levels of free amino acids and net release of amino acids from most tissues. Tissues with high rates of protein turnover are most affected, with the liver and gastrointestinal tract incurring the largest losses during short-term fasts. Skeletal muscle, which has lower rates of protein turnover, responds somewhat less dramatically, but because of its total mass, muscle is the predominate source of free amino acids during prolonged periods of food restriction.

Amino acids have been shown to play important roles in energy homeostasis during periods of high energy need or low energy intake. While the qualitative role is becoming clear, the quantitative level of this role remains uncertain. Most of the studies examining this role have been designed using leucine and alanine as metabolic tracers. These studies establish changes in protein turnover, increases in amino acid flux, and increase in leucine oxidation.

However, questions remain about the potential to generalize from these findings to other amino acids or to dietary protein requirements. Endurance exercise causes a reduction in muscle protein synthesis and net protein breakdown, but is there a real loss of amino acids; are there increases in urea production during exercise; are the effects unique to leucine or do they relate to other amino acids? These questions remain to be fully answered.

Using multiple isotope tracers, Wolfe et al.[627] examined amino acid metabolism during aerobic exercise. They found inhibition of protein synthesis, increased leucine oxidation, and increased flux of alanine. These findings are consistent with most earlier reports. However, using direct isotopic measures, they failed to find any increase in urea synthesis. Further, using lysine, a second indispensable amino acid, they demonstrated that the inhibition of protein synthesis was less than half that estimated by leucine (17% vs. 48%) and that there was no increase in lysine oxidation.

METABOLIC PATHWAYS PRODUCING ATP

- There are three basic ATP-synthesizing pathways in muscle. Two are anaerobic (or oxygen independent) and one is aerobic (or oxygen dependent).
- Phosphagen mobilization is the simplest mechanism for generating ATP. Creatine phosphate (PCr), catalyzed by creatine phosphokinase (CPK), forms ATP from ADP.

$$\text{PCr} + \text{ADP} + \text{H}^+ \leftrightarrow \text{ATP} + \text{creatine}$$

- anaerobic glycolysis, the partial catabolism of glucose to lactate is the second anaerobic means of forming ATP.

$$\text{glucose} + 2\ \text{ADP} \rightarrow 2\ \text{lactate} + \text{ATP}$$

- If glycogen is the substrate instead of glucose, an extra mole of ATP is generated.
- Not only carbohydrates but amino acids can be anaerobically catabolized to form ATP. Aspartate, for example, can be fermented to succinate or propionate. Unlike carbohydrates and protein, fats cannot be anaerobically reduced to form ATP.
- Oxygen is required for the complete oxidation of substrates such as glucose, glycogen, fatty acids, and amino acids. The pathways by which such complete oxidations are achieved are much more complex than the anaerobic pathways and involve the citric acid cycle.

The citric acid cycle is a series of intramitochondrial reactions through which acetyl residues are catabolized. This process liberates hydrogen equivalents, which, upon oxidation, lead to the release of most of the free energy of tissue fuels. The acetyl residues are in the form of acetyl-CoA, an ester of coenzyme A. CoA contains the vitamin pantothenic acid. The citric acid cycle is the final common pathway for the oxidation of carbohydrates, lipids, and proteins, since glucose, fatty acids, and many amino acids are all metabolized to acetyl-CoA or intermediates of the cycle. It also plays a major role in gluconeogenesis, transamination, deamination, and lipogenesis.

While several of these processes occur in most tissues, the liver is the only tissue in which they all occur. The citric acid cycle is the mechanism by which much of the free energy liberated during the oxidation of carbohydrates, lipids, and amino acids is made available. Thus, while energy-producing substrates may metabolize along several different pathways, the oxidation of common substrates formed in the metabolism of carbohydrates, fatty acids, and proteins (gluconeogenesis) terminate mainly in the citric acid cycle.

In general, the amount of adenosine triphosphate formed for each gram of protein that is oxidized is slightly less than that formed for each gram of glucose oxidized.

METABOLISM OF AMMONIA

Ammonia is formed in a number of reactions in the body during the degradation of amines, purines, and pyrimidines,[628-630] and the metabolism of amino acids. It seems, however, that the quantitatively important source of ammonia during exercise is the metabolism of amino acids.[631]

Skeletal muscle produces a large quantity of ammonia during prolonged submaximal (i.e., endurance) exercise, the source of which is the subject of some controversy. Ammonia production in skeletal muscle involves the purine nucleotide cycle and the amino acids glutamate, glutamine, and alanine and probably also includes the branched-chain amino acids as well as aspartate.[632]

Several authors have proposed that the degradation of amino acids, specifically, the branched-chain amino acids leucine, valine, and isoleucine, may be a source of ammonia during this type of activity. The ammonia response can be suppressed by increasing the carbohydrate availability and this may be mediated by decreasing the oxidation of the branched-chain amino acids.[633]

MacLean et al. performed a study in which the purpose was to examine the effects of oral BCAA supplementation on amino acid and ammonia metabolism in exercising humans.[634] Five men exercised the knee extensors of one leg for 60 min with and without (control) an oral supplement of BCAA. The subjects consumed 77 mg/kg of the supplement administered in two equal doses of 38.5 mg/kg at 45 and 20 min before the onset of exercise. According to the authors of the study, the 500-mg capsules of the commercially available BCAA supplement were reported to contain only the three BCAA in the following proportions: 220, 150, and 130 mg L-leucine, L-valine, and L-isoleucine, respectively. This was confirmed by dilution of the capsules in water and with analysis by high performance liquid chromatography.

The researchers concluded that their study clearly shows that BCAA supplementation results in significantly greater muscle ammonia production during exercise. Also, BCAA supplementation imposes a substantial ammonia load on muscle, as indicated by the consistently larger total alanine and glutamine releases observed during exercise. The elevated BCAA levels also suppress the degree of net protein degradation that normally occurs during exercise of this magnitude and duration.

Also of importance was the finding that the degree of contractile protein degradation was not increased during exercise for either trial. The authors noted that previous studies reported that muscle protein catabolism occurs primarily in noncontractile protein, while contractile protein catabolism is spared or even decreased. MacLean et al. found no significant elevations in the release of 3-methylhistidine (a marker of contractile protein catabolism — 3-methylhistidine is a muscle-specific amino acid that is produced and lost in the urine only when muscle protein is broken down) from muscle for either trial.

Since it is produced in degradation reactions, ammonia is usually considered an end product of metabolism which must be converted to urea, a nontoxic compound, for excretion. In most mammals, including humans, urea is produced in the liver by a cyclical series of reactions known as the urea cycle. The urea cycle, because of the intricacy of amino acid metabolism, and in particular the contribution of different tissues, is more complex than is generally thought.

In addition to its role in the urea cycle, ammonia can play a number of other roles in metabolism including:

- Acting as a substrate for the glutamate dehydrogenase reaction in the formation of nonessential amino acids and as a substrate for glutamine synthetase in the formation of glutamine in muscle;
- Acting as an important regulator of the rate of glycolysis in muscle, brain, and possibly other tissues;
- Regulation of acid/base balance by the kidney.

Ammonia, generated from glutamine within the tubule cells, acts as a third renal system to help the body cope with large acid loads. Once formed, ammonia diffuses into the tubule to combine with the protons as follows:

$$NH_3 + H^+ \rightarrow NH^{4+}$$

The hydrolysis of glutamine to glutamate in the distal tubules of the kidney, through the activity of the glutaminase enzyme, is the primary pathway for renal ammonia production, although additional ammonia can also be produced by the further conversion of glutamate to α-ketoglutarate, through the activity of the enzyme glutamate dehydrogenase. Furthermore, oxidation of glutamine carbons by the kidney gives rise to bicarbonate (HCO^{3-}) ion production for release into the blood stream, to further buffer hydrogen ion production. These processes allow the kidneys to effectively excrete excess protons and protect the body from acidosis.

Consequently, during acidosis major changes in renal glutamine metabolism occur to support ammoniagenesis. Renal uptake of glutamine has been shown to be accelerated by activation of the Na^+-dependent membrane transport system. The rate of glutamine hydrolysis and the maximal activity of the glutaminase enzyme were also increased, such that renal glutamine consumption was increased six- to tenfold, making the kidney the major organ of glutamine utilization during acidosis.

The glutamine is produced in muscle (although brain and liver may contribute small amounts) and transported to the kidney where the two nitrogen atoms are released as ammonia. Since glutamine release by muscle may be at the expense of alanine, the excretion of the nitrogen from amino acid metabolism in muscle is effectively switched from urea — which is produced from the metabolism of alanine in the liver — to ammonia, which is produced from glutamine metabolism in the kidney. In this way, the end product of nitrogen metabolism is put to good use by the body in achieving control of acidosis.

UREA FORMATION BY THE LIVER

The ammonia released during deamination is removed from the blood almost entirely by conversion into urea; two molecules of ammonia and one molecule of carbon dioxide combine in accordance with the following net reaction:

$$2NH_3 + CO_2 \longrightarrow H_2N - \underset{\substack{| \\ O}}{C} - NH_2 + H_2O$$

Practically all urea formed in the human body is synthesized in the liver. In pathological states such as serious liver dysfunction, ammonia can accumulate in the blood and become toxic. For example, high levels of ammonia can disrupt the functioning of the central nervous system, sometimes leading to a state called hepatic coma.

The stages in the formation of urea involve ornithine, citrulline, and arginine. Ornithine plus CO_2 and NH_3 forms citrulline which combines with another molecule of NH_3 to form arginine. Arginine plus water produces urea and reforms ornithine through the action of arinase. Once formed, urea diffuses from the liver cells into the body fluids and is excreted by the kidneys.

Chapter 4

DIETARY PROTEIN AND AMINO ACIDS

CLASSIFICATION OF PROTEINS

Depending on the composition, proteins may be divided into two main categories: (1) simple, and (2) conjugated. These two main categories can be further subdivided. The following lists the two main categories of proteins along with their distinguishing characteristics.

Simple proteins — simple proteins consist of only amino acids or their derivatives and include:

- Albuminoids (scleroproteins): these proteins are insoluble in water and are highly resistant to enzymatic digestion; some become gelatinous upon boiling in water or dilute acids or bases. They includes collagen, elastin, and keratin. They are found mainly in supporting tissues and are sometimes referred to as fibrous protein.
- Albumins: these proteins are readily soluble in water and coagulate upon heating. They are present in egg, milk, and serum.
- Globulins: these proteins have low solubility in water but their solubility increases with the addition of neutral salts. They coagulate upon heating. They are abundant in nature. Examples are serum globulins, muscle globulins, and numerous plant globulins.
- Glutelins: these proteins are insoluble in water but soluble in dilute acids or bases. They are abundant in cereal grains. Examples are wheat glutenin, rice oryzenin, and barley hordenin.
- Prolamines: these proteins are insoluble in water, absolute alcohol, or neutral solvents, but are soluble in 80% ethanol. On hydrolysis they give large quantities of proline and ammonia. Examples are zein in corn and gliadin in wheat. Wheat, because of its gluten content, occupies a unique position in food. Gluten is a mixture of two proteins, gliadin and glutenin; these two, when mixed with water, give the characteristic stickiness which enables the molecules present in wheat flour to be bound together by moderate heat with the production of dough from which bread is baked. Rye has a small content of gluten and so (with difficulty) can be made into a loaf. Oats, barley, maize, millet, and rice cannot be made into bread. The grains may be eaten after boiling or their flour made into porridge, bannocks, tortillas, etc.
- Protamines and histones: these basic polypeptides are soluble in water and not coagulated by heat. Large amounts are found in male fish roes and also in cellular nucleoproteins. Protamines have a practical use in the commercial production of delayed-action insulins.

Conjugated proteins — conjugated proteins are joined to various nonprotein substances and include:

- Chromoproteins: these are combinations of a protein and a pigmented (colored) substance. A common example is hemoglobin-hematin and protein.
- Lecithoproteins: these are combinations of protein and lecithin. They are found in fiber of clotted blood and vitellin of egg.
- Lipoproteins: these are water-soluble combinations of fat and protein. They act as vehicles for the transport of fat in the blood. They all contain triglycerides, cholesterol, and phospholipids in varying proportions. For example, low-density lipoprotein (LDL; "bad cholesterol") is the major carrier of cholesterol in the bloodstream.

- Metalloproteins: these are proteins that are complexed with metals. One example is transferrin, a metalloprotein that can bind with copper, iron and zinc. Various enzymes contain minerals.
- Mucoproteins or glycoproteins: these contain carbohydrate such as mannose and galactose. Examples are mucin from the mucus secretion, and some hormones such as human chorionic gonadotropin found in the urine of pregnant females.
- Nucleoproteins: these are combination of simple proteins and nucleic acids and are present in germs of seeds and glandular tissue.
- Phosphoproteins: these are compounds containing protein and phosphorus in a form other than phospholipid or nucleic acid. Examples are casein in milk and ovovitellin in eggs.

Possibly a third category, derived proteins, may be added to the two above. Essentially, derived proteins are the products of digestion. They are fragments of various sizes. From largest to smallest, in terms of the number of amino acids, derived proteins are proteoses, peptones, polypeptides, and peptides.

Proteins may also be classified according to their structure, an important property for their ability to function biologically. Some proteins are round to ellipsoidal and are called globular proteins. These are found in the tissue fluids of animals and plants in which they readily disperse, either in true solutions or colloidal suspension. Enzymes, protein hormones, hemoglobin, and globulins, including caseinogen in milk, albumin in egg white, and albumins and globulins of blood are all globular proteins. These proteins, while not easily digestible, are high-quality proteins and contain a good proportion of the essential amino acids.

Other proteins form long chains bound together in a parallel fashion, and are called fibrous proteins. These consist of long, coiled or folded chains of amino acids bound together by peptide linkages. They are the proteins of connective tissue and elastic tissue including collagen, elastin, and keratin, and are found in the protective and supportive tissues of animals such as skin, hair, and tendons. Many of the fibrous proteins are not very digestible, and if they are, they are usually poor-quality proteins.

While animal proteins can be divided into fibrous and globular, plant proteins are not so easily classified but, broadly speaking, most are glutelins or prolamines.

FUNCTIONS OF PROTEINS

Each distinctive protein performs a specific function in the body. In general, proteins may be classified as performing four basic functions:

1. Growth — The formation of new tissues requires the synthesis of protein. Such conditions occur during periods of growth — from infancy to adulthood, in pregnancy and lactation (each liter of human milk contains about 12 g of protein), and during adaptation to exercise. Wound healing requires the synthesis of new proteins, as do burns, fractures, and hemorrhage.
2. Maintenance — Protein in all humans, regardless of age, is continually being degraded and resynthesized — a process called protein turnover. Blood cells must be replaced every 120 days, while cells which line the intestine are renewed every 1 1/2 days. Moreover, as we'll see in detail later on, protein is lost from the body in the perspiration, hair, fingernails, skin, urine, and feces. This constant turnover and loss of protein requires that the body have a "pool" of amino acids upon which it can draw to replace losses. This "pool" is replenished by dietary protein.
3. Regulatory — Proteins in the cells and body fluids provide regulatory functions. Hemoglobin, an iron-bearing protein, carries oxygen to the tissues. Water balance and osmotic

pressure are regulated by the proteins of the blood plasma. Furthermore, the proteins act as buffers controlling the acid-base balance of the body, especially in the intracellular fluids. Many of the hormones which regulate body processes are proteins; for example, insulin, glucagon, growth hormone, and the digestive tract hormones. Enzymes, the catalysts for most all chemical reactions of the body, are proteins. Antibodies, which protect the body from infectious diseases, are proteins. The blood-clotting mechanism of the body is dependent upon proteins. Certain amino acids derived from dietary protein or synthesized in the body also perform important regulatory functions. For example, arginine participates in the formation of the final metabolic product of nitrogen metabolism — urea — in the liver, and glycine participates in the synthesis of purines, porphyrins, creatine, and glyoxylic acid.

4. Energy — The catabolism of amino acids yields energy — about 4 kilocalories (kcal) per gram of protein. In order for amino acids to be used for energy, the amino group (NH_2) must first be removed by a process known as deamination (see below). The carbon skeleton remaining following deamination — alpha keto acid residues — may be either converted to glucose (glycogenic pathway) or metabolized in fat pathways (ketogenic pathway). When energy consumption in the form of carbohydrates and fats is low, the energy needs of the body take priority and dietary and tissue proteins will be utilized at the expense of the building or repair processes of the body. In the body, amino acids may be used primarily for protein synthesis or energy production, depending upon (1) protein quality, (2) caloric level of the diet, (3) stage of development, including growth, pregnancy, and lactation, (4) prior nutritional status, and (5) stress factors such as fever, injury, and immobilization.

COAGULATION AND DENATURATION

Many water-soluble proteins coagulate when subjected to heat at about 100°C or above, as occurs in the normal process of cooking. A familiar example would be the change of the white of an egg on boiling. Once a protein has undergone this change its specific properties, e.g., enzymic, hormonal, or immunological, are permanently destroyed.

Proteins also undergo denaturation in which they become less soluble in water. This occurs when they are exposed to a variety of agents such as moderate heat, ultraviolet light, alcohol, and mild acids or alkalis. Proteins are most easily denatured at their isoelectric points, i.e., the particular pH at which the electric charges on their NH_2 and COOH groups precisely balance; this varies from one protein to another. The exact nature of the denaturation process is obscure although it involves some disorganization of the specific arrangement of the component amino acids. To a certain extent, it is reversible once normal conditions are restored; but most enzymes and allergens lose their specific properties once denatured.

PROTEIN DIGESTION, ABSORPTION, AND METABOLISM

Protein digestion is the mechanical, chemical, and enzymatic breakdown of the protein in food into smaller units. Digestion involves several stages including the mechanical extraction of the protein from the food, denaturation of the protein, and hydrolysis of the peptide bonds. Protein is mechanically extracted from the food in the process of mastication and by the action of the stomach. The low pH of the stomach plays a role in denaturation of the extracted protein, thus making it more accessible to the proteolytic enzymes of the gut. There is evidence that gastric emptying is delayed by the presence of proteinaceous food in the stomach, and this may be necessary to ensure effective extraction and denaturation of the protein prior to its entry in the duodenum.

In the small intestine enzymes from the pancreas and the small intestine split dietary protein into peptides (small groups of bonded amino acids) and individual amino acids. Protein must be digested to amino acids or di- and tripeptides before absorption can occur, although at times larger peptides can be absorbed. In the first few days of life and in certain disease states traces of polypeptides and undigested protein may be absorbed.[644]

There is some evidence that hydrolyzed protein fragments (i.e., peptides) cross the small intestine and reach peripheral tissue via the systemic circulation.[645] Dietary peptides can have specific actions locally on the gastrointestinal tract, or at more distant sites having an influence on physiological processes. These bioactive peptides can alter cellular metabolism and may act as vasoregulators, growth factors, releasing hormones, or neurotransmitters. The concept of dietary bioactive peptides offers an explanation for varying effects of diet on physiologic responses. Current experimental evidence indicates that diets that possess the capability of producing luminal peptides are superior to diets lacking this capacity. More research needs to be done to determine the anabolic and ergogenic effects of dietary bioactive peptides before they can be used effectively as nutritional supplements.

For the early stages of the digestion of protein, four types of enzymes are important: pepsins (secreted by serous cells in the gastric gland of the stomach), trypsin, elastase, and the chymotrypsins (all secreted by the acinar cells of the pancreas). The product of the action of these proteolytic enzymes is a series of peptides of various sizes. These are degraded further by the action of several peptidases (exopeptidases) that remove terminal amino acids, including carboxypeptidases A and B which hydrolyze amino acids sequentially from the carboxyl end of peptides. Aminopeptidases, which are secreted by the absorptive cells of the small intestine, hydrolyze amino acids sequentially from the amino end of peptides.

In addition, dipeptidases, which are structurally associated with the brush border of the absorptive cells, hydrolyze dipeptides into their component amino acids. The extent to which these act on substrates in the lumen, within the membrane of the cells, or within the cell itself is not known.

Protein digestion in the intestine results in the hydrolysis of both ingested protein and endogenous protein, in the form of digestive enzymes, other secreted proteins, and desquamated epithelial cells. Between 50 and 70 g of endogenous protein are digested daily, almost equal to the average daily amount ingested.

The final stages of the hydrolysis of peptides to dipeptides and amino acids, and their absorption, occur in the jejunum and ileum. The transport of amino acids and di- and tripeptides from the lumen into the cell is an active process (more on this later when discussing protein and amino acid supplements).

In general, animal proteins are more completely and rapidly absorbed than are vegetable proteins; possibly because of the cellulose covering in plant cells and the increased fiber associated with vegetable proteins.

Until the early 1950s, the absorption products of protein digestion were widely thought to be free amino acids for which there were several discernable transport mechanisms. There is now good evidence that small peptides containing two to six amino acid residues are absorbed from the gut lumen at least as rapidly as free amino acids.[646,647]

Measurements of the net absorption of amino acids after a meal containing 15 g of milk protein show that it is 70 to 80% complete in 3 h.

REQUIREMENT FOR DIETARY PROTEIN

The requirement for dietary protein consists of two components:

1. The requirement for the nutritionally essential amino acids (isoleucine, leucine, lysine, methionine, phenylalanine, threonine, tryptophan, and valine) under all conditions, and

for conditionally essential amino acids (arginine, cysteine, glutamine, glycine, histidine, proline, taurine, and tyrosine) under specific physiological and pathological conditions.
2. The requirement for nonspecific nitrogen for the synthesis of the nutritionally dispensable amino acids (aspartic acid, asparagine, glutamic acid, alanine, serine) and other physiologically important nitrogen-containing compounds such as nucleic acids, creatine, and porphyrins.

With respect to the first component, it is usually accepted that the nutritive values of various food protein sources are to a large extent determined by the concentration and availability of the individual indispensable amino acids. Hence, the efficiency with which a given source of food protein is utilized in support of an adequate state of nutritional health depends both on the physiological requirements for the indispensable amino acids and total nitrogen and on the concentration of specific amino acids in the source of interest.

PROTEIN QUALITY — AMINO ACID REQUIREMENTS

Early studies on protein quality demonstrated that some proteins supported growth and even survival better than others, and that a certain quantity of dietary protein was needed. This early work on the effects of feeding proteins of known amino acid composition, or diets containing specified pure amino acids, on the rate of growth or nitrogen balance of an experimental animal resulted in proteins being classified as complete, partially incomplete, and incomplete and also led to the concept of essential or nonessential or indispensable and dispensable amino acids. As well, it was found that the amino acid requirements vary according to the species and age of an animal and are determined in the last analysis by the amino acid composition of the tissue proteins formed during growth.[648]

Not all proteins are of equal nutritional value; this reflects their differing amino acid content. Although most proteins contain most of the 22 or so amino acids, these are present in widely differing proportions. Complete proteins contain all of the essential amino acids in sufficient amounts to maintain life and support growth in that animal. Partially incomplete proteins can maintain life, but cannot support growth. Incomplete proteins cannot maintain life or support growth. Since plant proteins may be deficient in one or more essential amino acids and meat contains all of the essential amino acids, the chances of developing a deficiency is greater for vegetarians than for meat eaters (see below). A lack of essential amino acids in the diet results in a variety of adverse effects that depend on the degree and length of deficiency. Dairy products, meat, fish, eggs, and poultry are examples of foods that contain complete proteins.

Essential amino acids are those which cannot be synthesized by the body or that cannot be synthesized at a sufficient rate to supply the normal requirements for protein biosynthesis.[649] These amino acids must therefore be present in the diet. The nonessential amino acids can be synthesized at a sufficient rate (provided, of course, that the supplies of amino nitrogen and carbon precursors are adequate). Thus an amino acid is nonessential if its carbon skeleton can be formed in the body, and if an amino group can be transferred to it from some available donor compound, a process called transamination (see above). For example, the body can make as much alanine as it needs quickly and easily because the carbon chain is pyruvate, a common metabolic product to which the amino group from another common nonessential amino acid can be added.

The use of the word essential, however, does not mean that the other nonessential amino acids are not equally as essential for formation of the proteins, but only that the others are not essential in the diet because they can be synthesized in the body. For protein synthesis to take place, all the amino acids required must be available. If the diet lacks one or more of these essential amino acids the body's ability to synthesize new protein is adversely affected.[650]

There are no recommended dietary allowances (RDAs) for any of the individual amino acids. Instead, since protein is made up of amino acids, RDAs are expressed in terms of amino acid patterns in protein intake.

Studies have shown that the currently accepted 1985 criteria for the amino acid requirement pattern is not capable of maintaining body amino acid homeostasis or balance.[651,652] Other diets, however, such as the Massachusetts Institute of Technology (MIT) requirement pattern (MIT diet), or the egg-protein pattern (egg diet) were capable of maintaining amino acid homeostasis. Thus it is hypothesized that current international estimations of essential amino acid requirements are far too low and must be modified in light of recent research.[653]

While the presence of essential amino acids is critical to protein synthesis, there is some evidence that lack of the nonessential amino acids can result in lower plasma levels of these amino acids,[654] which may ultimately compromise protein synthesis in situations where there is rapid growth.

During periods of active growth or tissue repair, more nitrogen is ingested than excreted (positive nitrogen balance). Conversely, in malnutrition or starvation, less nitrogen is ingested than excreted (negative nitrogen balance). To determine whether an amino acid is essential, it is omitted from the diet while all the other amino acids are included. If the omission results in negative nitrogen balance, the amino acid is deemed essential. In the absence of this single amino acid, the body has been unable to synthesize certain proteins so that the nitrogen that would have been used in this synthesis is excreted. By this criterion, the following amino acids are essential in humans: isoleucine, leucine, lysine, methionine, phenylalanine, threonine, tryptophan, and valine.

However, not all of the other amino acids can be considered nonessential at all times. In some cases of accelerated growth and other conditions, such as the nutritional support of the catabolic patient,[655] certain amino acids may become essential since the body cannot synthesize enough of the amino acid for that particular situation and the amino acid becomes rate limiting for protein synthesis. These amino acids are often referred to as conditionally essential.

For example, histidine is known to be required for normal growth in a child and is necessary for proper growth in the rat. It seems likely that histidine is also essential in human adults under certain conditions, and under conditions of dietary deficiency may be a limiting factor for growth.[656] Taurine may also be conditionally essential. The past 20 years have seen the status of taurine change from an end product of methionine and cysteine metabolism and a substance conjugated to bile acids to that of an important, and sometimes essential, nutrient. It is now added to most synthetic human infant formulas and pediatric parenteral solutions throughout the world.[657] Proline and glutamine are other examples of amino acids that may be conditionally essential. In one recent study the authors suggest that some nonessential amino acids such as proline and glutamate-glutamine may become limiting during lactation because of their unique contributions to milk protein synthesis.[658]

As well, there are other special considerations for certain of the nonessential amino acids. Although humans can synthesize most of the nonessential amino acids from glucose and ammonia, tyrosine synthesis requires the availability of phenylalanine, and cysteine requires the availability of methionine. Both phenylalanine and methionine are essential amino acids, and if they are available in the diet at or below minimal requirement levels, tyrosine and cysteine can become essential amino acids in that the lack of precursor amino acids decreases the ability of the body to produce these amino acids and they then become rate limiting for protein synthesis (see below).

For example, in some patients with liver disease the hepatic conversion of phenylalanine to tyrosine and methionine to cystine is inadequate, and unless sufficient cystine/tyrosine is administered[659] repletion of lean tissue (net protein synthesis) will be substantially limited and body function will be impaired.

However, while obtaining adequate amounts of the essential amino acids is important, the proportion of nonessential amino acid nitrogen has an influence on the essential amino acid requirements.[660,661] However, while increasing the amount of dietary nonessential amino acids may increase protein synthesis by increasing the level of dietary protein, it may not influence the overall requirements for the essential amino acids.[662] On the other hand, if the ratio of essential amino acids to the total nitrogen in a food is too high, essential amino acids will be used as sources of nitrogen for the nonessential amino acids.

Not only completeness, but digestibility as well are issues of concern with respect to protein quality. It's known that not all protein sources are utilized equally well and that the bioavailability of ingested protein varies according to the source of protein. A protein is digestible if a high proportion of its amino acids reach the body's cells so that they can synthesize the proteins they require. This indicates that the nitrogen in the protein is utilized with little waste. High-quality proteins are both complete and highly digestible, meaning that smaller quantities need to be ingested than would be the case for proteins of lower quality.

Egg protein is usually the standard against which other sources are often compared since it is utilized for growth in animals with an 85 to 90% efficiency (biological value). Plant proteins, because they are more difficult to digest and have a lower essential amino acid content, are utilized for growth only 50 to 80% as well as egg protein.

The quality or type of protein may also affect the absorption or utilization of other nutrients. In a recent study the influence of different protein sources on Zn absorption was evaluated.[663] The results of this study demonstrated that zinc absorption is inhibited by certain protein sources, such as bovine serum albumin and soybean-protein isolate, while other proteins have little or no effect.

VEGETARIAN DIETS

Vegetarians almost always abstain from eating red meat (mammalian) and usually abstain from eating poultry, fish, and other seafood. Depending on the type of vegetarian, the banned foods may also include any food of animal origin, whether "alive" or not. While there are many different kinds of vegetarians,[664] the following two basic types are the most common.

1. Lacto-ovo vegetarian — a vegetarian who combines milk products and eggs with a diet of vegetables, fruits, nuts, seeds, legumes, and grains. Vegetarians may also avoid milk products but consume eggs (ovo vegetarian) or vice versa (lacto vegetarian).
2. Vegan — this type excludes milk products, eggs and even honey. Their diet is derived exclusively from plants with all their protein intake being in the form of plant protein. The vegan also avoids any products derived from animals such as leather, wool, fur, down, silk, ivory, and pearl. Additionally, cosmetics and household items that contain animal ingredients or that are tested on animals are avoided. A fruitarian is even stricter, and avoids any plant products except those parts of the plant that are cast off or dropped from the plant and that do not involve the destruction of the plant itself.

Although humans have used some 300 plant species for food and at least 150 species have been cultivated for commercial purposes, most of the world's population depends on approximately 20 different plant crops, which are generally divided into cereals, vegetables (including legumes), fruits, and nuts. The most important groups for human nutrition are cereal grains and food legumes, including oil-seed legumes.

Because of completeness and digestibility some proteins are nutritionally better than others; they contain a more balanced range of the essential and conditionally essential amino acids. In general, proteins of animal origin contain adequate amounts of the essential amino acids and hence they are known as first class proteins. On the other hand, many proteins of vegetable origin are relatively deficient in certain amino acids, notably lysine and the sulfur-containing amino acids.

Mixtures of plant proteins can serve as a complete and well-balanced source of amino acids for meeting human physiological requirements.[665] However, combining the proper foods is necessary to obtain the necessary levels of both the essential or indispensable and conditionally indispensable amino acids.

The essential amino acid lysine is consistently at a much lower concentration in all major plant food protein groups than in animal foods. Since lysine is the limiting amino acid, the addition of limited amounts of lysine to cereal diets improves their protein quality. Studies in Peru and Guatemala have demonstrated that growing children benefitted by this addition.[666] In addition, the sulfur-containing amino acids are distinctly lower in legumes and fruits and threonine is lower in cereals compared with amounts found in proteins of animal origin.

COMPLEMENTARY PROTEINS

There are important differences among and between food products of vegetable and animal origin including the concentrations of proteins and indispensable amino acids that they contain. The concentration of proteins and the quality of the proteins in some foods of vegetable origin may be too low to make them adequate as sole sources of proteins. In some of the poorer parts of the world, diets are based predominantly on a single plant (e.g., corn) and frequently lead to malnutrition.

Fortunately, the amino acid deficiencies in a protein can usually be improved by combining it with another so that the mixture of the two proteins will often have a higher food value than either one alone. For example, many cereals are low in lysine but high in methionine and cysteine. On the other hand, soybeans, lima beans, and kidney beans are high in lysine but low in methionine and cysteine. When eaten together these types of proteins give a more favorable amino acid profile.

Another example would be the combination of soybean, which is low in sulfur-containing amino acids, with cottonseed, peanut, and sesame flour, and cereal grains, which are deficient mainly in lysine. In general, oilseed proteins, and in particular, soy protein, can be used effectively in combination with most cereal grains to improve the overall quality of the total protein intake. A combination of soy protein, which is high in lysine, with a cereal that contains a relatively good concentration of sulfur-containing amino acids results in a nutritional complementation; the protein quality of the mixture is greater than that for either protein source alone.

Some examples of complementary food proteins include beans and corn (as in tortillas); rice and black-eyed peas; whole wheat or bulgar, soybeans, and sesame seeds; and soybeans, peanuts, brown rice, and bulgar wheat. This kind of supplementation works when the deficient and complementary proteins are ingested together or within a few hours of each other.

Various nutritional responses are observed when two dietary proteins are combined. These have been classified by Bressani et al.[667] into one of four types.

Type I is an example where no protein complementary effect is achieved. For example, this occurs with combinations of peanut and corn, where each of the protein sources have a common and quantitatively similar lysine deficiency and are both also deficient in other amino acids.

Type II response is observed when combinations are made of two protein sources that have the same limiting amino acid, but in quantitatively different amounts. Corn and cottonseed flour, for example, are both limiting in lysine but cottonseed is relatively less inadequate than is corn.

The third type of response (Type III) demonstrates a true complementary effect because there is a synergistic effect on the overall nutritive value of the protein mixture; the protein quality of the best mix exceeds that of each component alone. This type of response occurs when one of the protein sources has a considerably higher concentration of the most limiting amino acid in the other protein. An example of this response, based on studies in children, is observed when corn and soy flour are mixed so that 60% of the protein intake comes from corn and the remainder from soy protein.

Finally, the Type IV response occurs when both protein sources have a common amino acid deficiency. The protein component giving the highest value is the one containing a higher concentration of the deficient amino acid. Combinations of some textured soy proteins and beef protein follow this type of response.

These nutritional relationships have been determined from rat bioassay studies. However, the more limited results available from human studies with soy and other legumes confirm the applicability of this general concept in human nutrition. This knowledge helps us to understand and evaluate how nutritionally effective combinations of plant protein foods can be achieved.

Even when combinations of plant protein foods are used there is still the concern of timing of ingestion of complementary proteins. Is there a need to ingest different plant proteins at the same time or within the same meal to achieve maximum benefit and nutritional value from proteins with different, but complementary, amino acid patterns? This concern may also extend to the question of the need to ingest a significant amount of protein at each meal, or whether it is sufficient to consume protein in variable amounts at different meals and even different days as long as the average daily intake meets or exceeds the recommended or safe protein intakes.

According to FAO/WHO/UNU,[668] estimates of protein requirements refer to metabolic needs that persist over moderate periods of time. However, as we'll see in the following chapters, the body does not store much protein outside of a meager free amino acid pool, and begins certain catabolic processes in the postabsorptive phase making the ingestion of regular amounts of protein critical for maximizing the anabolic effects of exercise.

There is a limited database that we can consult to make a definitive conclusion on the timing of consumption of complementary proteins or of specific amino acid supplements for proteins that are deficient in one or more amino acids. Earlier work in rapidly growing rats suggested that delaying the supplementation of a protein with its limiting amino acid reduces the value of the supplement.[669,670] Similarly, the frequency of feeding of diets supplemented with lysine in growing pigs affects the overall efficiency of utilization of dietary protein.[671] Studies in human adults showed that overall dietary protein utilization was similar whether the daily protein intake was distributed among two or three meals.[672,673]

In general, especially under conditions where intakes of total protein are high, it may not be necessary to consume complementary proteins at the same time. Separation of the proteins among meals over the course of a day would still permit the nutritional benefits of complementation.

However, in athletes trying to maximize protein synthesis and muscular hypertrophy it is necessary to have a full complement of amino acids present for every meal in order to maximize the anabolic effects of exercise. There is a meal-related decrease in proteolysis and increase in protein synthesis. In one study whole-body leucine and alpha-ketoisocaproate (KIC) metabolism were estimated in mature dogs fed a complete meal, a meal devoid of branched-chain amino acids, and a meal devoid of all amino acids.[674]

Using a constant infusion of [4,5-^{3}H]leucine and alpha-[1-^{14}C]ketoisocaproate (KIC), combined with dietary [5,5,5-$^{2}H_3$]leucine, the rate of whole-body proteolysis, protein synthesis, leucine oxidation, and interconversion of leucine and KIC were estimated along with the rate of leucine absorption. Ingestion of the complete meal resulted in a decrease in the rate of endogenous proteolysis, a small increase in the estimated rate of leucine entering protein, and a twofold increase in the rate of leucine oxidation. Ingestion of either the meal devoid of branched-chain amino acids or devoid of all amino acids resulted in a decrease in estimates of whole-body rates of proteolysis and protein synthesis, decreased leucine oxidation, and a decrease in the interconversion of leucine and KIC.

The decrease in whole-body proteolysis was closely associated with the rise in plasma insulin concentrations following meal ingestion. Together, these data suggest that the transition from tissue catabolism to anabolism is the result, at least in part, of decreased whole-body proteolysis. This meal-related decrease in proteolysis is independent of the dietary amino acid composition or content. In contrast, the rate of protein synthesis was sustained only when the meal complete in all amino acids was provided, indicating an overriding control of protein synthesis by amino acid availability.

FOOD PROCESSING

The processing of food with the use of heat and chemicals can adversely affect amino acid availability.[675] For example, lysine can be lost from mild heat treatment in the presence of reducing sugars such as glucose or lactose since these sugars react with free amino groups. This may also occur when the protein and sugar are stored together at low temperatures.

Under severe heating conditions, with or without the presence of either sugars or oxidized lipids, food proteins form additional chemical bonds and can become resistant to digestion so that availability of all amino acids is reduced. When protein is exposed to severe treatment with alkali, lysine and cysteine can be eliminated by the formation of lysinoalanine, which may be toxic. The use of oxidizing agents such as sulfur dioxide (SO_2) can result in a loss of methionine in the protein through the formation of methionine sulfoxide.

Heating can also have favorable effects. Heating soybean flour improves the utilization of protein by making the amino acid methionine more available, and heating raw soybeans destroys the inhibitor of the protein digestive enzyme trypsin. Cooking eggs destroys the trypsin inhibitor ovomucoid found in the white part of the egg.

MEASURING PROTEIN QUALITY

There are several ways to measure the protein quality of food. The three most quoted are the Protein Efficiency Ratio (PER), Biological Value (BV), and Protein Digestibility (PD).

Protein Efficiency Ratio

The Protein Efficiency Ratio is the best-known procedure for evaluating protein quality, and is used in the U.S. as the basis for food labeling regulations and for the establishment of the protein RDA. In this procedure, immature rats are fed a measured amount of protein and weighed periodically as they grow. The PER is then calculated by dividing the weight gain (in grams) by the protein intake (also in grams).

While simple and economical, the PER procedure is time-consuming. Also, evidence from studies with rats indicate that the pattern of amino acids required for maintenance and tissue protein accretion is quite different. Thus, the amino acid requirements of growing rats are not the same as for those of mature rats, much less mature human beings. Indeed, the intracellular muscle free amino acid pool of rats is probably less suitable for the investigation of amino acid metabolism, due to the great differences in their distribution in human and rat muscle.[676]

Nevertheless, the PER is used widely today. A recent study compared the protein quality of different animal foods and of their mixtures with vegetable foods, mainly cereals, at the 30:70 animal:vegetable protein proportion with experiments performed under the same conditions.[677] The animal foods were eggs, beef, pork, barbecued lamb, chicken, ham, sausage, and milk powder. The vegetable foods used in the mixtures were rice, lime-treated corn flour, wheat flour and cooked black beans. The protein concentrations in the raw and cooked materials were analyzed. The PER and digestibilities were determined in Fisher 344 weanling rats. Based on the corrected PER, the foods with the best protein quality were egg (3.24), sirloin beef (3.16), lamb (3.11) and chicken breast (3.07), which were significantly different from milk powder (2.88) and beef liver and beef round (2.81 and 2.70, respectively). Ham (2.63) and pork loin (2.57) had a similar protein quality to that of casein (2.50). The lowest protein quality was found in sausages (2.14). In most of the mixtures of animal and vegetable protein (30:70), the PER was similar to or higher than that of the animal food alone. Beans were the vegetable food that showed the lowest response to the addition of animal food. The conclusion of the study is that some 30:70 mixtures of animal:vegetable protein, such as chicken, beef round, and pork with cereals, could be utilized for regular meals because of their high PER and low cost.

Biological Value

To determine the relative utilization of a protein by the body, it is necessary to measure not only urinary but also fecal losses of nitrogen when that protein is actually fed to human beings under test conditions. Even under these circumstances, small additional losses from sweat, sloughed skin, hair, and fingernails will be missed. This kind of experiment determines the biological value (BV) of proteins, a measure used internationally.

The BV test involves two nitrogen balance studies. In the first, no protein is ingested and fecal and urinary nitrogen excretions are measured. It is assumed that under these conditions nitrogen lost in the urine is the amount the body always necessarily loses by filtration into the urine each day, regardless of what protein is fed (endogenous nitrogen). The nitrogen lost in the feces (called metabolic nitrogen) is the amount the body invariably loses into the intestine each day, whether or not food protein is fed. In the second study, an amount of protein slightly below the requirement is ingested, and intake and losses are measured. The BV is then derived using the following formula:

Biological Value = 100 times the equation

food N – (fecal N – metabolic N) – (urinary N – endogenous N)/food N – (fecal N – metabolic N)

The denominator of the BV equation expresses the amount of nitrogen absorbed: food N minus fecal N (excluding the N the body would lose in the feces anyway, even without food). The numerator expresses the amount of N retained from the N absorbed: absorbed N (as in the denominator) minus the N excreted in the urine (excluding the N the body would lose in the urine anyway, even without food). Thus, it can be more simply expressed as:

$$BV = N\ retained/N\ absorbed \times 100$$

The BV method has the advantages of being based on experiments with human beings and of measuring actual nitrogen retention. Its disadvantages are that it is cumbersome, expensive, sometimes impractical, and it is based on several assumptions that may not be valid.

For example, the subjects used for testing may not be similar physiologically or in terms of their normal environment or typical food intake (e.g., dietary protein intake history) to those for whom the test protein may ultimately be used. Also, that the protein is retained in the body does not necessarily mean that it is being well utilized.

There is considerable exchange of protein among tissues (protein turnover) that is hidden from view when only N intake and output are measured. One tissue could be shorted, and the test of biological value would not detect this. At present, the relationship between protein intakes and optimum organ function and health is poorly understood. Nevertheless, it would appear that the results obtained by the BV method would be more applicable to humans.[678]

As examples we can compare the BV of two proteins that are on the opposite end of the scale — vegetable proteins and hydrolyzed whey protein. Plant proteins have a low BV and therefore supplementation is a necessity for most plant-based vegetarian (as against lacto-ovo and lacto vegetarians) athletes who wish to increase lean body mass.[679] A recent study measured the effects of a diet made up of plant protein in rats. The results demonstrate the insufficiency of vegetable sources of food with respect to proteosynthesis and the content of limiting amino acids (decisive for the synthesis of peptide chains) in the period of the organism development.

On the other hand, whey protein has a higher BV and is much more suitable for athletes wishing to increase muscle mass. As well, the BV of whey protein increases once it has been predigested (i.e., its high molecular weight protein fractions have been broken down into more efficiently absorbed short-chain peptides such as di-, tri-, and oligopeptides).

Protein Digestibility-Corrected Amino Acid Score (PDCAAS)

The latest way to assess dietary protein quality is PDCAAS, recommended by the FAO/WHO Joint Expert Commission on Protein Evaluation in Rome in 1990. Several factors such as inadequacies of the protein efficiency ratio method (PER, the poorest test) and other animal assays, advancements made in standardizing methods for amino acid analysis and protein digestibility, availability of data on digestibility of protein and individual amino acids in a variety of foods, and reliability of human amino acid requirements and scoring patterns make the amino acid score, corrected for true digestibility of protein, the most suitable routine method for predicting protein quality of foods for humans.[680]

The protein digestibility-corrected amino acid score method is a simple and scientifically sound approach for routine evaluation of protein quality of foods. The PDCAAS is directly applicable to humans, and incorporates factors for more real-life variables than either PER or BV. The amino acid pattern for humans aged 2 to 5 years is used as the basis for determination of PDCAAS, since this age group matches or exceeds amino acid requirement patterns of older children and adults. Corrections for digestibility of protein are also taken from human data. PDCAAS scores range from 1.0 to 0.0, with 1.0 being the upper limit of protein quality (able to support growth and health).

Interestingly, using PDCAAS results in a score of 1.0 for isolated soy protein, identical to other proteins with scores of 1.0 (such as casein, lactalbumin, or ovalbumin).[681] This finding reflects the successful, long-term use of soy protein as the exclusive protein source for infants, who have even higher amino acid requirements than children or adults.

Discrepancies between the PER and PDCAAS are related to the differences between young growing rats and humans. Growing rats have a larger requirement for sulfur-containing amino acids to generate the larger amounts of keratin for whole-body coats of hair, which humans do not possess.

Thus soy protein can be added to the list of complete proteins for humans, along with milk and egg proteins. Other vegetable proteins (pea, beans, peanuts, wheat, oats, etc.) still have less than adequate protein scores.

DIETARY PROTEIN REQUIREMENTS

The term protein requirement means that amount of protein which must be consumed to provide the amino acids for the synthesis of those body proteins irreversibly catabolized in the course of the body's metabolism. The dietary requirement for protein comprises two components: (1) a requirement for total nitrogen, and (2) a requirement for the nutritionally indispensable amino acids. The nutritionally indispensable amino acids alone do not maintain body nitrogen balance; a source of "nonspecific" nitrogen from dispensable amino acids, such as from glycine and alanine or other nitrogen compounds, is also required.[682]

The recommended allowances for protein (nitrogen) are based upon experiments in which normal requirement is defined as the intake necessary to achieve zero balance between intake vs. output. Most estimates assume normal digestion and absorption and normal metabolism. In some cases, estimates of daily turnover are used to determine the amount of nutrient required to maintain body stores.

Thus the intake of nitrogen from protein must be sufficient to balance that excreted; this basic concept is called nitrogen balance.

THE RECOMMENDED DAILY ALLOWANCE (RDA)

The minimum daily requirement, that is, the minimum amount of dietary protein which will provide the needed amounts of amino acids to optimally maintain the body, is impossible to determine for each individual without expending a good deal of time and effort for each person.

To eliminate the necessity of determining individual nutrient requirements, a system called the recommended daily allowance (RDA) has been devised. As research accumulates for each of the many essential nutrients, its associated RDA is revised. How is the RDA established? Ideally, sufficient research is conducted to show (1) that a given nutrient is needed by the human, (2) that certain deficiency signs can be produced, (3) that these signs can be avoided or reversed if the missing nutrient is administered, and (4) that no further improvement is observed if the nutrient is administered at levels above that which reversed the deficiency symptoms.

Next, studies are conducted on a variety of subjects to determine their minimal need. Since humans vary so much, it is not possible to measure the requirements over a broad range of human variability. To allow for this variability, a safety factor is added on to the determined minimum needs of the group of subjects studied. As more subjects are studied and more data accumulated, the added safety factor becomes smaller.

In the case of protein and amino acid requirements, the RDA was set at twice the minimum value of the subject who required the most protein and/or amino acid in all the studies conducted. By greatly increasing the recommended intake figure over that experimentally determined, it was hoped that the protein and amino acid needs of the majority or 95% of the U.S. population would be met. The RDA for protein was originally quite high. For many years, it was set at 1 g/kg body weight for the average adult male. The average adult male was assumed to weigh 70 kg (about 155 lb) so the RDA was 70 g/d. With an ever-increasing data base which the Nutrition Board of the National Research Council can use for its recommendations, the RDA for protein has been adjusted downward every 5 years.

Presently (as of 1993) the protein RDA for an adult male is set at 56 g/d. This presumes that the dietary protein is coming from a mixed diet containing a reasonable amount of good-quality proteins. For persons subsisting on mixtures of poor-quality proteins, this RDA may not be adequate.

RDAs are set not only for the individual nutrients but also for age groups within each nutrient. For some age groups the data base is very poor, e.g., preadolescents, toddlers, young children, and pregnant females; there is a continual revision as data become available.

Guidelines of nutritional requirements in health have been formulated in the reports, updated periodically, of the Food and Nutrition Board of the National Research Council of the United States.[683] These recommended dietary allowances, expressed for age and sex and modified for such conditions as pregnancy and lactation, are designed to cover the requirements of virtually all healthy individuals. With the exception of energy, the allowances are not average requirements but rather a recommended intake sufficient to meet the needs of all healthy individuals.

Proper nitrogen balance studies are laborious and are performed over a period of several days. A shortcut is often taken and an estimate of nitrogen balance is made by collecting and measuring nitrogen in the urine since the end products of protein metabolism leave the body mainly via this route, and by estimating other losses.

Estimations are made of the nitrogen lost in the feces and the small losses of protein from skin, hair, fingernails, perspiration, and other secretions.

About 90% of the nitrogen in urine is urea and ammonia salts — the end products of protein metabolism. The remaining nitrogen is accounted for by creatinine (from creatine), uric acid (products of the metabolism of purines and pyrimidines), porphyrins, and other nitrogen-containing compounds.

Urinary nitrogen excretion is related to the basal metabolic rate (BMR). The larger the muscle mass in the body, the more calories are needed to maintain the BMR. Also, the rate of transamination is greater as amino acids and carbohydrates are interconverted to fulfill energy needs in the muscle. About 1 to 1.3 mg of urinary nitrogen are excreted for each kilocalorie required for basal metabolism. Nitrogen excretion also increases during exercise and heavy work.

Fecal and skin losses account for a significant amount of nitrogen loss from the body in normal conditions, and these may vary widely in disease states. Thus, measurement of urinary nitrogen loss alone may not provide a predictable assessment of daily nitrogen requirement when it is most needed. Fecal losses are due to the inefficiency of digestion and absorption of protein (93% efficiency). In addition, the intestinal tract secretes proteins in the lumen from saliva, gastric juice, bile, pancreatic enzymes, and enterocyte sloughing.

Taking all these losses into consideration and using nitrogen balance as a tool, the recommended daily dietary allowance for protein may be derived on the following basis:

1. Obligatory urinary nitrogen losses of young adults amount to about 37 mg/kg of body weight.
2. Fecal nitrogen losses average 12 mg/kg of body weight.
3. Amounts of nitrogen lost in the perspiration, hair, fingernails, and sloughed skin are estimated at 3 mg/kg of body weight.
4. Minor routes of nitrogen loss such as saliva, menstruation, and seminal ejaculation are estimated at 2 mg/kg of body weight.
5. The total obligatory nitrogen lost — that which must be replaced daily — amounts to 54 mg/kg, or in terms of protein lost this is 0.34 g/kg (0.054×6.25).
6. To account for individual variation the daily loss is increased by 30%, or 70 mg/kg. In terms of protein, this is 0.45 g/kg of body weight.
7. This protein loss is further increased by 30%, to 0.6 g/kg of body weight, to account for the loss of efficiency when consuming even a high-quality protein such as egg.
8. The final adjustment is to correct for the 75% efficiency of utilization of protein in the mixed diet of North Americans. Thus, the recommended daily allowance (RDA) for protein becomes 0.8 g/kg of body weight for normal healthy adult males and females, or 63 g of protein per day for a 174 lb (79 kg) humans and 50 g/d for a 138-lb (63 kg) woman.

The need for dietary protein is influenced by age, environmental temperature, energy intake, gender, micronutrient intake, infection, activity, previous diet, trauma, pregnancy, and lactation.

RECOMMENDED DAILY INTAKES FOR ATHLETES

The recommended dietary allowances make little provision for changes in nutrient requirements for the athlete. Energy requirements increase with exercise as the lean (muscle) mass increases and as resting metabolic energy expenditure increases. Increased physical activity at all ages promotes the retention of lean muscle mass and requires increased protein and energy intake.

HISTORICAL OVERVIEW

The history of protein requirements for athletes is both interesting and circular. In the mid-1800s the popular opinion was that protein was the primary fuel for working muscle.[684] This was an incentive for athletes to consume large amounts of dietary protein.

In 1866 a study based on urinary nitrogen excretion measures (in order for protein to provide energy its nitrogen must be removed and subsequently excreted, primarily in the urine) suggested that protein was not an important fuel, and contributed about 6% of the fuel used during a 1956-m climb in the Swiss Alps.[685] This study and others, led to the perception that exercise does not increase one's need for dietary protein. This view has persisted to the present.

Recently, however, there is some evidence to show that protein contributes more than is generally believed today. The data in the 1866 study likely underestimated the actual protein use for several methodological reasons. For example, the subjects consumed a protein-free diet before the climb, postclimb excretion measures were not made, and other routes of nitrogen excretion may have been substantial.

However, based largely on these data, this belief has persisted throughout most of the twentieth century. This is somewhat surprising because Cathcart[686] in an extensive review of the literature prior to 1925 concluded "the accumulated evidence seems to me to point in no unmistakable fashion to the opposite conclusion that muscle activity does increase, if only in small degree, the metabolism of protein." Based on results from a number of separate experimental approaches, the conclusions of several more-recent investigators support Cathcart's conclusion.[687]

We believe that current dietary protein recommendations are insufficient for athletes and those wishing to maximize lean body mass and strength. These athletes may well benefit from protein supplementation. With exercise and under certain conditions, the use of protein and amino acid supplements may have significant anabolic and anticatabolic effects.

In a recent work, Peter Lemon, of the Applied Physiology Research Laboratory, Kent State University, addressed the issue of the protein requirements of athletes.[688] Lemon remarked that current recommendations concerning dietary protein are based primarily on data obtained from sedentary subjects. However, both endurance and strength athletes, he says, will likely benefit from diets containing more protein than the current RDA of 0.8 g/kg/d, though the roles played by protein in excess of the RDA will likely be quite different between the two sets of athletes.

For strength athletes, Lemon states that protein requirements will probably be in the range of 1.4 to 1.8 g/kg/day, whereas endurance athletes need about 1.2 to 1.4 g/kg/d. There is no indication that these intakes will cause any adverse side effects in healthy humans. On the other hand, there is essentially no valid scientific evidence that protein intakes exceeding about 1.8 to 2.0 g/kg/d will provide an additional advantage, he adds.

PROTEIN BALANCE

Protein balance is a function of intake relative to output (utilization and loss). Body proteins are in a constant state of flux with both protein degradation and protein synthesis constantly going on. Normally, these two processes are equal, with no net loss or net gain of protein taking place. Protein intake usually equals protein lost.

However, if protein synthesis (anabolism) is greater than protein degradation (catabolism), then the overall result is anabolic with a net increase in body protein. If protein degradation is greater than protein synthesis then the overall result is catabolic with a net decrease in body protein.

Protein catabolism is necessary to eliminate proteins that are no longer required by the cell, or that have become dysfunctional, and to provide substrates for energy production.

Thus degradation of proteins involves enzymes, hormones, and structural and contractile proteins.

As well, protein and amino acids are lost from the body through the urine; feces; sweat; seminal, vaginal, buccal, and menstrual fluids; the desquamation of skin and mucosal areas; and hair and nail growth and loss. Nitrogen derived from amino acids is mainly lost in urine and feces and from sweat.

Unlike the fats and carbohydrates that can be stored in the form of triglycerides and glycogen, there is no storage form of protein or amino acids. All of the protein and amino acids (except for a very small amount of free amino acids that make up the plasma and intracellular amino acid pool) serve either a structural or metabolic function. Excess amino acids from protein are transaminated and the nonnitrogenous portion of the molecule is transformed into glucose and used directly, or into fat or glycogen. The unneeded nitrogen is converted to urea and excreted in the urine.

The larger the body muscle mass, the more transamination of amino acids occurs to fulfill energy needs. Each kilocalorie needed for basal metabolism leads to the excretion of 1 to 1.3 mg of urinary nitrogen. For the same reason, nitrogen excretion increases during exercise and heavy work.

Obligatory Nitrogen Losses and Protein Requirements

Urea accounts for over 80% of urinary nitrogen. The remaining nitrogen is excreted as creatinine, porphyrins, and other nitrogen-containing compounds. Thus total urine loss of nitrogen = urinary urea nitrogen (mg/dl) × daily volume (dl)/0.8. Urinary nitrogen is related to the resting metabolic rate.

Fecal and skin losses account for a large proportion of nitrogen loss from the body (about 40%) in normal circumstances. The magnitude of these losses, however, varies in disease states. Thus, measurement of urinary nitrogen often provides a useful index of daily nitrogen requirement.

Minimal nitrogen loss (in grams per day) from a 70-kg person on a diet that is nitrogen free but energy adequate approximates 1.9 to 3.1 in urine, 0.7 to 2.5 in stool, and 0.3 from skin, for a mean total loss of 4.4 g/d and a maximum total loss of 5.9 g/d.

Equivalent protein loss can be calculated by multiplying nitrogen loss by 6.25 so that mean total loss by metabolism of protein is 4.4 × 6.25 or 27.5 g/d or about 0.4 g/kg body weight for a 70-kg person, and maximum total loss by metabolism of protein is 5.9 × 6.25 or 36.9 g/d or about 0.5 g/kg body weight for a 70-kg person. The recommended protein allowance for adults varies from 0.6 to 0.9 g/kg to allow for a margin of safety.

This protein allowance is raised considerably if low-quality protein is the main source of protein. Low-quality proteins, including certain vegetable proteins, do not support growth as well as protein from milk, eggs, or meat. The differences in the nutritional value of protein are largely due to the higher content of essential amino acids in animal proteins and to differences in digestibility.

Protein requirements are highest during growth spurts and it is during these times that protein deficiency is most harmful.

As well, protein requirements are raised if other energy sources are not ingested in adequate amounts — as is sometimes seen in persons and athletes who are dieting to decrease their body fat levels. Amino acids ingested without other energy sources are not efficiently incorporated into protein partly because of the energy lost during amino acid metabolism. Moreover, incorporation of each amino acid molecule into peptides requires three high-energy phosphate bonds. Consequently, excess of dietary energy over basal needs improves the efficiency of nitrogen utilization.

Effects of Exercise on Dietary Protein Requirements

High protein intake has been the mainstay of most athletes' diets. Athletes in general, and strength athletes and bodybuilders in particular, consume large amounts of protein.[689] One reason for their increased protein consumption is their increased caloric intake. Another is that most athletes deliberately increase their intake of protein-rich foods and often use protein supplements.

Many scientific and medical sources feel that protein supplementation and high-protein diets are unnecessary and that the recommended daily allowance suggested by government research committees supplies more than adequate amounts of protein for the athlete.[690] In fact overloading on protein is felt to be detrimental because of the increased load to the kidneys of the metabolic breakdown products formed when the excess protein is used as an energy source.

In recent years the results of a number of investigations involving both strength and endurance athletes indicate that, in fact, exercise does increase protein/amino acid needs.[691-695] In a recent review the overall consensus has been that all athletes need more protein than sedentary people, and that strength athletes need the most.[696]

Recently, researchers at McMaster University in Hamilton, Ontario concluded that the current Canadian Recommended Nutrient Intake for protein of 0.86 g/kg/d is inadequate for those engaged in endurance exercise.[697] Moreover, their results indicated that male athletes may have an even higher protein requirement than females.

Butterfield performed a review of the literature and recommended high protein intakes (up to 2 to 3 g/kg) for physically active individuals.[698] She found evidence for the existence of an intricate relationship between protein and energy utilization with exercise. "When energy intake is in excess of need, the utilization of even a marginal intake of protein will be improved, giving the appearance that protein intake is adequate. When energy intake and output are balanced, the improvement in nitrogen retention accomplished by exercise seems to be fairly constant at protein intakes greater than 0.8 g/kg/d, but falls off rapidly at protein intakes below this. When energy balance is negative, the magnitude of the effect of exercise on protein retention may be decreased as the activity increases, and protein requirements may be higher than when energy balance is maintained."

Somewhat in agreement with Butterfield's conclusions are the results of another study by Piatti et al.[699] They investigated the effects of two hypocaloric diets (800 kcal) on body weight reduction and composition, insulin sensitivity, and proteolysis in 25 normal obese women. The two diets had the following compositions: 45% protein, 35% carbohydrate, and 20% fat (high-protein diet); and 60% carbohydrate, 20% protein, and 20% fat (high-carbohydrate diet). The results, said the authors, suggest that (1) a hypocaloric diet providing a high percentage of natural protein can improve insulin sensitivity; and (2) conversely, a hypocaloric high-carbohydrate diet decreases insulin sensitivity and is unable to spare muscle tissue.

In another study it was shown that a protein intake as high as four times the recommended RDA (3.3 g/kg of body weight per day vs. RDA of 0.8 g/kg/d) resulted in significantly increased protein synthesis even when compared to a protein intake that was almost twice the RDA.[700] This observation that a protein intake of approximately four times the RDA, in combination with weight training, can promote greater muscle size gains than the same training with a diet containing what is considered by many to be more than adequate protein, is in tune with what many bodybuilders and other weight-training athletes believe.

In another study the effects of two levels of protein intake (1.5 or 2.5 g/kg/d) on muscle performance and energy metabolism were studied in humans submitted to repeated daily sessions of prolonged exercise at moderate altitude.[701] The study showed that the higher level of protein intake greatly minimized the exercise-induced decrease in serum branched-chain amino acids.

Thus the protein needs of athletes are substantially higher than those of sedentary subjects because of the oxidation of amino acids during exercise and gluconeogenesis, as well as the retention of nitrogen during periods of muscle building.[702] Intense muscular activity increases both protein catabolism and protein utilization as an energy source.[703] Thus a high-protein diet may decrease the catabolic effects of exercise by several means, including the use of dietary protein as an energy substrate, thus decreasing the catabolism of endogenous protein during exercise.

Athletes have for years maintained that a high-protein diet is essential for maximizing lean body mass. And even though there have been attempts to discourage it, the popularity of high-protein diets has not waned. Athletes seem to feel intuitively that they need higher levels of protein than the average sedentary person. This intuitive feeling is backed up by their claims of the ergogenic effects of high-protein diets. Are these effects simply psychological? Not according to studies that have shown the anabolic effects of increased dietary protein intake. For example, in one recent study done in rats,[704] dietary energy had no identifiable influence on muscle growth. In contrast, increased dietary protein appeared to stimulate muscle growth directly by increasing muscle RNA content and inhibiting proteolysis, as well as increasing insulin and free T3 levels.

Supplements that may work through a placebo effect but have no intrinsic effects, although perhaps popular for a while, eventually fall by the wayside and are abandoned by the majority. High-protein diets are used because they work. As well, the use of protein supplements is also popular because of their effectiveness above and beyond a whole-food high-protein diet.

Although there has been some concern about the effects of a high dietary protein intake on the kidney, there seems to be no basis for these concerns in healthy individuals.[705,706] In fact, some animal studies have pointed to a beneficial effect of high-protein diets on kidney function.[707]

As well, there has been some concern about the adverse effects of high-protein diets on the serum lipid profile. However, it would seem that these concerns also have little basis in facts. In one study a diet higher in lean animal protein, including beef, was found to result in more favorable HDL ("good" cholesterol) and LDL ("bad" cholesterol) levels.[708] The study involved 10 moderately hypercholesterolemic subjects (6 women, 4 men). They were randomly allocated to isocaloric high- or low-protein diets for four to five weeks, after which they switched over to the other. Protein provided either 23% or 11% of energy intake; carbohydrate provided 65% or 53%; and fats accounted for 24%. During the high-protein diet, mean fasting plasma total cholesterol, LDL, and triglycerides were significantly lower, HDL was raised by 12%, and the ratio of LDL to HDL consistently decreased.

EFFECT OF DIETARY PROTEIN ON PROTEIN METABOLISM

The dietary history of the individual is an important factor affecting protein turnover. This would include not only the long-term effects of the previous diet, but also the short-term effects of recent prior meals. Anabolic and catabolic activities can be influenced by the amount as well as the frequency and timing of protein intake.

The overall and specific metabolic effects of diets containing inadequate amounts of protein have been extensively studied.[709-719] Following short-term restriction of dietary protein there is a decrease in the rates of whole-body and organ protein synthesis and turnover.[720-724] Amino acids are catabolized less and used more as precursors for endogenous compounds such as nucleic acids and creatine and for necessary protein synthesis.

High levels of protein in the diet usually result in increased hepatic amino acid catabolism, especially in the beginning when there is a dramatic increase in the level of dietary protein or individual amino acids. The liver, because of its ability to adapt intracellular metabolizing enzyme[725-727] and transport processes,[728] has a major role in maintaining serum amino acid levels within a certain physiological range.[729] However, even with this increased catabolic effect, higher protein diets or diets modified for their amino acid content result in higher serum and tissue levels of amino acids.[730-735] Supplementation with amino or keto acids also usually results in increased serum and tissue levels.[736-739] For more information on the effects of oral supplementation of amino acids please see below under the individual amino acids.

Altered intakes of protein and amino acids modulate the rates of the major systems (protein synthesis, protein degradation, and amino acid oxidation) responsible for the maintenance of organ and whole-body protein and amino acid homeostasis. Switching from a low-protein diet to a high-protein diet or a high-protein diet to a low protein diet results in adaptive responses that reflect the metabolic state of the organism. Protein deficiency results in decreased proteolysis and decreased protein synthesis, changes that spare amino acids. Switching from a low- to a high-protein diet results in an adaptation phase in which there is a high rate of protein synthesis (a catch-up phase) and increased amino acid oxidation.[740-742] Similarly, supplementing the diet with certain amino acids can also increase protein synthesis and amino acid oxidation.[743,744]

A recent review looked at the mechanisms and nutritional significance of metabolic responses to altered intakes of protein and amino acids, with reference to nutritional adaptation in humans.[745] They concluded that for oxidation amino acid availability is a primary determinant and protein synthesis is affected, particularly at the initiation phase. Thus the immediate response to a change in dietary protein levels is often the opposite that occurs once the body has adapted to the change. For example, the rate of degradation of myofibrillar protein in skeletal muscle rises just after the beginning of fasting,[746] but decreases once the body is accustomed to the dietary change (see below).

Studies have shown that the body feels the amino acid pinch after only two protein-restricted meals. In one study[747] the mechanism governing short-term adaptation to dietary protein restriction was investigated in nine normal adults by measuring their metabolic response to a standard mixed meal, first while they were adapted to a conventional high-protein diet (day 1), and then again after they had eaten two low-protein meals (day 2). Urea appearance (measured as the sum of its urinary excretion and the change in body urea pool size), body retention of ^{15}N-alanine included in each test meal, and whole-body protein turnover were calculated over the 9 h following meal consumption on each day. Postprandial urea nitrogen appearance decreased on day 2. Whole-body N flux, protein synthesis, and protein breakdown all decreased significantly on day 2.

The authors concluded that short-term metabolic adaptation occurs within two meals of reduced protein intake. The mechanism appears not to involve selectively in increased "first-pass" retention of dietary amino acids, but rather a general reduction in fed-state whole-body protein breakdown. It was also shown in the study that inadequate protein intake for as few as two meals induces a prompt compensatory increase in body protein retention when protein is returned to the diet.

The authors of another study[748] relate: "The argument here is that body protein is lost in the post-absorptive state and that the extent of these losses is likely to be variable according to the extent to which changes in protein synthesis and degradation in response to fasting is conditioned by dietary protein intake."

Thus, if there is an induction of protein-oxidizing enzymes and a high rate of protein turnover as dietary protein intake rises, and if this effect persists for an appreciable period of time when the diet is changed, then after a period on a high-protein diet a switch to a low-protein diet "should result in a marked negative balance with insufficient fed-state gain for balance while the high post-absorptive losses persist."

AMINO ACID METABOLISM

Amino acids are not stored in the body other than as integral parts of protein. However, there is a small amount of extracellular and intracellular free amino acids that is referred to as the free amino acid pool. This free amino acid pool in muscle is labile, i.e., constantly changing, and is affected by the quantity and quality of dietary protein which, in turn, affects protein metabolism.[749]

During exercise most protein synthesis is suppressed in muscle, although the synthesis of certain proteins remains unchanged or even increases. The general suppression of protein synthesis in muscle leaves much of the free amino acid pool unused. As a result of the suppression and an increase in muscle protein catabolism, an increased pool of available free amino acids is created. The main use of free amino acids is connected with the energy requirement of muscular activity, through the oxidation of branched-chain amino acids and the use of alanine in gluconeogenesis (see below).[750]

The increases in the free amino acid pool, in the rate of the glucose-alanine cycle, and in the use of amino acids in the liver are stimulated by an increased level of glucocorticoids and a decreased level of insulin during exercise. During recovery after exercise, the use of amino acids for adaptive protein synthesis is intensified.

Should any amino acids required for the synthesis of new contractile proteins be limiting in availability, the training response may suffer as a result. Moreover, as the dietary provision of amino acids is always inefficient[751] the need for a continuous and ready supply of amino acids may be of particular importance to those individuals hoping to maximize training-induced lean tissue gains.

Fasting causes energy levels to drop. Catabolism of muscle proteins is enhanced at first, and then amino acids such as alanine and glutamine are liberated which can be metabolized for energy via the citric acid cycle or be used to form glucose via gluconeogenesis.

In the postabsorptive state, amino acids are released from the periphery to provide precursors for protein synthesis in the splanchnic organs. In skin, for instance, integrity is maintained in the absence of amino acid intake by using amino acids resulting from the net breakdown of muscle protein as precursors for synthesis.

The importance of the prevailing amino acid concentration has been suggested by studies showing that increased amino acid availability alone may augment skeletal muscle protein synthesis in healthy men.[752,753] It appears that increasing amino acid availability is a major component in the resulting increase seen in protein synthesis.

The hormonal response to protein and to amino acids, and the direct effects of these substrates, constitute the two mechanisms by which feeding influences amino acid turnover and oxidation. In rats it has been shown that the anabolic drive from dietary proteins and amino acids is mediated in part by their effects on insulin, thyroid hormone, and IGF-1.[754] In humans an increase seen in insulin secretion, along with increased levels of amino acids, has been shown to result in an overall increase in protein deposition. The hyperinsulinemia decreased proteolysis but did not stimulate protein synthesis, and the hyperaminoacidemia stimulated protein synthesis but did not suppress endogenous proteolysis.[755,756]

A recent study found that amino acids fed alone, which exert a minor stimulus to insulin secretion, increase plasma amino acid levels, markedly stimulate protein synthesis and oxidation, and inhibit protein degradation in humans.[757] The authors of this study concluded that the feeding response of protein synthesis, degradation and amino acid oxidation, reflects the combined impact of insulin, inhibiting degradation, and tissue amino acids both inhibiting degradation and stimulating synthesis and oxidation.

In another study the authors concluded that in the human adult amino acid catabolism is necessarily the major fate of dietary protein at low concentrations, with the shift to deposition requiring increasing dietary protein concentrations.[758] Thus with lower protein intake the stimulus for protein synthesis is depressed while with higher protein intakes there is an increase in protein synthesis. In this study the regulatory influence of dietary amino acids on anabolic processes only occurred with higher protein intakes. It would appear that the anabolic drive induced by low-protein (0.36 g/kg/d) and medium-protein (0.77 g/kg/d) diets was inadequate.

Changes in dietary protein or amino acid intake may alter transport of certain neutral AA into skeletal muscle via changes in plasma amino acid pools. In one study amino acid transport systems A and L, which preferentially transfer small neutral amino acids and large neutral amino acids, respectively, were studied in the isolated soleus muscle.[759] Selective differences were observed in transport by skeletal muscle of model amino acids for the A and L systems: increased transport resulting from various stimuli was limited to the model for the A system, and transport of either model was depressed with mixtures containing physiological levels of amino acids.

THE DIETARY PROTEIN PARADOX — PROBABLE NEED FOR PROTEIN AND AMINO ACID SUPPLEMENTS EVEN IN DIETS HIGH IN DIETARY PROTEIN

Simply increasing dietary protein through the use of increased amounts of whole protein-containing foods may not be enough. Some studies have suggested that increased dietary intake of protein may inhibit growth. In one study 28-day-old male Sprague Dawley rats were fed, either *ad libitum* or in restricted amounts, isoenergetic diets containing 2, 5, 10, 15, 25, or 50% lactalbumin protein and 5, 11.9, or 21.1% fat for 8 weeks and were then killed.[760] Weekly food consumption and body weight, terminal weight, body water and lipid; and liver weight, DNA, RNA, protein, and lipid were measured. The growth rate increased progressively with each increase in the level of dietary protein up to 25% protein and then declined. Growth was also accelerated by a high-fat diet but was retarded by restriction of energy intake. Total body lipid correlated directly with the level of fat in the diet. Multiple regression analysis showed that the maximum rate of weight gain of 58.8 g/week occurred when the diet contained 23% protein. Growth rate declined when the diet contained a higher protein level.

More recently, Moundras et al.[761] found that increasing the dietary protein level in rats led to a reduced availability of some amino acids for peripheral tissues. This was accompanied by a depressed weight gain in animals fed the highest protein diet (60% casein). The authors suggested that the depression in growth rate might be due to energy wastage caused by catabolism of excess amino acids, the reduction in the availability of certain amino acids, or decreased insulinemia in rats fed the high-protein diets.

In this study, set up to evaluate the effect of changes in dietary protein level on overall availability of amino acids for tissues, rats were adapted to diets containing various concentrations of casein (7.5, 15, 30, and 60%) and were sampled either during the postprandial or postabsorptive period. In rats fed the protein-deficient diet, glucogenic amino acids (except threonine) tended to accumulate in plasma, liver, and muscles. In rats fed high-protein diets, the hepatic balance of glucogenic amino acids was markedly enhanced and their liver concentrations were consistently depressed. This response was the result of a marked induction of amino acid catabolism (a 45-fold increase of liver threonine-serine dehydratase activity was observed with the 60% casein diet). The muscle concentrations of threonine, serine, and glycine underwent changes parallel to plasma and liver concentrations, and a significant reduction of glutamine was observed.

During the postabsorptive period, adaptation to high-protein diets resulted in a sustained catabolism of most glucogenic amino acids, which accentuated the drop in their concentrations (especially threonine) in all the compartments studied. The time course of metabolic adaptation from a 60% to a 15% casein diet was also investigated. Adaptation of alanine and glutamine metabolism was rapid, whereas that of threonine, serine, and glycine was delayed and required 7 to 11 days. This was paralleled by a relatively slow decay of liver threonine-serine dehydratase (T-SDH) activity, in contrast to the rapid adaptation of pyruvate kinase activity after refeeding a high-carbohydrate diet.

Thus in a high-protein diet in which the protein is obtained from high-protein whole foods, the decreased availability of amino acids, specifically threonine, glycine, and serine as well as glutamine and alanine, may result in a decrease in protein synthesis. The use of these AAs in a protein supplement may correct the relative deficiency and increase the amount and efficiency of protein synthesis.[762]

It also seems that some amino acid deficiencies may result from the use of different protein foods in both isocaloric and hypocaloric diets. For example, in one study the substitution of soybean protein for casein in a high-protein diet resulted in a taurine deficiency in cats.[763] When a casein-based diet containing either 25 or 50% protein was given to cats for 6 weeks, no difference in plasma taurine concentration was observed; however, substituting soybean protein for casein resulted in a significant decrease in plasma taurine concentration of cats in the 50% soybean protein group, but not in the 25% soybean protein group. In a second part of this study when the food intake of cats was limited, cats fed 60% soybean protein or casein diets had significantly lower plasma taurine concentrations than cats fed a 30% casein diet, with the 60% soybean protein diet causing the greater decrease.

In high-protein diets there is an increased intake of BCAAs which have been shown to stimulate protein synthesis (see below or above). However, with a high-protein diet the BCAAs are quickly catabolized to alanine and glutamine in muscles, which in turn are used for gluconeogenesis and by the gut and immune system, respectively (see below).

Even with the formation of glutamine from BCAAs a feature of high-protein whole-food diets is the decrease in hepatic, plasma and muscle glutamine concentrations. This decrease may have important implications for effective protein synthesis. Increasing the endogenous levels of glutamine by the use of exogenous glutamine might have important effects on increasing protein synthesis in high-protein whole-food diets.

Low levels of alanine between high-protein meals results in low levels of plasma alanine.[764] This decrease in plasma alanine may result in an increase in protein catabolism and decrease in protein synthesis. Supplemental alanine may be important for the regulation of protein metabolism and increasing the anabolic drive.

High-protein diets may also result in decreased levels of threonine, glycine, and serine in liver, plasma, and muscle (see below). Since threonine is an essential amino acid, its decrease might cause severe metabolic alterations and significant decreases in protein synthesis.

PROTEIN NEEDS IN CALORIE-RESTRICTED DIETS

Because of the increased oxidation of endogenous protein during weight loss, an increased level of exogenous protein is needed to minimize the autophagy (breakdown of muscle protein) that occurs. In a randomized trial in 17 healthy obese women, a diet containing 1.5 g protein per kilogram ideal body weight was found to result in significantly better protein-sparing than an isocaloric diet providing only 0.8 g protein per kilogram ideal body weight.[765] Patients lost weight at the same rate on the two diets, but since there was less nitrogen loss on the diet without carbohydrate, it can be assumed that more fat loss occurred than on the diet where carbohydrate replaced some of the protein.

Bodybuilders who are dieting down to a contest and undergoing glycogen depletion would oxidize more protein for energy and thus likely need even higher dietary protein to prevent muscle catabolism. As well, since it has been shown that individuals with lower glycogen stores oxidized more than twice the protein than those with high initial stores, this would further increase the need for dietary protein.[766]

Bodybuilders preparing for competition cut calories to lose body fat. In order to maintain and perhaps even build muscle tissue, dietary protein must be increased even further than with their normally high-protein diets. As well, as has been stated above, those on calorie-restricted diets and those with increased muscle mass need more protein in their diets than normal.

In order to increase dietary protein but minimize the caloric increase, foods must be chosen that are low in energy and high in protein. This leads to a diet that is traditionally high in chicken breasts, egg whites, and white fish. This type of restricted diet is a common dietary practice among competing bodybuilders and some other athletes involved in sports with weight classes.[767]

Unfortunately a diet that consists mainly of these foods may be counterproductive. One of the reason lies in the nonessential amino acid alanine.

THE GLUCOSE-ALANINE CYCLE

Alanine, like glutamine, is considered a nonessential amino acid, an important interorgan nitrogen carrier and energy substrate. Alanine efflux increases in the postabsorptive state, under stress, in fasting and starvation, and during exercise resulting in an increase in hepatic gluconeogenesis.[768-770]

As well, glucose taken up from plasma can be converted to pyruvate and then to alanine in many tissues including liver, kidney, splanchnic, and muscle. The use of the alanine carbon chain to produce glucose which is subsequently released into the systemic circulation for use by the rest of the body is known as the glucose-alanine cycle.[771-774] The glucose-alanine cycle permits the catabolism of skeletal muscle tissue amino acids (BCAAs in particular) and cellular protein and results in a direct energy output for work and a net increase of glucose for anaerobic oxidation which is especially important during anaerobic muscle contraction.

The glucose-alanine cycle, induced by exercise, is also hypothesized to serve as a nontoxic, water-soluble carrier of amino groups produced through protein catabolism.[775-777] The carrier, alanine, moves these groups out of the tissue and prevents the buildup of toxic ammonia molecules. Once in the blood, alanine is picked up by the liver. At this organ, the amino groups enter the urea cycle with formation of urea which is then excreted by the kidneys. What remains is the carbon skeleton of the carrier; it is converted to glucose via gluconeogenesis. This glucose is released into the bloodstream from the liver, and the skeletal muscle picks it up during circulation. To complete the cycle, the glucose in the skeletal muscle is converted to pyruvate and is then transaminated to form alanine.

While the stimulus for alanine metabolism during exercise involves several hormones, the results of a recent study support the view that the stimulation of the glucose-alanine cycle by glucocorticoids promotes alanine supply and utilization in liver during exercise.[778] As well, in this study hepatic arginase activity was decreased during exercise in adrenalectomized rats as against normal rats, and no elevation of urea levels was found in blood, liver, or skeletal muscles. Consequently, the use of products of the deamination of alanine (and other amino acids) for urea formation also depends on glucocorticoids.

Studies have shown that muscle is the major source of plasma alanine and lactate in postabsorptive humans.[779] The source of the alanine released from muscle is from the catabolism of skeletal muscle tissue and from *de novo* synthesis from branched-chain amino acids and pyruvate. Lactate and pyruvate can also be released from skeletal muscle and used as substrates for hepatic gluconeogenesis (Cori cycle). It has been shown that the contribution of the Cori cycle can be substantial, accounting for up to 35% of hepatic glucose output.[780,781]

However, the contribution to hepatic gluconeogenesis from the glucose-alanine cycle is also significant, and may be even more so with exercise when amino acid flux is increased.[782,783] In one study the rates of alanine incorporation into glucose by isolated liver cells of fed rats was fivefold higher than those observed when lactate was used as substrate.[784] Studies have shown that glycolytic and oxidative enzyme responses are significantly altered by both endurance and sprint training. Skeletal muscle has an increased capacity to form alanine from pyruvate after exercise, and after short-term exercise such as sprinting, there is a substantial increase in plasma alanine levels.[785]

This exercise-induced synthesis of alanine allows the use of amino acids as an energy substrate, decreases the ammonia buildup in skeletal muscle secondary to the catabolism of muscle, and provides a substrate for hepatic gluconeogenesis and thus provides extra energy, especially for anaerobic muscular contraction.[786,787]

Studies have shown that alanine flux and *de novo* synthesis increase significantly when protein intake is restricted, and are significantly reduced with high protein intake.[788] Alanine can be formed from the BCAAs and other AAs, and by the transamination of pyruvate. Thus alanine can be derived not only from other amino acids but from glycolysis. The glucose in the muscle cell is metabolized to pyruvate (producing ATP for muscular contraction). To complete the cycle the pyruvate then provides the carbon skeleton from which alanine is synthesized — the amino groups coming from the deamination of amino acids, especially the BCAAs. In the liver, alanine's amino group is used to form urea which is excreted, and the resulting pyruvate is used to form glucose that is released into the blood and taken up by muscle cells. The sequence of the glucose-alanine cycle is summarized in Figure 1.

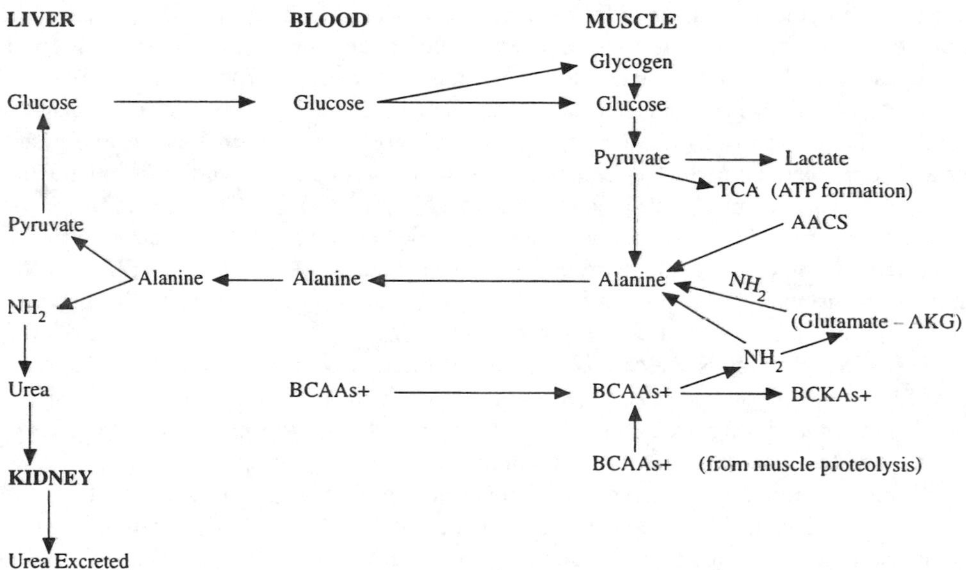

FIGURE 1 The glucose–alanine cycle in exercise.

Some of the carbon skeleton of alanine produced in muscle is from amino acid precursors derived from leucine, glutamate, valine, isoleucine, methionine, aspartate, and asparagine via a pathway involving phosphoenolpyruvate (PEP) carboxykinase and pyruvate kinase, and/or NADP-malate dehydrogenase (malic enzyme). While some researchers feel that a large portion of the carbon skeletons for *de novo* alanine synthesis comes from amino acids,[789] others feel that neogenic flux from amino acids is unlikely to be of major quantitative importance for provision of the carbon skeleton of alanine.[790]

However, it is obvious that since significant alanine production continues even after the limited circulating glucose and glycogen stores have been depleted, this alanine owes both the carbon skeleton and amino group to the amino acids that result from the catabolism of protein.

As noted above, alanine is released from the catabolism of alanine-containing muscle protein. This source of alanine can be significant. In one study the rate of appearance of alanine, the *de novo* synthesis of alanine, and rate of alanine release from protein breakdown were determined in five healthy subjects at rest and during exercise.[791] The low-intensity exercise was performed for 120 min on a treadmill at 45% of the subject's VO_2max. The total rate of appearance of alanine, calculated with the ^{15}N-alanine tracer, increased significantly during exercise. The amount of alanine derived from pyruvate also significantly increased during exercise, but the proportion of the total decreased from 65% at rest to 57% during exercise. Consequently, the alanine derived from protein breakdown significantly increased and was also increased as a percent of total alanine flux. With higher-intensity exercise the amount of alanine derived directly from protein breakdown would increase even further.

The differences seen in the plasma AAs of trained athletes may play a physiologically relevant role in accommodation to the metabolic demands of exercise. Trained athletes exhibit significantly higher plasma concentrations of alanine after a bout of intensive exercise, while at rest they exhibit significantly higher plasma concentrations of leucine, isoleucine, and tyrosine.[792] Alanine plays a central role as a primary gluconeogenic substrate (along with lactate, glycerol, and glutamine) and as an ammonia carrier (transferring NH_3 groups, produced by transamination and deamination of other amino acids, to the splanchnic tissues).[793]

Overall, it is felt that the purpose of protein degradation during exercise is not only as a direct energy source, but also as an indirect energy source by providing alanine (and other amino acids such as glutamine, see below) directly and also amino acid precursors for alanine production, for glucose production in the liver.[794,795]

ALANINE NEEDS AND BODYBUILDERS

However, although yielding much-needed energy, this catabolism of BCAAs and cellular protein (to produce glutamine and alanine) is counterproductive. Any loss of amino acids is detrimental if they could have been used to maintain or increase skeletal muscle mass.

Alanine is found in appreciable levels in many foods including beef, lamb, milk products, corn meal, peas, and potatoes. However, there is no appreciable alanine in many foods including chicken, fish, eggs, and bacon. Now while bacon is not a common food consumed by bodybuilders, chicken, fish, and eggs are the staple of many bodybuilding diets.

Many bodybuilders are on a restrictive diet that may include little else besides large quantities of these three foods for months at a time, and some bodybuilders stay on this kind of restricted diet almost year round. Even noncompeting bodybuilders may run into problems with obtaining enough dietary alanine. Today, low-fat diets are recommended in order to decrease saturated fat intake. This usually means decreased consumption of beef, lamb, and milk products. Again, overall alanine intake may be low.

Thus some diets, especially calorie-restricted diets, may be moderately or even severely alanine deficient, making high-quality protein and/or alanine supplementation a necessity. Since alanine is a nonessential amino acid, can't the body make it as it needs it? Yes it can, but alanine synthesis by the body is part of the problem.

One way to increase the availability of a specific amino acid, whether essential or nonessential, is to cannibalize cellular structural and contractile proteins and use the needed amino acid as it's released. In the case of nonessential amino acids, they can also be formed from other released amino acids. As noted above, both processes contribute to alanine production.

In general, if there is a deficiency of or need for any one amino acid (AA) then the body will catabolize body proteins in an effort to supply the needed AA, regardless of why the AA is needed: whether for protein synthesis of needed proteins and enzymes, or for gluconeogenesis (the conversion of amino acids and other substrates into glucose). Thus, the use of exogenous alanine prior to and after exercise might be expected to decrease exercise-induced proteolysis and increase the availability of intracellular AAs for protein synthesis.

It has been shown that the amino acid alanine has effects on both insulin and glucagon and raises plasma glucose concentrations in diabetics,[796] and can produce sustained glucose recovery from hypoglycemia.[797] As well, it has been shown that alanine decreases proteolysis[798] and is a potent stimulus for protein synthesis. Although the mechanism of this action has not yet been determined, it is felt that this increase in protein synthesis might be secondary to the provision of an energy source[799] or an increase in cellular hydration (see below). The uptake of alanine increases the intracellular content of K^+ and the cell volume.[800]

The use of exogenous alanine would decrease the need for catabolism of muscle and provide a stimulus for protein synthesis, both directly and by helping to maintain the intracellular pool of free amino acids by decreasing the use of other amino acids for alanine production. As well, exogenous alanine would provide extra energy for anaerobic muscular contraction both by allowing BCAAs to be oxidized if need be rather than used to produce alanine, and by providing an increase in hepatic and systemic, and thus intracellular, glucose availability.

A diet low in alanine should be supplemented with alanine-rich protein foods or supplements. The supplements that consist of whole protein, hydrolyzed protein, or mixtures of amino acids offer a low-calorie source of alanine and other amino acids. These supplements are not merely useful, convenient alternative food choices, but necessary for protein synthesis and the maintenance of lean body mass.

Because of its anabolic and anticatabolic effects, a case could be made for alanine supplementation for all athletes wishing to maximize lean body mass, regardless of dietary alanine intake.

Chapter 5

PROTEIN FOODS VS. PROTEIN AND AMINO ACID SUPPLEMENTS

INTRODUCTION

The source of dietary protein can be whole foods, especially eggs, meat, fish, soy, and dairy products, whole protein supplements that usually are inexpensive and contain one or more of soybean, milk and egg protein, hydrolyzed protein containing variable amounts of di-, tri-, and polypeptides, and amino acid mixtures.

The usual consensus is that there are no valid scientific or medical studies to show that supplements of intact protein have an anabolic advantage over high-quality protein foods. The advantages usually cited for the use of whole protein supplements include:

1. Convenience of preparation and storage, and long shelf life.
2. Replacement of dietary protein for those wishing to decrease dietary fat.
3. Ability to raise protein intake by those who wish to minimize caloric intake.
4. Increasing dietary protein by those who cannot eat the volume of food necessary to insure adequate or increased protein intake.
5. In some cases the cost of protein supplements is lower than corresponding high-protein foods.

While these are valid points, protein supplements have other distinct advantages over whole food protein in hypocaloric, isocaloric, and hypercaloric diets.

For example, several studies involving Refit (a milk powder containing about 90% proteins and 5% mineral salts — Ca, P, K, Na) have shown the ergogenic effects of this protein supplement.[801,802] In one study, 9 male and 8 female top Olympic athletes were given 1.2 to 1.5 g of milk protein daily per kilogram of body weight during a period of 6 months.[803] The milk proteins were consumed in addition to 2.2 to 2.5 g of proteins per kilogram body weight in their diets. A control group with the same number of athletes and from the same sports was fed on the same diet, but without extra addition of milk protein.

The effects of the addition of extra milk proteins were monitored by estimating some parameters such as lean body mass, fat mass, muscle strength, protein and lipid composition in the blood serum, calcium metabolism, urinary mucoproteins, and liver and kidney functional tests. All the athletes had been under medical supervision during the experiment and no side effects were registered. The results indicated that extra milk proteins significantly improved physiological condition and led to better sports performance, even when compared to the controls.

In another study, 66 Romanian Olympic endurance athletes (30 kayak-canoe, 36 rowing; 45 males and 21 females) participated in a trial to determine the possible biological effects of an isolated soy protein supplement given at 1.5 g/kg/d, for 8 weeks.[804] A control group was used that did not receive the supplemental protein. The soy protein supplementation resulted in significant increases of lean body mass and strength. The same authors also found significant effects from the use of a combination vitamin supplement compound that contained amino acids.[805]

A recent study examined the effects of food supplements designed to foster muscular gains when combined with weight training.[806] The study included 28 weight-training subjects, who took 1 of 3 supplements daily: 190 g maltodextrin, a carbohydrate source that acted as a source of calories only (about 760 cal); Gainer's Fuel 1000, a weight-gain powder providing both calories and protein (just over 1400 cal and 60 g protein per day); and Phosphagain, a powder advertised to help increase muscle gains without gaining excess body fat, providing less calories and more protein in the form of whole food protein and high levels of creatine monohydrate and of certain amino acids such as glutamine and taurine (about 600 cal and 80 g of whole food protein and amino acids per day).

Results showed that those on either Phosphagain or Gainer's Fuel gained more lean mass compared to those consuming maltodextrin, showing that increasing dietary protein and other nutrients resulted in a superior gain in muscle as compared to those who simply took in the equivalent amount of calories. In addition those on Phosphagain gained more lean body mass and less fat than those on Gainer's Fuel. Why the difference?

Phosphagain contains nutrients not found in the Gainer's Fuel product. These nutrients include creatine monohydrate, taurine, and L-glutamine. These three nutrients may have, along with the differences in the macronutrients, made the difference. For more information on them see the relevant sections in this book. Besides having more protein (due mainly to the large amounts of taurine and glutamine), Phosphagain also had a much lower carbohydrate content — 69 vs. 290 g per daily serving. Both had low levels of fat. The increased carbohydrate and subsequent calorie content is likely responsible for the increased fat gain seen with Gainer's Fuel, a problem that is also seen when whole foods are used to increase protein intake and other nutrients.

Gainer's Fuel, Phosphagain 2, Myoplex Plus, Met-Rx, Hot Stuff, and a host of others contain a large number of nutrients and can be used as meal replacements or as a source of extra nutrients beyond the three squares a day. Some of these products are advertised as weight gainers while others are more specific and claim to be lean body mass weight gainers. While the difference in products may not be as extreme as the advertiser's claim, there is some validity to the differentiation of the two product types and their effect on fat accretion and gains in lean body mass.

The meal replacement products, whether for weight loss or for weight gain, provide the standard macro- and micronutrients at different calorie levels. They may be convenient and can either be more or less costly than whole foods available at the supermarket, but as an all-in-one package they are usually more convenient and provide better nutrition than many of us get with junk food meals and calorie-full but nutrient-deficient snacks. But on the whole, those who are conscientious about what they buy and eat and are willing to put in the time and energy can do as well or better by just buying the whole foods and planning their own diets for weight gain or weight loss.

However, some of the newer complete nutrient supplements such as Myoplex Plus and Phosphagain 2 definitely have an edge over even the most meticulously prepared diets. In order to get pharmacological levels of some of the nutrients present in these products, it would be necessary to consume an unrealistic amount of certain foods resulting in a much larger than desired calorie intake and increase in body fat.

HYDROLYSATES — COMPARISON TO WHOLE PROTEIN AND INTACT WHOLE PROTEIN SUPPLEMENTS

Special processing can make certain protein supplements more effective and less problematic than whole foods. One example is the whey protein presently on the market.

About 20% of the protein in milk (milk has about 6.25% protein) is whey protein. In the course of production of cheese, quargs, and casein, a lot of whey results. At one time the whey was considered waste and was often dumped into ponds. Whey is rich in branch-chain amino acids (BCAA), lactose, minerals, and vitamins, and contains lactalbumin (similar to serum albumin) and traces of fat.

Milk and milk products (including whey) can cause intestinal bloating and gas in certain individuals. This is due to the lactose content and the fact that soon after birth the production of the enzyme lactase, responsible for hydrolysis of lactose into galactose and glucose (its constituent monosaccharides), is reduced. By age 3 to 7 years in most humans the ability to digest lactose is substantially decreased.[807] Because of the possibility of lactose intolerance, the manufacturers of some whey proteins remove the lactose from the whey. As well, most whey proteins on the market are low in fat since the fat is extracted through centrifugation.

In the past decade it has been shown that whey and whey protein may possess special properties not seen in other proteins including casein, the other milk protein.[808,809] In one study, a whey protein diet appeared to enhance the liver and heart glutathione concentration in aging mice and to increase longevity.[810] As well, undenatured whey protein has been shown to enhance the immune system,[811-813] and to lower serum cholesterol[814] as compared to casein and soy proteins. Conversely, a recent study has shown that casein, but not whey or soy protein, has antimutagenic effects[815] and may thus be protective against certain cancer-producing genotoxic compounds.

A study done this year compared the effects of four isoenergetic and isonitrogenous diets on the nitrogen utilization, total serum protein concentration, and serum amino acid profile in starved rats at weaning.[816] These diets differed only in the molecular form of two milk proteins, whey protein and casein, which were either native or partly hydrolyzed. Nitrogen retention was higher in the two groups of rats given the protein hydrolysate-based diets compared with those given the intact protein-based diets. This was associated with a lower urinary nitrogen excretion in rats given the whey protein-hydrolysate and the casein hydrolysate diets. Despite this fact, the serum amino acid pattern of rats given the hydrolyzed protein diet was very similar to those given the corresponding native protein diet.

In conclusion, the study proved that enzymic hydrolysates from milk proteins have equivalent effects to native proteins in recovery after starvation in rats at weaning on nitrogen absorption, total serum protein concentration, and serum amino acid profile, and even give a higher nitrogen retention. The study did not show any harmful effect in using protein hydrolysates instead of native proteins.

On the other hand, another study using the same four nitrogenous diets done by the same authors evaluated the effect of the molecular form of dietary protein (native or enzymatically hydrolyzed) on the total serum protein concentrations and the serum amino acid profile of growing rats at weaning.[817] In this study, differences in the serum amino acid profiles exclusively related to the amino acid composition of the protein (casein or whey proteins), but differences due to their molecular forms were not observed.

The authors concluded that the use of enzymatic hydrolysates of whey proteins and casein has the same effects as their native proteins on nitrogen intake, body weight gain, and serum amino acid profile of growing rats at weaning. The higher nitrogen retention seen in the previous study might have been due to the poor nutritional state of the starved rats. It is possible that some athletes on low-calorie fat-reducing diets might also have a higher nitrogen retention with the use of enzymatic hydrolysates of whey proteins and casein. An example would be competitive bodybuilders who are often on semistarvation diets when preparing for a competition.

WHEY PROTEIN HYDROLYSATES AND THE ATHLETE

Whey protein, because of its increased bioavailability and solubility, and its higher percentage content of branched-chain amino acids, is felt to be a superior form of protein supplementation for athletes. A study done a decade ago pointed out the possible ergogenic effects of whey protein.[818]

Recently, a number of improved whey protein concentrates have become available at a reasonable, although still relatively expensive price. The predigested whey protein powder that is made by low-temperature, high-speed sonic drying is one of the best protein powders available. These powders contain protein that has not been denatured due to high-temperature preparations (as are many of the protein powders now on the market). Some whey proteins have the lactose removed through the use of micropore membrane filters and ion-exchange columns and therefore are better tolerated than many milk (either casein or whey) proteins that contain variable amounts of lactose.

Protein powders with a high BV and improved solubility may be worth the extra bucks because they're so convenient to use and it doesn't take as much to significantly increase protein intake. Another advantage of the hydrolyzed ion exchange whey proteins is that they are much more soluble than the others and thus can be prepared with a minimum of fuss. As well, for those who are lactose intolerant, the use of whey protein supplements allows them to use this quality source of protein.

In diets that are low calorie and relatively protein deficient, whey protein may offer some advantages over whole food proteins and other kinds of protein supplements. We'll discuss some of these points in more detail below.

BV of Whey Hydrolysates

In a recent study it was shown that whey protein hydrolysate has a significantly higher BV than the whole protein.[819] This corroborates an earlier study that found a higher nitrogen balance in rats fed a diet containing whey protein hydrolysate compared with the native protein.[820]

In this earlier study the effects of alimentary whey proteins given as whole proteins (WP), controlled trypsin and chymotrypsin hydrolysate oligopeptides (WPH), or a free amino acid mixture (AAM), on growth, nitrogen retention, and steatorrhea, were assessed in 24 Wistar rats after 72 h of starvation and 24 to 96 h of realimentation, and in 24 controls. The three diets had the same caloric, nitrogen, vitamin, and mineral contents. Rats had free access to the liquid diets. Only rats which ate the whole diet (90 cal) were included in the study.

No differences in steatorrhea and fecal nitrogen were observed. The absorption rate was over 95% on the three diets. In contrast, weight gain was statistically better on WPH than on WP or AAM. This was associated with a statistically higher nitrogen retention at all time periods studied, which was a result of a significant lower nitrogen urinary excretion. The authors concluded that this better growth was a result of a better protein synthesis and lower ureagenesis.

WHEY PROTEIN AND THE IMMUNE SYSTEM

Arginine, the branched-chain amino acids, and glutamine are the most important amino acids involved in immune system function.[821] Whey protein is naturally high in BCAA, and certain whey protein powders currently available are said to be fortified with glutamine. Glutamine supplementation may also be beneficial in the treatment of athletes affected by exercise-induced stress and overtraining.

EFFECTS OF WHEY PROTEIN ON GLUTATHIONE LEVELS

Glutathione is a peptide that contains one amino acid residue each of glutamic acid, cysteine, and glycine. Glutathione occurs widely in plant and animal tissues, and plays a major role in protecting skeletal muscle and other body tissues from oxidative damage.[822] The author of a recent review stresses the importance of an augmented antioxidant defense system and suggests that all athletes, especially the "weekend" ones, regularly or occasionally ingest foods rich in antioxidants.[823]

The muscular injury models in which reactive oxygen species are supposed to play a role are ischemia/reperfusion syndrome, exercise-induced myopathy, heart and skeletal muscle diseases related to the nutritional deficiency of selenium and vitamin E and related disorders, and genetic muscular dystrophies. These models provide evidence that mitochondrial function and the glutathione-dependent antioxidant system are important for the maintenance of the structural and functional integrity of muscular tissues.

Studies have shown that exhaustive physical exercise causes a change in glutathione redox status in blood. It has also been found that antioxidant administration, i.e., oral vitamin C, *N*-acetyl-L-cysteine, and/or glutathione is effective in preventing oxidation of the blood glutathione pool after physical exercise in rats.[824] Cysteine is rate limiting for glutathione synthesis, and can become conditionally essential in intensive care unit (ICU) patients under physiological stress.

In one study, researchers, realizing that protein in enteral products may be the sole source of cysteine, decided to determine the effects of two different proteins, casein and whey, on glutathione status in ICU patients.[825] The results indicated that mean glutathione concentration increased in those fed whey protein, but not in those fed casein.

According to the authors, casein contains 0.3% cysteine, whereas whey protein contains 2.0 to 2.5% cysteine. It was concluded that protein sources containing high levels of cysteine may be effective in maintaining or repleting whole-blood glutathione.

WHEY AND CASEIN AND ANTIGENICITY — ADVANTAGES OF HYDROLYSATES

As well as superior absorption and higher BV, protein supplements may be superior to whole foods for use in people who have certain food allergies.

For example, it has been shown that early introduction to formula instead of breast feeding can lead to allergic reactions against milk proteins as well as other foods. All the major cow milk proteins in their native states are potential allergens in infants with milk allergy. A lot of research has gone into finding solutions to this problem so that hypoallergenic formulas could be used for infants, nursing mothers, and for allergic children and adults, and also for enteral nutrition.[826-829] For example, studies have shown that there are significant effects of even a partial whey hydrolysate formula on the prophylaxis of atopic disease.[830]

Heat treatment can reduce the antigenicity of whey proteins considerably, but it has virtually no effect on the antigenicity of casein. Infants allergic to milk still react to heat-denatured whey proteins. Therefore, heat denaturation alone cannot produce a formula with low allergenicity. Enzyme hydrolysis reduces the antigenicity and allergenicity of protein. Partial hydrolysis produces hydrolysate consisting mainly of large peptides, whereas extensive hydrolysis produces hydrolysate containing a mixture of large and small peptides and free amino acids.

When hydrolysate formula is made, casein or whey protein hydrolysate is ultrafiltered to remove large residual peptides. Certain amino acids are fortified to provide a balanced amino acid profile. In the U.S. the final formulation must comply with the recommendations of the Codex Alimentarius Commission (FAO/WHO) and the U.S. Infant Formula Act to provide adequate infant nutrition. Protein hydrolysate-based formulas can be improved by further reducing the residual allergenicity, increasing the small peptide content, and improving the taste.

Thus protein hydrolysates, if properly prepared, are much less antigenic. Hypoallergenic protein hydrolysates are prepared in such a way that the quantity of antigenic material is drastically reduced and thus can be used by those who are normally allergic to milk proteins. The enzymatic hydrolysis of proteins coupled with ultrafiltration is the best way to reduce their antigenicity, and also preserving the nutritional qualities of the amino acids and the peptides produced.

In one recent study two milk protein (whey protein and casein) hydrolysates were obtained by enzymatic hydrolysis.[831] In the casein hydrolysate, an ultrafiltration stage was performed to remove all the peptides with molecular weights >2500. A nutritional value study of both hydrolysates was undertaken. No differences were found between the native proteins and their enzymatic hydrolysates. The casein hydrolysate, after being ultrafiltered, was devoid of sensitizing capacity by the oral route and was also ineffective in producing local or systemic anaphylaxis in previously sensitized animals, as shown by *in vivo* assays.

Amino acid formulas, because of their decreased antigenicity, would likely be useful for those who have severe cows' milk intolerance and who have already reacted to a whey or casein hydrolysate formula.[832]

WHEY PROTEIN — CONCLUSIONS

From the above it can be seen that there are substantial possible benefits of whey protein use by athletes including increased protein synthesis, enhanced immune system performance, and antioxidant activity.

FREE-FORM AMINO ACIDS VS. DI- AND TRIPEPTIDES

A controversy exists in the athletic community over the absorption of free amino acids vs. small peptides. The process by which protein is degraded and absorbed provides us with the answer to this controversy.

Less than 1% of total protein that passes through the GI tract is lost in the stool, usually in the form of tough fibrous and indigestible protein. The makeup of the protein as presented to the digestive tract determines how much is absorbed and how much is lost. For example, whole peanuts may pass right through, while the protein from peanut butter is almost totally absorbed.

Protein digestion is traditionally thought to proceed to hydrolyzation of protein to free amino acids which are subsequently absorbed and enter the circulation. Current research, however, has shown that protein fragments, mainly small peptides, are absorbed intact and transported by the systemic circulation to peripheral tissues.

Several studies have shown that hydrolysates made up mostly of di- and tripeptides are absorbed more rapidly than AAs and hydrolysates containing larger peptides, and much more rapidly than whole foods.[833,834] There are transport systems in the gut for both individual amino acids (usually, functionally similar amino acids such as the neutral ones will share a carrier) and for small peptides. The considerably greater absorption rate of amino acids from the dipeptide than from the amino acid mixture appears to be the result of uptake by a system that has a greater transport capacity than amino acid carrier systems, thus minimizing competition among its substrates.[835] The di- and tripeptides are absorbed intact, hydrolyzed intercellularly and released as free amino acids, or released intact into the circulation.

It is the kinetics of the absorption and not the net absorption of AAs from whole protein, a small peptide mixture (produced by enzymatic hydrolysis), and a mixture of amino acids that determines the greater nutritive value of the mixture of small peptides.

In one study, six nonanesthetized pigs were used to study the intestinal absorption of AA from either an enzymic hydrolysate of milk (PEP) containing a large percentage of small peptides (about 50% with less than five AA residues) and very few free AAs (8%), or from a mixture of free AAs with an identical pattern (AAL) infused intraduodenally.[836] The absorption of AAs was greater, more rapid, and more homogeneous after PEP infusion than after AAL infusion, independent of the amount infused. Thus enzymic hydrolysates are superior to a mixture of an equivalent pattern of free AA.

A more recent study has shown similar results.[837] In this study the nutritive value of two nitrogen-containing mixtures, one formed from small peptides (milk protein mild enzymatic hydrolysates) and the other consisting of a mixture of free amino acids having the same pattern except for glutamine, was measured in rats. In this study protein utilization was found to be greater for the mixtures of small peptides than for the mixture of free amino acids. The authors felt that under conditions of discontinuous enteral feedings, a mixture of small peptides is of greater nutritive value than a mixture of AAs having a close composition, probably because some amino acids from peptides (especially leucine and arginine) are more rapidly absorbed and may produce greater insulin reaction. In another study it was found that this greater rate of absorption appears to be buffered, although not abolished, if carbohydrates are present.[838]

Human studies have been done on surgical or trauma patients. In a prospective study, 12 intensive-care patients, after abdominal surgery, received three alternate 6-day courses of two enteral diets with identical nitrogen (0.3 g/kg N per day) and energy (60 kcal/kg per day) supply.[839] The protein hydrolyzate (PH) diet contained enzyme-hydrolysed casein and lactoserum (60% small peptides), while the nondegraded protein (NDP) diet contained a nitrogen source of similar amino acid composition, but in the form of nondegraded proteins.

The patients were randomized to receive either PH-NDP-PH or NDP-PH-NDP. Parameters reflecting protein metabolism were assessed in the plasma, urine, and stomal effluent on days 1, 6, 12, and 18, 3 h after stopping the nutrition (t0), and 1 h after restarting it (t1). Comparisons of t1 and t0 values showed that 13 amino acids (including the 8 essential amino acids) increased significantly with the protein hydrolysate diet, but only two increased with the nondegraded protein diet. Similarly, with protein hydrolysate, insulinemia at t1 was significantly higher than at t0 and correlated with plasma leucine, phenylalanine, alanine, and lysine concentrations. In addition, significant improvements in plasma albumin, transferrin, and retinol binding protein concentrations were seen with protein hydrolysate, together with a significant decrease in the plasma phenylalanine/tyrosine ratio and urinary 3-methylhistidine excretion.

The authors of this study concluded that in patients in intensive care after abdominal surgery, enteral support containing small peptides is more effective than an equivalent diet containing whole proteins in restoring plasma amino acid and protein levels.

On the other hand, another study compared the effects on nitrogen balance. Diets containing lactalbumin whole protein, its peptide-rich enzymic hydrolysate, or an equivalent mixture of free amino acids as the sole source of dietary nitrogen were fed to two healthy subjects, each studied for 38 days on two separate occasions.[840] The results of this study showed no significant differences in the effect of the three nitrogen sources on nitrogen balance. The authors concluded that there is no nutritional evidence to support the current practice of prescribing expensive enteral diets containing peptides or amino acids rather than the much cheaper whole protein to patients with normal gastrointestinal function. As we have seen, however, this conclusion does not apply to those under trauma, surgery, or exercise-induced catabolic stress.

The bottom line is that hydrolysates containing a mixture of small peptides and free amino acids are absorbed faster and produce more pharmacological effects (increasing GH and insulin response) than mixtures of free amino acids, and much faster than whole food protein. However, this still doesn't give us the complete picture since commercial preparations have confused the issue. Most peptide-bound amino acids are formed from whole protein foods, usually by either enzyme or acid hydrolysis. Both processes create some free-form amino acids along with the some small-chain peptides. Although any protein containing foods or tissues (including skin, hair, hooves, etc.) can be used as a starting point for hydrolysis, the most commonly used are the milk proteins casein and lactalbumin, and egg.

Although it's possible to produce a hydrolysate that is made up of mostly di- and tripeptides along with some free amino acids, such is not usually the case. Many preparations state that they have small peptides when in fact the amount of these peptides is very low, with most of the preparations being in the form of large oligopeptides. Free-form AA preparations are absorbed more rapidly than most of the peptide preparations now on the market. On the other hand, amino acids are more expensive than the most costly whole protein supplements and some free-form amino acids are difficult to take because of their bad smell and taste.

Notwithstanding the misrepresentation that can occur with some commercial preparations and the possible problems with palatability, in order to make the best use of the few hours of hypermetabolism that exist after training a protein supplement high in di- and tripeptides would seem to be absorbed fastest and thus give the most immediate anabolic and anticatabolic effects.

A PRACTICAL GUIDE TO COMMERCIAL AMINO ACID PREPARATIONS

A large number of products are commercially available that contain amino acids in one form or another. Amino acids are commercially available in both free and peptide-bonded forms. The athlete is often confused both by the large variety and the claims made for various products. Some basic facts are outlined below that will help the buyer make better choices.

FREE-FORM AMINO ACID MIXTURES

These crystalline amino formulations can consist of individual or combinations of two or more amino acids. They should be reserved for those times when rapid absorption can make a difference or for their pharmacological effects (as outlined below).

Comprehensive mixtures of free-form amino acids can be used as an adjunct to food or as an alternative to whole food protein supplements to increase dietary protein. There is no evidence, however, that shows any advantage to using the much more expensive free-form amino acid mixtures simply to augment protein intake.

There are times when the use of a free-form amino acid mixture or a product that contains free-form AAs together with di- and tripeptides may be more useful than either high-protein foods and whole food protein supplements. The free-form amino acid and small peptides are absorbed much faster and more expeditiously from the GI tract than whole food protein and even than mixtures of free amino acids. As well, the use of specific combinations of free-form AA mixtures before, during, and after training may be useful because of their pharmacological effects (as discussed below).

The kind and quantity of AA ingested, and the form it is in, have an effect on the portion that enters the systemic circulation. Normally, most of the AAs, except for the BCAAs, entering the liver from the digestive tract via the portal vein are deaminated and the resulting ammonia is converted to urea. A lesser amount is released into the general circulation as free AAs.

Large amounts of oral, powdered crystalline AAs present a bolus of AAs to the liver, allowing a larger portion of AAs to escape processing by the liver and reach the systemic circulation. Less would reach the systemic circulation if the same amount were ingested as whole protein powder or tablets of free AAs, because although the same quantity of AAs is presented to the liver, it is presented over a longer period of time so that more of the AAs are catabolized to urea.

If the powder is held in the mouth before swallowing, some of the AAs are absorbed from the buccal mucosa directly into the systemic circulation, bypassing the liver; the rest is absorbed through the gastric and intestinal mucosa. The overall result of buccal and gastrointestinal absorption of powdered AAs is a relatively higher level of the AAs in the systemic circulation. This results in higher tissue levels and a more pronounced systemic effect.

PEPTIDE-BONDED AMINO ACIDS

Peptide-bonded amino acids are useful for increasing dietary protein intake and for improving the protein efficiency ratio of dietary protein at specific times after training (as explained below). Since they are a mixture of amino acids, they cannot be used for pharmacological effects.

General protein supplements and mixtures of multiple amino acids can be used to increase dietary protein intake, and after training to make use of the "window of opportunity". They're used by all athletes but more are used by strength athletes — track and field, Olympic and power lifters, and bodybuilders to maximize lean body mass and strength. Taken by themselves or mixed with a variety of other supplements and foods they can be a valuable, easy to use, palatable addition to the athletes' diets.

The better, higher-priced, products usually offer more value. These products usually have a higher biological value, are more palatable, hypoallergenic, and are more natural, usually containing no chemical additives, artificial colors, or sweeteners.

FACTORS AFFECTING AMINO ACID BIOAVAILABILITY

The length of time it takes to digest a protein food and for the digested amino acids to be available for use by the body are determined by a number of factors, which include:

- Cooking — Amino acids are sensitive to heat although the degree of sensitivity varies with each amino acid. For example, arginine is extremely stable and will decompose only if exposed to sustained temperatures above 470°F. Carnitine decomposes at temperatures of 284°F. Cooking, in addition to killing micro-organisms, makes the long spiral polypeptide chains unwind, causing the amino acid to become more exposed when it reaches the digestive system.
- Physical nature of the food — Whether solid, liquid, powder, or tablet, whether and to what extent it is chemically predigested, and the type and amounts of binders, fillers, and other nutritive and nonnutritive materials.
- Status of the digestive system — Genetics, age, overall health, and specific diseases and illnesses.
- Metabolism or utilization by the intestine before absorption — Such as occurs with glutamine.
- Metabolism or utilization in the liver before transfer to the general circulation — For maximal directed effects, amino acids should be taken on an empty stomach and in a dosage that enables significant quantities to reach the target tissues.

ROLE OF AMINO ACID SUPPLEMENTATION IN MUSCLE HYPERTROPHY AND STRENGTH

The use of commercial amino acid supplements by athletes has increased dramatically in the past decade. While a certain amount of research has been done to determine the amount of dietary protein needed by strength and endurance athletes (see above), less is known about how the quality of protein or specific amino acid supplements affect metabolic and physiological responses to strength and endurance training.

Amino acids serve two rather different functions. Dietary amino acids are metabolized in a number of ways and are used to replenish the free amino acid pools in tissues and plasma. Oxidative losses of free amino acids occur both during and after feeding. The oxidative losses occur during feeding because they are consumed at a rate which is usually in excess of the rate in which net protein synthesis can occur, so that oxidation occurs as part of the process of maintaining the relatively small but important tissue-free amino acid pools. Any excess amino acids above the amounts needed for immediate protein synthesis and replenishment of the free amino acid pool are oxidized, transformed, or metabolized and stored as glycogen or fat.

As well, amino acids exert an important regulatory influence on growth, development, and protein turnover through their activation of various hormonal and metabolic responses. This effect is primarily aimed at the stimulation of growth but also includes the stimulation of oxidative losses. These anabolic influences may be exerted for short periods after feeding and/or under the influence of specific hormones. With the manipulation of diet and of the hormonal milieu, the anabolic influences can be prolonged.

Chapter 6

PHYSIOLOGICAL AND PHARMACOLOGICAL ACTIONS OF AMINO ACIDS

INTRODUCTION

Amino acids are the building blocks of body proteins including structural and contractile proteins, enzymes, and certain hormones and neurotransmitters. They also function in many other metabolic activities; are used as substrates for energy production; are involved in immune function, ammonia detoxification, and the synthesis of nucleic acids; and also function as antioxidants. Amino acids, either free form or in the form of small peptides, are potent physiological and pharmacological agents. For example:

Amino acid availability rapidly regulates protein synthesis and degradation. In one recent study endogenous leucine flux, reflecting proteolysis, decreased, while leucine oxidation increased in protocols where amino acids were infused.[841] As well, nonoxidative leucine flux reflecting protein synthesis was stimulated by amino acids.

Increasing amino acid concentrations stimulate protein synthesis in a dose-dependent manner at the level of mRNA translation-initiation and inhibits protein degradation by inhibiting lysosomal autophagy. Supplying energy alone (i.e., carbohydrate and lipids) cannot prevent negative nitrogen balance (net protein catabolism) in animals or humans; only the provision of certain amino acids allows the attainment of nitrogen balance.[842]

Certain neurotransmitters (i.e., acetylcholine, catecholamines, and serotonin) are formed from dietary constituents (i.e., choline, tyrosine and tryptophan). Changing the consumption of these precursors alters release of their respective neurotransmitter products. As well, many amino acids have been shown to act as CNS neurotransmitters.[843-859]

Acute dietary indispensable amino acid deficiency may increase vulnerability to seizures by repeated activation of the anterior piriform cortex of the brain.[860]

Glutamine[861] and taurine[862] have hepatoprotective and antihepatotoxic effects.

Several amino acids, such as cysteine (decreases cross linkage of proteins) and histidine,[863] have significant antioxidant effects.

Several AAs, including the essential BCAAs, especially leucine, are used directly as oxidizable fuels during exercise. Depending on the duration and intensity of exercise and other factors such as glycogen stores and energy intake, AAs can provide from a few to approximately 10% of the total energy for sustained exercise.[864]

Arginine, glycine, and methionine are AAs that are required for the hepatic synthesis of creatine. Creatine is taken up by skeletal muscle, where it is phosphorylated to form phosphocreatine (PC), a high-energy phosphate compound and an important energy source for cellular energy and muscular contraction.

Lysine has been shown useful for treating herpes infections in some patients, although there is considerable controversy on its effectiveness, perhaps because other factors such as dietary intake have not been taken into account.[865]

Cysteine, a precursor for reduced glutathione, may be of some use in reducing hepatotoxicity secondary to drugs (such as alcohol and anabolic steroids) and infections.[866,867]

Studies have shown that muscle wasting postoperatively can be countered by the use of enteral or parenteral glutamine, alpha-ketoglutarate, and the BCAAs.

Intravenous or oral feedings rich in branched-chain amino acids are said to improve nutrition in chronic liver disease and to exert anticatabolic effects on protein degradation, thus sparing muscle protein.[868]

All amino acids have the capacity to accept or release hydrogen ions. Only glutamate, aspartate, histidine, and perhaps arginine serve as buffers with respect to regulation of hydrogen ions in the body. Glutamine is especially important as a buffer in the kidney.

Studies have shown a dose-related suppression of food intake by phenylalanine and an anorexic effect of aspartame.[869]

Some of the amino acids may also be effective for the treatment and prevention of certain diseases. For example, a study in rabbits has shown that L-arginine, the precursor of endothelium-derived relaxing factor (EDRF), decreases atherosclerosis in hypercholesterolemic animals.[870]

It has even been shown that certain amino acids may have protective effects on lactational performance against toxic compounds.[871] In this study, glycine, which increases growth hormone release, and tryptophan, which enhances and mimics prolactin secretion, negate the harmful effects of 7,12-dimethylbenzanthracene by stimulating mammary gland growth and secretion.

Apart from acting as a protein supplement, AAs alone or in various combinations can have specific and different pharmacological and physiological effects including effects on immunomodulation, neurotransmitters, hormones, control of protein turnover, renal function, and maintenance of gut trophicity.[872] Certain amino acids exert pharmacological effects similar to hormones and drugs. Thus amino acids (and their metabolites and analogues) can transcend their roles of being just the building blocks of protein and can actually regulate protein synthesis by acting as anabolic and anticatabolic agents and affect hormonal functions.

For example, in one study examining the effects of certain amino acid groups on renal hemodynamics, the glomerular filtration rate and renal plasma flow were increased by infusion of mixed gluconeogenic amino acids (arginine, glycine, proline, cysteine, methionine, and serine) but not by either alanine, another gluconeogenic amino acid, or the BCAAs.[873]

In another study synthesis and degradation of globular and myofibrillar proteins across arm and leg muscles were examined during stepwise increased intravenous infusion of amino acids (0.1, 0.2, 0.4, and 0.8 g/kd/d of nitrogen) to healthy volunteers.[874]

In this study, protein dynamics were measured by a primed constant infusion of L-phenylalanine and the release of 3-methylhistidine from skeletal muscles. Amino acid infusion caused a significant uptake of the majority of amino acids across arm and leg tissues, except tyrosine, tryptophan, and cysteine, probably due to low concentrations of these amino acids in the formulation. The balance of globular proteins improved significantly due to stimulation of synthesis and attenuation of degradation across arm and leg tissues despite insignificant uptake of tyrosine, tryptophan, and cysteine. Degradation of myofibrillar proteins was uninfluenced by provision of amino acids.

Arterial concentrations and flux of glucose, lactate, and free fatty acids were unchanged despite increasing concentrations of plasma amino acids from 2.6 to 5.8 m*M*. Plasma insulin, IGF-1, and plasma concentrations of IGF-1 binding proteins-1 and -3 remained at fasting levels throughout the investigation. The results of this study demonstrate that neither insulin nor circulating IGF-1 explained improved protein balance in skeletal muscles following elevation of plasma amino acids. Rather, some amino acids in themselves trigger cellular reactions that initiate peptide formation. In this study the limited availability of some extracellular amino acids was overcome by increased reutilization of the intracellular amino acid.

There is evidence that specific amino acids play a role in the etiology of fatigue and the overtraining syndrome in athletes because their flux during exercise causes a change in certain metabolic kinetics. The metabolism of BCAAs, glutamine, and tryptophan may be the key to understanding some aspects of central fatigue and some aspects of immunosuppression that are very relevant to athletic endeavor.[875]

Complex AA mixtures do not give the same pharmacological effects as do the use of individual or combinations of a few or more select AAs. In the case of the effects on the CNS (in regulating hypothalamic and pituitary function, and in affecting the level of certain neurotransmitters) the reason is partly due to the nature of the transport mechanism that carries the AAs across the blood-brain barrier into the specific central nervous system (CNS) neurons.

The large neutral AAs (LNAA) such as tryptophan, tyrosine, the BCAAs (valine, leucine, isoleucine), phenylalanine, and methionine compete with each other for the same available transport molecules. Thus the presence in plasma of several of these AAs in any significant amounts results in a decrease in the amounts of each AA that are transported into the body and the CNS.[876] On the other hand, if only one or a small number of specific AAs were ingested, then serum levels of these AAs would rise appreciably over the serum levels of the other AAs so that more of the ingested AAs would enter the CNS.

It follows that individual or selectively combined AAs should be taken by themselves on an empty stomach. If taken with food, the AAs derived from natural sources compete with any individual or combination of specific AAs, thus diluting the physiological and pharmacological effects of these AAs.

CENTRAL NERVOUS SYSTEM EFFECTS OF AMINO ACIDS

The amount of neurotransmitter released when a neuron fires varies and is dependent to some degree on changes in neurotransmitter synthesis resulting from the metabolic consequences of normal activities such as eating and exercise.[877] These activities produce their effects by varying the plasma levels of nutrients that are the precursors of the neurotransmitter. It has been shown that increasing the precursors for the neurotransmitters often leads to an increased synthesis of the specific neurotransmitter.[878-880] Other studies have shown that specific brain regions may respond uniquely to amino acid ingestion and that dietary composition may influence the amino acid profiles of the extracellular fluid in brain.[881]

Thus many individual or combinations of AAs may enhance athletic performance when used to produce pharmacological changes in behavior and physiological functions that precursor-dependent neurons happen to subserve. For example, tyrosine and phenylalanine (which can be converted to tyrosine), are precursors for the neurotransmitters dopamine, epinephrine, and norepinephrine, thus potentially possessing some antidepressant, stimulating, and anorexic properties. Studies have shown that the use of exogenous tyrosine can transiently increase plasma and CNS catecholamines.[882]

Tryptophan can be converted by the body to niacin. Also, along with other nutrients, it is a precursor for the neurotransmitter serotonin. There seems to be some evidence that large doses of tryptophan may act as a relaxant, and may be useful as a mild nighttime sedative[883] and antidepressant.[884]

The AAs alanine, asparagine, gamma-aminobutyrate (GABA), glutamine, glycine, and taurine have been shown to act as CNS neurotransmitters.[885,886] GABA also stimulates growth hormone secretion, likely mediated via dopamine release at a suprapituitary level.[887]

EFFECTS OF AMINO ACIDS ON GROWTH HORMONE RELEASE

Amino acid (AA) supplements are popular among bodybuilders and other athletes because of claims that pharmacologic dosages of one or combinations of AAs can increase growth hormone release. Studies have shown that indeed pharmacologic dosages of some

AAs can increase the release of growth hormone. Histidine, arginine, L-dopa, tryptophan, valine, leucine, ornithine, tyrosine, phenylalanine, lysine, methionine and GABA all may potentiate GH secretion.[888-894] The amino acids can also stimulate other hormones. For example, arginine, like other dibasic AAs, stimulates pituitary release of growth hormone and prolactin, and pancreatic release of glucagon and insulin.[895] Ornithine, on the other hand, while stimulating GH release does not stimulate insulin release even in relatively high dosages.[896]

While several studies have shown that certain amino acids increase GH secretion, others studies have not. In general, however, larger doses of the GH-stimulating amino acids show more of a GH response than some of the doses used in studies that have not shown this effect.[897]

For example, in one study the authors used quantities of various amino acids as recommended by the manufacturers. Unfortunately, most manufacturers, because of the expense, recommend less than therapeutically effective dosages. In this study 7 male bodybuilders fasted for 8 h and then were given in random order either a placebo, a 2.4-g arginine/lysine supplement, a 1.85-g ornithine/tyrosine supplement, or a 20-g Bovril® drink.[898] Blood was collected before each treatment and again every 30 min for 3 h for the measurement of serum GH concentration. On a separate occasion, subjects had an intravenous infusion of 0.5 μg GH-releasing hormone per kilogram of body weight to confirm that the GH secretory response was normal. The main finding was that serum GH concentrations were not consistently altered in healthy young males following the ingestion of the amino acid supplements in the quantities recommended by the manufacturers.

Athletes often use combinations of growth hormone stimulators in hopes of increasing growth hormone secretion even further. There is in fact some basis for this belief — the synergistic effect of clonidine, propanolol, L-dopa, and others has been documented.[899] The GH-releasing effect of both arginine and pyridostigmine is mediated via the same mechanism, namely, by suppression of endogenous somatostatin release. Combined administration of either arginine or pyridostigmine with GHRH has a similar striking GH-releasing effect which is clearly higher than that of GHRH alone.[900] On the other hand, the mechanisms by which insulin-induced hypoglycemia, L-dopa, and arginine stimulate GH secretion are all different.[901]

The effect of various amino acids on GH will also be discussed below under the specific amino acid.

HEPATOPROTECTIVE AND CYTOPROTECTIVE EFFECTS OF AA

Glycine has been shown to have important specific and general hepatoprotective effects. One study showed the importance of glycine in protecting hepatocytes from noxious insult in general, as well as from valproate (VPA), an antiepileptic drug that causes hepatotoxicity, in particular.[902] In this study VPA caused a dose-dependent increase in leakage of lactic acid dehydrogenase (LDH), and glycine prevented this toxic response. L-Carnitine, L-alanine, and L-cysteine did not protect hepatocytes from VPA. Glycine also partially antagonized inhibition of fatty acid beta-oxidation by VPA, as estimated by the generation of acid-soluble products from [^{14}C]palmitic acid.

These results are consistent with the hypothesis that glycine prevents VPA toxicity by removing acyl-CoA esters, which accumulate during VPA exposure and interfere with fatty acid beta-oxidation. In this same study, glycine also antagonized the toxic effects of acetaminophen on hepatocytes, although at higher concentrations than required to protect hepatocytes from VPA. Because the mechanism of toxicity of acetaminophen probably is different from that of VPA, a nonspecific cytoprotective effect may contribute to glycine antagonism of VPA toxicity.

One study investigating the mechanism by which glycine protects against hepatocyte death during anoxia, found that glycine may exert its cytoprotective activity during lethal anoxic hepatocyte injury, in part by inhibiting Ca^{2+}-dependent degradative nonlysosomal proteases, including calpains.[903] The results also pointed to the hepatoprotective effects of alanine since glycine and alanine (but not valine) markedly improved cell viability during anoxia in a concentration-dependent manner.

Glycine has been shown to have some cytoprotective effect when administered to recipients of livers preserved for 24 or 48 h. In a recent study glycine suppressed some hepatocellular injury, as reflected in a reduction in the concentration of serum enzymes.[904]

Glycine has also been shown to protect renal tubule cells and hepatocytes from ischemia, ATP depletion, and cold-storage injury. For example, some protection against hypoxic injury by supraphysiological glycine and alanine concentrations has been found in the isolated perfused rat kidney.[905]

Intravenous glutamine protects liver cells from oxidant injury by increasing intracellular glutathione (GSH) content. In one study, oral glutamine supplementation was shown to enhance the selectivity of antitumor drugs by protecting normal tissues including liver, from and possibly sensitizing tumor cells to chemotherapy treatment-related injury.[906] Another study has alluded to the hepatoprotectant effects of an arginine-aspartate mixture.[907]

In the following chapters we'll cover some of the relevant biological and pharmacological effects of each amino acid in detail. We'll limit our coverage to those amino acids that may have an effect on anabolic and catabolic processes in the body and that may influence athletic performance.

L-DOPA

L-Dopa or levodopa (Larodopa, Prolopa, and Sinemet — used in the treatment of Parkinson's disease) is used by some athletes to stimulate endogenous growth hormone production. L-Dopa is the levorotatory isomer of dihydroxyphenylalanine and the metabolic precursor of the neurotransmitter dopamine. It is commercially available either by itself (Larodopa) or in combination with compounds which increase the concentration of levodopa in the brain, such as carbidopa (Sinemet), or benserazide (Prolopa).

A useful growth hormone stimulator with potentially serious adverse effects, it is only available by prescription in many countries.

ANALOGUES AND DERIVATIVES OF AMINO ACIDS

A number of analogues and derivatives of amino acids have been found to have significant effects on protein metabolism even though many of these analogues cannot replace their parent compounds in protein. Current concepts for explaining the effects of amino acids on protein turnover in skeletal muscle are based on the assumption that the amino acids might become rate limiting for protein synthesis in muscle under catabolic conditions. However, since most amino acid analogues cannot replace any of the amino acids in protein, the present thoughts on protein synthesis appear to be incomplete.

In one study, the effect of L-norleucine, an isomer of leucine, on protein metabolism *in vivo* was studied in suckling rats. Rats were injected subcutaneously with various doses of L-norleucine (0.5 and 5.0 μmol/g body weight) every 12 h from 3 to 15 days postpartum. Protein concentration, amino acid concentrations, and incorporation of $[^3H]$tyrosine into protein were analyzed in liver, muscles of thigh, and small intestine. Amino acid concentrations and insulin levels in serum were also measured. At 5 days of age, norleucine induced an increase in protein concentration of skeletal muscle with an increased incorporation of [^{3}H]tyrosine into protein, indicating an accelerated protein synthesis. Changes in protein metabolism were paralleled by alterations in the amino acid pattern of this tissue.

Another study looked at the analogues and derivatives of six of the amino acids which most effectively inhibit protein degradation in isolated rat hepatocytes (leucine, asparagine, glutamine, histidine, phenylalanine, and tryptophan) to see if they could antagonize or mimic the effect of the parent compound.[1463] No antagonists were found. Amino alcohols and amino acid amides tended to inhibit protein degradation strongly, apparently by direct lysosomotropic effect as indicated by their ability to cause lysosomal vacuolation.

Amino acid alkyl esters and dipeptides inhibited degradation to approximately the same extent as did their parent amino acids, possibly by being converted to free amino acids intracellularly. Of several leucine analogues tested, four (L-norleucine, L-norvaline, D-norleucine, and L-allo-isoleucine) were found to be as effective as leucine in inhibiting protein degradation.

Although none of the analogues in this study had any effect on protein synthesis, there is a possibility that certain amino acid derivatives or analogues might be found that have significant effects on both protein degradation and protein synthesis and that could be used to counter cachexia and increase the anabolic effects of exercise.

THE EFFECTS OF PROTEIN ON DIETARY INTAKE AND APPETITE

Studies have been rather inconclusive regarding the effect of dietary protein on protein intake and appetite. Until recently, the effect of dietary protein on the level of free essential amino acids in brain and on serotonin levels has been the focus of these studies.[635-641] In a review of these studies[642] the authors concluded that analysis of evidence of associations among dietary protein content, brain amino acid and serotonin concentrations, and protein self-selection by rats suggests that:

1. Protein intake is not regulated precisely, although rats will select between low- and high-protein diets to obtain an adequate, but not excessive, amount of protein;
2. Associations between brain serotonin concentration and protein intake are weak, although consumption of single meals of protein-deficient diets will elevate brain serotonin concentration;
3. The nature of signals that drive rats to avoid diets containing inadequate or excessive amounts of protein remains obscure;
4. Whole-brain amino acid and serotonin concentrations are quite stable over the usual range of protein intakes, owing to competition among amino acids for uptake across the blood-brain barrier and effective metabolic regulation of blood amino acid concentrations;
5. Protein intake and preference are not in themselves regulated, but what appears to be regulation of intake and preference is a reflection of the responses of systems for control of plasma amino acid concentrations; and
6. The relative stability of the average protein intake of groups of self-selecting rats (which gives the appearance of regulation) results from averaging the variable behavioral responses — learned aversions and preferences — of rats to the variety of sensory cues arising from diets that differ in protein content.

Studies in humans have shown that high-protein versions of the same food systems show more sensory-specific satiety and decrease hunger more than lower-protein versions.[643]

Chapter 7

ESSENTIAL AMINO ACIDS

INTRODUCTION

Essential amino acids, also called indispensable amino acids, must be supplied in the diet either as free amino acids or as constituents of dietary proteins. By this criterion, the following eight amino acids are essential in humans:

Isoleucine	Phenylalanine
Leucine	Threonine
Lysine	Tryptophan
Methionine	Valine

Note: Leucine, isoleucine, and valine are branched-chain amino acids.

THE BRANCHED-CHAIN AMINO ACIDS: ISOLEUCINE, LEUCINE, AND VALINE

The branched-chain amino acids (BCAAs) are so named because they have a carbon chain which deviates or branches from the main linear carbon backbone.

The BCAAs isoleucine, leucine, and valine have been investigated for their anticatabolic and anabolic effects. In heart and skeletal muscle *in vitro*, increasing the concentration of the three BCAAs or of leucine alone reproduces the effects of increasing the supply of all AAs in stimulating protein synthesis and inhibiting protein degradation.[908]

Several studies have indicated that leucine acts as an *in vivo* regulator of protein metabolism by decreasing protein degradation and increasing protein synthesis. In one study leucine infusion decreased plasma concentrations of several amino acids.[909] The authors concluded that leucine decreases protein degradation in humans and that this decreased protein degradation during leucine infusion contributes to the decrease in plasma essential amino acids.

In another study with rats, excessive intake of a single BCAA led rapidly to elevated plasma concentrations of both the amino acid administered and its corresponding alpha-keto acid and, if the rats had previously been fed a low protein diet, to an increase in liver branched-chain alpha-keto acid dehydrogenase activity.[910] Leucine caused decreased plasma isoleucine, valine, alpha-keto-beta-methylvaleric acid, and alpha-keto isovaleric acid concentrations. These decreases were not caused by increased degradation of these metabolites to carbon dioxide as BCAA oxidation rates *in vivo* were unchanged by leucine loading and the degradative enzymes were unchanged in adequately fed rats. The authors suggest that the decreased concentrations of these amino and keto acids may be the result of decreased protein degradation or increased protein synthesis, possibly mediated by insulin.

In a recent study, the mechanisms of protein gain during protein feeding were investigated using a combination of oral and intravenous labeled leucine in healthy young men.[911] The oral labeled leucine was administered either as a free oral tracer (^{13}C- or $^{2}H_3$-leucine) added to unlabeled whey protein, or as whey protein intrinsically labeled with L-[1-^{13}C]leucine. When the oral tracer was free leucine, it appeared in the plasma more rapidly than the unlabeled leucine derived from the whey protein, and this resulted in an artifactual 88%

decrease of protein breakdown. When the oral tracer was protein bound, protein breakdown did not change significantly after the meal. By contrast, nonoxidative leucine disposal (i.e., protein synthesis) was stimulated 63% by the meal.

The authors concluded that:

1. An intrinsically labeled protein is more appropriate than an oral free tracer to study postprandial leucine kinetics under nonsteady-state conditions.
2. Protein gain after a single whey protein meal solely results from an increased protein synthesis with no modification of protein breakdown.

Louard et al. examined the effects of infused BCAA on whole-body and skeletal muscle amino acid kinetics in ten postabsorptive normal subjects.[912] Ten control subjects received only saline. Infusion of BCAAs caused a fourfold rise in arterial BCAA levels and a two-fold rise in BCAA keto acids. Plasma insulin levels were unchanged from basal levels. The results implied that BCAA infusion results in a suppression of whole-body and forearm muscle proteolysis. Since insulin levels were unaffected by the infusion of BCAAs, the observed alterations in muscle and whole-body amino acid kinetics appear to be independent of insulin, and are probably mediated by the elevated BCAA concentrations themselves.

Another recent study looked at the effects of long-term BCAA administration on metabolic and respiratory parameters.[913] The authors concluded that the physical fitness of BCAA-treated subjects improved, and that BCAA seemed to promote protein synthesis in the fat-free body mass.

As well, leucine has been shown to increase the release of acetoacetate and 3-hydroxybutyrate (as a result of the partial oxidation of leucine).[914] The ketone bodies, beta-hydroxybutyrate and acetoacetate, are known to be useful sources of energy, and also show a glucose-sparing effect.[915] It has been shown experimentally that oral or parenteral intake of beta-hydroxybutyrate decreases the amount of protein catabolized in obese people on starvation diets.[916] Both KIC and HMB (see below) also seem to have some ketone-like anticatabolic effects.

In a recent review the authors concluded that:[917]

1. The ketone bodies, D-beta-hydroxybutyrate and acetoacetate, inhibit glycolysis thereby reducing pyruvate availability, which leads to a marked inhibition of BCAA metabolism and alanine synthesis in skeletal muscles from fasted mammalian and avian species.
2. The rate of glutamine release from skeletal muscles from fasted birds is increased at the expense of alanine in the presence of elevated concentrations of ketone bodies because of an increase in the availability of glutamate for glutamine synthesis.
3. Ketone bodies inhibit both protein synthesis and protein degradation in skeletal muscles from fasted mammalian and avian species *in vitro*. The mechanisms involved remain unknown.
4. Inhibition of amino acid metabolism and protein turnover in skeletal muscle by ketone bodies may be an important survival mechanism during adaptation to catabolic states such as prolonged fasting.

Alvestrand et al.[918] found leucine to decrease the net degradation of muscle protein even in normal resting subjects, something Blomstrand and Newsholme[919] suggested might aid repair and recovery and be of importance for athletes doing regular physical training. Alvestrand's group found that approximately 40% of the leucine taken up by muscle was accumulated in the intracellular free pool, some 20% could have been incorporated into protein, and 40% was probably oxidized.

Studies using BCAAs have found them to have a beneficial effect on the synthesis of proteins under special circumstances. For example, one study showed that BCAAs have a specific effect on the synthesis of plasma proteins by cultured hepatocytes.[920] Another study found a positive benefit from BCAAs as the protein component of total parenteral nutrition in cancer cachexia.[921]

On the other hand, the role of the BCAAs in protein synthesis is not completely clear. Current concepts for explaining the effects of BCAA on protein turnover in skeletal muscle are based on the assumption that the BCAA or leucine alone might become rate limiting for protein synthesis in muscle under catabolic conditions. However, in one study using suckling rats, the use of the leucine analogue norleucine was found to stimulate protein synthesis even though norleucine cannot replace any of the BCAA in protein.[922]

Several amino acids show changes in intracellular and extracellular concentrations in response to exercise, suggesting that skeletal protein, amino acid catabolism, and gluconeogenesis is increased by exercise.[923] The branched-chain amino acids (BCAAs) (leucine, isoleucine, and valine) are specifically utilized by muscle metabolism, although some evidence indicates their use by other organ tissues.[924]

Leucine and other BCAAs, unlike most other amino acids, are oxidized (used as energy) by muscle cells, and are a source of cellular energy in the form of ATP and PC. They are also involved in the glucose-alanine cycle (see section on alanine). There is a significant activation of BCAA metabolism with prolonged exercise, and current studies indicate that this is more pronounced in endurance-trained subjects than in untrained controls.[925]

Plasma concentrations of the BCAAs (leucine, isoleucine, and valine) are more prominently affected than the concentrations of other amino acids by changes in caloric, protein, fat, and carbohydrate intake in humans.[926]

BCAA administration before exercise affects the response of some anabolic hormones, mainly growth hormone, insulin and testosterone.[927] A study conducted by Carli et al.[928] examined the effects of BCAA administration on the hormonal response in male marathon runners to a 1-h running test at constant speed.

In this study using 14 male long-distance runners, 2 trials were carried out at 1-week intervals. In each trial 1 h of running was performed at a predetermined speed for each athlete. In the first trial (E) the athletes were given a commercial diet product containing BCAAs (5.14 g leucine, 2.57 g isoleucine, 2.57 g valine) with milk proteins (12 g), fructose (20 g), other carbohydrates (8.8 g), and fats (1.08 g) — the total energy content being 216 kcal. In the second trial (P), the athletes received a similar mixture with the same energy content but without BCAAs, which were replaced by additional milk proteins (10 g). In both trials the mixture was taken approximately 90 min before the running test.

The BCAA mixture ingested by the athletes in the E trial elicited, in resting conditions, a sustained elevation in plasma BCAA levels which lasted several hours. In the whole-milk protein without the BCAA trial there was a decrease in serum free testosterone (as measured by the decreased testosterone:SHBG ratio) and sex hormone-binding globulin (SHBG). This was thought to have been an indication of increased metabolic clearance of testosterone.

In the E trial testosterone was unchanged at the end of the exercise period and it actually increased in the following rest period. The authors concluded, "We would suggest that exogenous administration of BCAA and their uptake by muscle fibers could limit endogenous amino acid oxidation and indirectly prevent testosterone muscle clearance." This suggestion is also supported by the direct anabolic effect of BCAA, mainly leucine, on muscle proteins.[929] In this study the authors suggest that branched-chain amino acids may be rate limiting for muscle protein synthesis.

An anticatabolic effect of BCAA administration was also indicated by the values of the testosterone:cortisol ratio, an indicator of changes in the anabolic-androgenic activity of the body,[930] in the last sample.

In summary, the study showed that the hormone response to exercise was modified by BCAA ingestion and that the anabolic hormones insulin and, especially, testosterone were favorably affected when BCAAs were substituted for equivalent amounts of whole-milk proteins. These findings are extremely important and point out the advantages of BCAA supplementation over the use of whole food proteins and even whole food protein supplements.

In a recent study, 25 competitive wrestlers restricted their caloric intake for 19 days, using a hypocaloric control, hypocaloric high-protein, hypocaloric high-branched-chain amino acid, and hypocaloric low-protein diet to determine the effects of caloric restriction on body composition and performances versus control diet (C, n = 6).[591] Anthropometric parameters (weight, percent body fat) and adipose tissue (AT) distribution measured by magnetic resonance imaging (MRI) obtained before and after diet, were compared. A significant highest body weight loss and decrease in the percent of body fat were observed for subjects of the hypocaloric high BCAA group. Subjects in this group exhibited a significant reduction in abdominal visceral adipose tissue (VAT). There was no change in aerobic (VO_2max) and anaerobic, and in muscular strength. The authors concluded that under our experimental conditions, the combination of moderate energy restriction and BCAA supplementation induced significant and preferential losses of VAT, and allowed maintainance of a high level of performance.

Of the BCAAs, leucine appears to be the most important for athletes. Leucine affects various anabolic hormones and has anabolic and anticatabolic effects. It's also involved in nitrogen metabolism and ammonia removal. A study in 1994 found that leucine infusion depressed muscle proteolysis.[931] The use of large amounts of leucine, and not valine and isoleucine, while decreasing the serum levels of valine and isoleucine does not adversely affect the rate of protein synthesis.[932]

In another study the plasma and muscle concentrations of tyrosine, phenylalanine, and BCAAs were measured before and after two types of sustained intense exercise during which the subjects were given a mixture of BCAAs or a placebo.[933] An increase in the muscle concentration of tyrosine and/or phenylalanine could be an indication of net protein degradation in skeletal muscle since these amino acids are neither taken up nor metabolized by this tissue. The investigation comprised two separate studies, both involving male subjects.

In one aspect of the study 26 subjects participated in a 30-km cross-country race. In a second aspect, 32 subjects participated in a full-length marathon race (42.2 km). All subjects were well trained. In both races, the subjects were randomly divided into two groups. One group, the test group, was given a drink containing a mixture of BCAAs in a 5% (cross-country) or 6% (marathon) carbohydrate solution. The other group (placebo) was given 5% and 6% carbohydrate solutions in the cross-country and marathon races, respectively. The total amount of BCAAs given to each subject in the cross-country race was 7.5 g (2.6 g leucine, 3.8 g valine, 1.1 g isoleucine) and in the marathon race 12 g (4.2 g leucine, 4.8 g valine, 3.0 g isoleucine).

The results of the study showed that an intake of the BCAA mixture prevented an exercise-induced increase in the muscle concentration of tyrosine and phenylalanine, which was found in the placebo groups. This, the authors remarked, might indicate an inhibitory effect of BCAAs on the net rate of protein degradation in the working muscles during exercise. Furthermore, they added "... a decreased net rate of protein degradation during exercise might improve physical performance and would probably aid repair and recovery after such intense exertion. Hence, this finding could be of some importance for athletes doing regular physical training."

The authors suggest that the intake of BCAAs during exercise might decrease the protein degradation that occurs in human skeletal muscle during that exercise.

The intake of BCAAs during exercise might also alleviate some of the fatigue seen in prolonged exercise. Plasma levels of free tryptophan have been shown to increase during exercise and the levels of BCAAs to decrease. Thus the ratio of free tryptophan to BCAAs increases markedly with some forms of exercise. It is thought that this increased ratio may lead to an increase in the transport of tryptophan across the blood-brain barrier, and hence to an increase in the synthesis of 5-hydroxytryptophan (5-HT or serotonin) in specific areas of the brain. This may be responsible for the development of some of the physical/mental fatigue seen during prolonged exercise.[934]

There are a number of compounds that potentially may have more of an anticatabolic and anabolic effect than the BCAA, but which at present are not generally commercially available. For example, one study on amino acid metabolism with exercise[935] found that plasma concentration of glutamine, the branched-chain keto acids (BCKA), and short-chain acyl carnitines were elevated with exercise. Utilization of these compounds may spare muscle glutamine and BCAAs and thus may have a greater muscle-sparing effect than any other amino acid combination.

The significance of the serum changes of amino acids with exercise has not been fully explored. Serum amino acid levels can change for a number of reasons. For example, increases in the serum level of any amino acid could be due to decreased use, increased release, or increased formation of that amino acid, and might be associated with increased use of that amino acid by other tissues. Thus in some instances of increased levels of an amino acid such as glutamine, supplementation of that amino acid might be necessary to decrease protein catabolism and increase protein synthesis. In other instances, increased levels of an amino acid might simply show decreased use of that amino acid and supplementation would not be of any value.

In one study the quantitative relationship between insulin and plasma amino acid (AA) levels were characterized in five healthy young men during a number of euglycemic insulin infusions.[936] While eight of the ten amino acids measured decreased in a dose-responsive pattern to increasing levels of insulin, alanine and glycine concentrations remained unaffected. In this instance the use of exogenous alanine would not likely affect protein metabolism whereas the use of some of the other amino acids, such as the BCAA, would. Alanine supplementation (since it is a major gluconeogenic precursor) might be useful before and/or during exercise since alanine flux would increase as exercise time and intensity increased.

BCAAs AND PROTEIN METABOLISM

Protein synthesis is the process in which amino acids are linked together by peptide bonds to form one or more long polypeptide chains. Once a chain or group of chains has achieved a stable three-dimensional configuration and is biologically active as a result, it is termed a protein.

In a given cell, all proteins are fabricated from a common pool of free amino acids. As synthesis proceeds, the required amino acids are obtained from this cellular pool and are carried to the growing polypeptide chain by transfer RNA (tRNA) molecules. When the intracellular free amino acid pool is limiting, protein synthesis would therefore be expected to suffer. Indeed, the apparent importance of the prevailing amino acid concentration has been demonstrated by several recent studies which found that increased amino acid availability alone may augment skeletal muscle as well as whole-body protein synthesis in young healthy men.[956-958] Thus, supplemental BCAAs, by helping to maintain the free amino acid pool in skeletal muscle fibers, could conceivably increase the rate of protein synthesis beyond that achievable by foodstuffs alone.

BCAA supplements may also be helpful in reducing protein catabolism. The degradation of muscle proteins is a normal part of animal metabolism. An important early adaptation to fasting is the mobilization of amino acids from skeletal muscle protein for gluconeogenesis or direct oxidation.[959] This net loss of muscle protein in fasting is due to both a decrease in the overall rate of protein synthesis and an enhancement of proteolysis.

Several hormones, in particular glucocorticoids (e.g., cortisol) and insulin, appear to be involved in mediating these changes in protein turnover. Interestingly, some researchers have suggested that anabolic steroids may exert some of their observed muscle-building effects by antagonizing the catabolic effects of glucocorticoids. Insulin deprivation also leads to activated muscle protein catabolism, and this effect likely plays a role in mediating the increased proteolysis seen during fasting.

During exercise, a greater availability of BCAAs in muscle tissue could help to maintain a more favorable testosterone:cortisol ratio. This would be expected to enhance the productivity of the training session in terms of its growth-stimulating capacity. Additionally, leucine (as well as arginine) are potent insulin secretagogues, and so in this way may be of help in reducing the catabolism of muscle protein. The transamination of leucine to alpha-ketoisocaproic acid appears to be important for its anticatabolic effects on muscle protein. Hence, supplements containing this compound may prove more effective in this regard.

Muscle protein accretion is the net difference between protein synthesis and degradation and results in muscle hypertrophy during growth and development. Hence, in order to achieve optimal gains in muscle mass it would seem prudent to optimize muscle protein synthesis while minimizing muscle protein catabolism. As the results of the aforementioned studies suggest, the use of BCAAs could prove helpful in this regard.

BCAAs AND HYPOXIA

Exposure to high altitude often results in a loss of body mass. This has been shown to be largely due to a reduction of lean body mass attributable to skeletal muscle wasting.[955] On the ultrastructural level, it has been shown that the muscle fibers apparently shrink, causing the relative capillary density to increase. This effectively reduces the distance that oxygen must diffuse to reach the site of cellular respiration (i.e., the mitochondria), thereby effectively enhancing the performance of the muscle fiber under conditions of chronic hypoxia.[954] The cause of muscle wasting under hypoxic conditions is not entirely understood. Reduced caloric intake and/or a direct effect of hypoxia on protein metabolism could play a role.[955] Another possible explanation for high-altitude muscle loss could be a relative lack in the intake or absorption of some essential amino acids, which would therefore be mobilized from skeletal muscles.[955] Since this can be limited by a dietary supplement of branched-chain amino acids, Schena and co-workers[955] thought that this may also be the case for subjects exposed to chronic hypoxia. To test the hypothesis, they administered BCAAs to a group of healthy human subjects during a 21-day trek through the Peruvian Andes.

In all, 16 subjects (11 men, 5 women) participated in the study. The subjects were subdivided into two groups for age, sex, and fitness by an independent researcher unaware of the aim of the study and not involved in the project. All members of the two groups received, in a double-blind manner, envelopes containing either a mixture of BCAAs (per envelope: 1.2 g leucine, 0.6 g isoleucine, 0.6 g valine) or an inert substance with the same appearance and taste (placebo). The dosage was two envelopes three times a day for the duration of the trek (total per day: 7.2 g leucine, 3.6 g isoleucine, 3.6 g valine).

Upon return from the trek, all subjects (with the exception of one subject from the BCAA group) had lost a significant amount of body mass. In the placebo group, the loss amounted to 1.8 kg, which skin-fold measurements revealed was partitioned as 90% fat mass and 10% lean body mass. In the BCAA group, the loss of body mass was less (1.07 kg), but still significant compared to pre-trek values. In this group, however, the decrease in body mass was only due to loss of fat, whereas the lean mass tended to increase by 0.71 kg. The increase was nonsignificant. The authors remarked, "From the differences in lean body mass one may conclude that on the whole the placebo group was catabolizing, whereas the BCAA group was synthesizing muscle tissue."

BRANCHED-CHAIN KETO ACIDS

Branched-chain keto acids (BCKAs) are very similar to BCAAs, the only difference being the presence of a "keto" group instead of an "amino" group. In essence, BCKAs can be viewed as ammonia-free sources of BCAAs.

BCKAs (like BCAAs) can increase lean body mass and improve nitrogen retention. They are also essential for energy production in muscle and for the removal (detoxification) of ammonia.[937] The most pronounced results are obtained in athletes during strenuous and/or prolonged bouts of exercise, as well as in individuals consuming high-protein diets.

BCKAs are both made from, and converted into, BCAAs. Thus, BCKAs can function as dietary supplements for the essential branched-chain aminos, although their capacity to generate BCAAs is well below 100%. In one study, for example, the efficiency for conversion in normal rats (and in rats with impaired kidney function) was 50% (meaning that only half of the ingested BCKAs were made into BCAAs).[938] Others have reported similar findings in both humans and animals (between 35 and 65% conversion). The likely reason that this value is so low is that BCKAs are picked up and burned (oxidized) in various organs before they can be made into BCAAs.

Exercise has profound effects on the intracellular and extracellular levels of amino acids and their metabolites. In one study using rats, plasma concentration of glutamine, the BCKAs and short-chain acyl carnitines were elevated with exercise. Ratios of plasma BCAAs/BCKAs were dramatically lowered by exercise in the trained rats. A decrease in plasma-free carnitine levels was also observed. The data from this study suggest that amino acid metabolism is enhanced by exercise even in the trained state. As well, BCAAs may only be partially metabolized within muscle and some of their carbon skeletons are released into the circulation in the forms of BCKAs and short-chain acyl carnitines.

It's possible that supplying these compounds may decrease the catabolism of BCAAs so that they can be used for protein synthesis.

ALPHA-KETOISOCAPROIC ACID (KIC)

Alpha-ketoisocaproate (KIC), the keto acid of leucine, is clearly the most important BCKA. KIC is anabolic, and anticatabolic, particularly during catabolic states. Since any intensive, strenuous activity is also catabolic, there is every reason to believe that the BCKAs will prove to be of value to bodybuilders, power lifters, and aerobic athletes.

Both leucine and KIC are metabolized further to alpha-amino-n-butyrate and beta-hydroxy-beta-methylbutyrate. These compounds have not as yet been investigated in humans for their anabolic and protein-sparing properties. However, they may have some anabolic and anticatabolic effects.

Although KIC is the transamination product of the BCAA leucine, and both tend to increase in parallel in the serum when exogenous leucine is used,[939] there is substantial evidence that it has anabolic and protein-sparing properties separate from leucine.[940,941] On the other hand, leucine has properties apart from its transamination to KIC.

In one study the effects of leucine, its metabolites, and the 2-oxo acids of valine and isoleucine on protein synthesis and degradation in incubated limb muscles of immature and adult rats were investigated.[942] The results of this study seemed to point to an anabolic and anticatabolic effect of leucine which was found to stimulate protein synthesis and reduce protein catabolism. However, the anticatabolic effects of leucine, in contrast to its anabolic effects, required its transamination to the 2-oxo acid 4-methyl-2-oxopentanoate or KIC. While the oxo acid of leucine was found to have significant effects, the 2-oxo acids of valine and isoleucine did not affect protein synthesis or degradation.

Interestingly, the authors of this 1984 study felt that the effect of KIC in preventing muscle degradation was likely due to the accumulation within cells of a metabolite of KIC (such as HMB). They also felt that it is KIC rather than leucine that reduced the catabolic process. Supplements containing KIC in pharmacological doses have been shown to decrease the rate of 3-methylhistidine excretion by patients with Duchenne's muscular dystrophy.[943] 3-Methylhistidine, which occurs only in the myofibrillar proteins, is often used as an indicator of contractile protein degradation.[944]

The results of these studies confirmed the results obtained from an earlier study that concluded that KIC showed anticatabolic but not anabolic effects.[945] That is, KIC reduced muscle catabolism but did not stimulate protein synthesis. Leucine, on the other hand, seemed to have effects on protein synthesis. Interestingly enough, the authors concluded that neither of the other two BCAAs (isoleucine and valine) promoted protein synthesis.

Perhaps one of the more important actions of KIC (and also leucine) is its enhancement of the anabolic drive via stimulation of insulin secretion. Both leucine[946] and KIC (and other AA compounds such as arginine, ornithine, and OKG) stimulate insulin secretion. Insulin increases the intercellular transport of amino acids (AAs) and has both anabolic and anticatabolic effects.

BETA-HYDROXY-BETA-METHYLBUTYRATE (HMB)

One of the newest anabolic/anticatabolic supplements to hit the market is beta-hydroxy-beta-methylbutyrate (HMB), a leucine catabolite. The classical pathway of leucine metabolism involves conversion to alpha-ketoisocaproate, transport into the mitochondria and oxidation to HMG-CoA, which can then be converted to ketones. An alternative leucine metabolic pathway has been described. In this pathway leucine is converted to KIC and KIC is oxidized to HMB by a cytosolic enzyme called KIC-dioxygenase.[947]

The HMB produced is further metabolized in at least three ways. The first fate is further metabolism to HMG-CoA. This cytosolic source of HMG-CoA plays at least some role in cholesterol synthesis. A second fate of HMB produced in the cell is loss in the urine. Previous feeding studies indicate that up to 40% of the HMB fed is lost in the urine and likely accounts for the relative short half-life of HMB of about 1 h. The third fate of HMB appears to be further use by the cell.

HMB meets the criteria of a dietary supplement because it is found in some foods in small amounts (such as catfish and some citrus fruits), it is found in breast milk, and it is used and produced by body tissues. As yet there has been no evidence that HMB is a necessary nutrient and that the body utilizes it preferentially for modulating protein synthesis. However, it seems to have effects on protein synthesis and may help maximize the anabolic effects of exercise.

HMB has been seriously studied in the past five years and found to have an effect on protein synthesis and lean body mass. Animal studies have shown that HMB appears to be nontoxic and may counteract the effects of stress and increase growth and health of animals.[948-951]

One study looked at effects of leucine and its catabolites on *in vitro* mitogen-stimulated DNA synthesis by bovine lymphocytes.[952] The results of the study suggest that leucine is necessary for mitogen-induced DNA synthesis by bovine lymphocytes, and that this requirement for leucine can be partially met by KIC. When leucine was not limiting, KIC, HMB, and HMG at concentrations that might occur *in vivo* did not alter lymphocyte DNA synthesis *in vitro*. Thus it would appear that in some circumstances and in some tissues HMB is lower down on the anabolic and anticatabolic scale than either leucine or KIC.

However, a few recent studies suggest that HMB has significant anticatabolic potential in skeletal muscle. Especially promising is a study that has been accepted for publication in which supplementation with either 1.5 or 3 g of HMB per day was shown to partly prevent exercise-induced proteolysis/muscle damage and result in larger gains in muscle function associated with resistance training in humans.[953]

In this study, the effects of dietary supplementation of HMB were studied in two experiments. In Study 1, 41 untrained (no participation in a resistance training program for at least 3 months) subjects were randomized among 3 levels of HMB supplementation (0, 1.5, or 3.0 g HMB per day) and 2 protein levels and weight lifted (WL) 1.5 h 3 days a week for 3 weeks. In Study 2, subjects were fed either 0 or 3.0 g HMB per day and WL for 2 to 3 h 6 days a week for 7 weeks.

In Study 1, HMB significantly decreased the exercise-induced rise in muscle proteolysis, as measured by urine 3-methylhistidine, during the first two weeks of exercise. Plasma creatine phosphokinase (CK), was also decreased with HMB supplementation. WL was increased by HMB supplementation when compared with the unsupplemented subjects during each week of the study.

After a 1-week adaptation period, the 3-week supplementation/exercise protocol was started. After only 1 week of training/supplementation, muscle protein breakdown in the group fed 3 g HMB was decreased 44% (compared to placebo). Muscle protein breakdown continued to be lower in the HMB group for the entire 3-week study. A second indicator of muscle damage and muscle breakdown is the muscle-specific enzyme called creatine phosphokinase (CPK). This enzyme was also markedly decreased with HMB supplementation.

The biochemical indicators of muscle damage were also accompanied by demonstrable increases in muscle strength and muscle mass. Lean body mass increases for the 0, 1.5, and 3.0 g HMB per day study were 0.4, 0.8, and 1.2 kg/3 weeks, respectively. Strength increases for the 0, 1.5, and 3 g HMB per day study were 10, 23, and 29%, respectively.

In Study 2, in which the intensity of exercise was much higher, fat-free mass was significantly increased in HMB-supplemented subjects compared with the unsupplemented group at 2, 4, 5, and 6 weeks of the study. This second part of the study may be of even more significance than the first part in that proteolysis would ordinarily be expected to be higher, with a danger of overtraining, and therefore the anticatabolic effects of HMB would be even more prominent.

Nissen et al. subsequently carried out another study to see if HMB has similar effects in trained subjects.[953] In this 4-week, double-blind study, 3 g of HMB per day in capsules were given in three divided doses to trained and untrained subjects while they participated in an intense weight-training program.

HMB was equally effective for both the previously trained and untrained groups, so results were pooled for HMB supplementation. Overall, HMB increased lean body mass 4.44 lb or 3.1% and decreased body fat by 2.17 lb or 7.3% (both significantly better than control groups). The HMB-supplemented subjects also showed an increase in their bench-press strength of 22 lb, which represents a 37% absolute increase over that of controls; and similar results were found for other exercises.

Although it seems from the available studies that HMB has some influence on protein metabolism, the mechanisms behind any effects are unknown. HMB may be a compound that regulates protein synthesis either through hormonal receptor effects (cortisol, testosterone, GH, IGF-1, insulin) or by modulating the enzymes responsible for muscle tissue breakdown. HMB may have effects on the metabolism of leucine and glutamine and perhaps other anabolic and anticatabolic amino acids, or may decrease gluconeogenesis and the subsequent oxidation of amino acids in the intracellular amino acid pool and catabolism of skeletal muscle cellular protein.

There are several studies in progress involving HMB. At the Federation of American Societies for Experimental Biology (FASEB) annual meeting April 6th to April 9th, six abstracts on HMB were presented.[953a] Three of the studies investigated the effects of HMB supplementation on body composition in females, in the elderly, and in horses. In all studies, supplementation with HMB led to increases in lean-body mass, decreased body fat, and increased strength and stamina. An *in vitro* study investigated the way in which HMB decreases body fat. The authors concluded that HMB increased the utilization of fat, sparing protein and carbohydrates.

The two remaining studies examined the possible synergistic effects of the combined intake of creatine monohydrate and HMB. While the results of these two studies did not reach statistical significance, the results did show some positive changes. Further studies combining these two, perhaps with glutamine or some other compound, using a longer period of supplementation may show changes in lean body mass, body fat, and strength and stamina that are statistically significant.

LYSINE

Low levels (as seen in some vegetarian diets — see above) can slow protein synthesis, affecting muscle and connective tissue. It has an inhibitory effect on viral growth and is used in the treatment of herpes simplex.[996] Information on effects of lysine have been documented in other sections of this book. In this section we will concentrate on the lysine-carnitine connection and the effects of carnitine and acetyl-L-carnitine.

L-CARNITINE

L-carnitine (gamma-trimethylamino-3-hydroxybutyrate), an endogenous compound widely distributed in mammalian tissues, is metabolized from lysine and methionine, although its true point of origin is trimethyllysine. This molecule is either obtained from the diet or is synthesized in the body from L-lysine which is methylated three consecutive times by an S-adenosyl-methionine. Trimethyllysine is transformed into hydroxy-trimethyllysine, then into trimethylaminobutyraldehyde, and finally into trimethylaminobutyrate (or gamma-butyrobetaine). The gamma-butyrobetaine is hydroxylated into carnitine. This reaction chain only functions well when three vitamins — ascorbic acid, pyridoxine, and niacin — are present.[997] Studies on rat have shown that skeletal muscle, heart, intestines, testis, and especially kidneys, insure the transformation of trimethyllysine into gamma-butyrobetaine, but that only the testis, and especially the liver, can hydroxylate gamma-butyrobetaine into carnitine.

However, in the rat the relative importance of the kidneys and liver in total carnitine synthesis has not yet been determined. The situation is the same in humans, although it has been proven that human brain and kidneys, as liver, have gamma-butyrobetaine hydroxylase. It is known that the rate of carnitine synthesis depends on three factors — the amount of trimethyllysine available, the rate of gamma-butyrobetaine transfer to tissue(s) hydroxylating it, and gamma-butyrobetaine hydroxylase activity.[998] Butyrobetaine undergoes hydroxylation in the liver, brain, and kidney to form carnitine, which in turn is transported via the plasma to the heart and skeletal muscle where it is important for allowing beta oxidation of fatty acids. Carnitine is synthesized in liver and kidney, stored in skeletal muscle, and excreted mainly in urine.

Dietary lysine deficiency results in tissue carnitine deficiency.[999-1003] Vitamin C deficiency results in decreased carnitine synthesis in the liver and decreased carnitine levels in heart and skeletal muscle.[1004,1005]

Most of the carnitine needed is ingested by the diet, in particular from meat and dairy products. The rest is biosynthesized. In most cases endogenous synthetic pathways are sufficient to provide adequate amounts of carnitine to meet the needs of the body. However, circulating carnitine levels of strict-vegetarian adults and children, and of infants fed carnitine-free formulas, are significantly lower than normal. In one study, excess amounts of the carnitine precursors lysine plus methionine, epsilon-N-trimethyllysine, or gamma-butyrobetaine were fed as supplements to a low-carnitine diet for 10 days.[1006]

In this study dietary gamma-butyrobetaine dramatically increased carnitine production, epsilon-N-trimethyllysine had a somewhat smaller effect, and lysine plus methionine had even less effect on carnitine synthesis. The authors concluded that carnitine synthesis is not limited by the activity of gamma-butyrobetaine hydroxylase but that carnitine synthesis from exogenous epsilon-N-trimethyllysine is limited either by enzymatic processes that lead to the final intermediate, gamma-butyrobetaine, or by the ability of this substrate to enter tissues capable of carrying out these transformations.

The carnitine acyltransferases (acetyl-, octanoyl-, palmityl-, and possibly others) esterify tissue acyl-CoA to carnitine producing acylcarnitine, which readily passes into mitochondria. Once in the mitochondria the long-chain fatty acids are oxidized and used as an energy substrate for many tissues, and are also metabolized to ketones in the mitochondria of liver cells. The main consequence of carnitine deficiency is impaired energy metabolism.

L-Carnitine is present in plasma, skeletal muscle, and to a lesser extent in other tissues, and is necessary for the transport of long-chain fatty acids across the inner mitochondrial membrane. Besides being necessary for the beta-oxidation of long-chain fatty acids at the mitochondrial level, L-carnitine seems also to have a role in the metabolism of the branched-chain amino acids, in ammonia detoxification, and in urea production.[1007-1009]

One study concluded that carnitine stimulates decarboxylation of branched-chain amino acids by increasing the conversion of their keto analogues into carnitine esters, and that a greater carnitine acyltransferase activity in muscle than in liver may be responsible for the greater carnitine effect in muscle.[1010]

Although carnitine has the ability to be ketogenic,[1011] once formed, ketones are carnitine-independent energy carriers for different tissues. The ketone bodies, beta-hydroxybutyrate and acetoacetate, are known to be useful sources of energy, and also show a glucose-sparing effect.[1012] It has been shown experimentally that oral or parenteral intake of beta-hydroxybutyrate decreases the amount of protein catabolized in obese people on starvation diets.[1013]

The CNS can use only glucose and ketones for its energy requirements. Ketones are products of lipid metabolism and can be readily oxidized in muscle, and in case of glucose deficiency, in the CNS. The two ketones which are biologically important are acetoacetic acid and beta-hydroxybutyric acid. During fasting and/or sustained exercise, once the initial glycogen store is used up by the body the serum glucose must be kept within certain safe limits until the ketones can be formed in adequate amounts. The processes involved in producing sources of energy for the body are all hormonally regulated, with insulin, glucagon, growth hormone, epinephrine, and cortisol involved (see above).

Exercise, fasting, and hypoglycemia increase glucagon, growth hormone, and epinephrine levels. These higher levels stimulate adipose lipase,[1014] which cleaves triglyceride into glycerol and three FFA molecules. This process leads to increased free fatty acid and ketone production, thus sparing the skeletal muscle protein from catabolism. Glucagon, which increases when insulin decreases, causes a rise in hepatic carnitine concentration and thus activates the ketone-forming machinery of the liver. Once activated, the rate of ketone formulation is dependent on, and proportional to, the amount of free fatty acid derived from the breakdown of storage fat.

In rats, plasma and hepatic carnitine deficiencies have been associated with steatosis and retarded growth.[1015,1016] In human infants, systemic carnitine deficiency is characterized by hepatic steatosis, hypoglycemia, and a defect in fasting-induced ketogenesis. In this disorder, hepatic carnitine deficiency leads to a defect in the transport of long-chain fatty acids into the mitochondria, limiting fatty acid oxidation and resulting in increased reesterification of fatty acids to triglyceride. Carnitine deficiency can result in muscle weakness and hypotonia in patients with cystinosis and renal Fanconi syndrome who are carnitine deficient.[1017]

Carnitine deficiencies are common. Currently, these deficiencies are classified into two groups.[1018] In deficiencies with myopathy, only the muscles are deficient in L-carnitine, perhaps as a result of a primary anomaly of the L-carnitine transport system in muscles. In systemic deficiencies, L-carnitine levels are low in the plasma and in all body tissues. Systemic L-carnitine deficiencies are usually the result of a variety of disease states including deficient intake in premature infants or long-term parenteral nutrition, renal failure, organic acidemias, and Reye's syndrome. Modifications in L-carnitine metabolism have also been reported in patients with diabetes mellitus, malignancies, myocardial ischemia, and alcohol abuse.[1019]

Synthetic carnitine is available in oral and parenteral forms and usually used in doses ranging from 100 to 5000 mg daily. Oral carnitine supplementation results in increased plasma and tissue levels of carnitine[1020,1021] and trimethyllysine.[1022] The higher doses of carnitine lead to increased systemic and hepatic carnitine, and may lead to increased ketone production, free fatty acid utilization, and increased adipose tissue breakdown. It is possible that ketones inhibit essential protein catabolism. These facts may be useful to athletes wishing to reduce their weight and fat content and retain maximum muscular size and strength. Utilization of these substances might not increase the rate of weight loss, but might increase the ratio of fat to lean tissue loss.

These compounds might also be useful in reducing muscle breakdown during strenuous prolonged exercise. Thus, the most useful feature of exogenous carnitine and ketones is their postulated ability to increase the production and utilization of free fatty acids and ketones and thus preserve muscle protein while fasting or exercising.

There may be a synergistic effect of L-carnitine and androgens, although no studies have linked effects of carnitine on fat metabolism with the anabolic and lipolytic effects of testosterone. Testosterone injections, however, have been shown to raise some tissue levels of carnitine,[1023] but not that in liver, heart, and skeletal muscle, although testosterone decreases the urinary excretion of carnitine.[1024]

L-Carnitine is used by some athletes because of its supposed antifatigue effect (thus increasing exercise capacity and enhancing performance) and in an attempt to minimize the loss of essential muscle cellular protein during prolonged exercise and in dieting. Although some that feel that there is no evidence supporting the concept that acute administration of carnitine is associated with increased physical performance in athletes,[1025] L-carnitine administration has been shown to (1) increase lipid turnover in working muscles leading to glycogen saving and, as a consequence, allow longer performances for given heavy work loads; and (2) contribute to the homeostasis of free and esterified L-carnitine in plasma and muscle, the feeling being that the levels of one or more of these compounds decrease in the course of heavy repetitive exercise.[1026]

Although exogenous L-carnitine has been shown to be useful in treating carnitine deficiency and the sequelae of this deficiency (such as cardiomyopathy and skeletal muscle pain and weakness[1027-1029]), and in cases of deficient tissue perfusion,[1030] there is limited evidence that it is useful in normal individuals.[1031]

However, since carnitine is an essential cofactor in the catabolism of fats as an energy source, studies have been carried out to see if carnitine loading has effects on plasma and tissue carnitine and on performance. Studies have shown that there is an increased urinary excretion of esterified and total carnitine after physical exercise (due to an increased overflow of short-chain carnitine esters in urine) and that both these potentially unfavorable effects were prevented by oral administration of L-carnitine.[1032]

There are studies that show the possible beneficial effects of L-carnitine on athletic performance[1033-1036] perhaps by stimulating pyruvate dehydrogenase activity, thus diverting pyruvate from lactate to acetylcarnitine formation,[1037,1038] and by allowing a larger quantity of FFA to enter the mitochondria and to be more extensively used as an energy source.[1039] Studies have shown that carnitine may induce an increase of the respiratory chain enzyme activities in muscle, probably by mechanisms involving mitochondrial DNA.[1040]

It is also possible that carnitine may have a hypertrophic effect on skeletal muscle.[1041] In this study the authors investigated the effect of long-term i.v. administration of L-carnitine on human muscle fibers. They found that in patients undergoing hemodialysis, the use of carnitine for 12 months resulted in a marked increase in serum and muscle carnitine levels together with hypertrophy and predominance of type 1 fibers. The authors suggest that carnitine has a specific trophic effect on type 1 fibers which are characterized by an oxidative metabolism.

In one study, running a marathon caused a fall in the plasma content of unesterified carnitine and an increase in the level of acetylcarnitine present.[1042] Loading of the athletes with L-carnitine for 10 days before running a marathon abolished the exercise-induced fall in plasma-free carnitine while amplifying the production of acetylcarnitine. However, in this study carnitine loading of the athletes made no detectable improvement in performance of the marathon.

A recent study examined the effect of diet supplementation of oxaloacetate precursors (aspartate and asparagine) and carnitine on muscle metabolism and exercise endurance in rats.[1043] The results suggest that the diet supplementation increased the capacity of the muscle to utilize FFA and spare glycogen. Time to exhaustion was about 40% longer in the experimental group compared to the control, which received a commercial diet only. These findings suggest that oxaloacetate may be important to determine the time to exhaustion during a prolonged and moderate exercise.

Hyperammonia has been shown to alter lipid metabolism and decrease body fat content in rats.[1044] However, ammonia can be toxic. L-carnitine and its analogues such as acetyl-L-carnitine, however, have been reported to have protective effects against ammonia toxicity.[1045] Studies are needed to explore the possible anabolic potential of the ammonia and L-carnitine/ALCAR interaction.

Thus, while some studies have pointed to the possible ergogenic effects of carnitine, other studies have found that L-carnitine supplementation does not seem to enhance athletic performance.[1046,1047] The different findings may be due to the dose and length of carnitine supplementation since the effects of L-carnitine seem to be dependent on these two factors.

Carnitine, however, might have more to offer athletes under certain conditions. In one study, ten moderately trained male subjects were submitted to two bouts of maximal cycle ergometer exercise separated by a 3-day interval.[1048] Each subject was randomly given either L-carnitine (2 g) or placebo orally 1 h before the beginning of each exercise session. At rest, L-carnitine supplementation resulted in an increase of plasma-free carnitine without a change in acid-soluble carnitine esters. Treatment with L-carnitine induced a significant postexercise decrease of plasma lactate and pyruvate and a concurrent increase of acetylcarnitine.

Carnitine might be an effective supplement in high-fat, high-protein diets. Certainly, carnitine appears to be an important nutrient for newborns whose main energy fuel is constituted by fat (colostrum is particularly rich in carnitine).[1049] As well, it has been shown that carnitine excretion increases on a high-fat diet.[1050]

While on a high-fat, low-carbohydrate diet the skeletal muscles use lipids for energy during rest and exercise. Activated fatty acids are transferred across muscle mitochondrial membranes by esterification with carnitine. Several transferase enzymes, including carnitine palmityltransferase, release the fatty acids in the mitochondria, where they then undergo β-oxidation.

Endogenous carnitine levels may be enhanced to some extent by the use of the AAs lysine and methionine (see above), and the use of some of the essential nutrients involved in carnitine synthesis such as iron and vitamins C, B_6, and niacin.

ACETYL-L-CARNITINE

When L-carnitine is introduced in the body an increase in the level of acetylcarnitine (acetyl-L-carnitine, ALC, ALCAR), the acetyl ester of carnitine also occurs. However, despite this biochemical connection, acetylcarnitine seems to have some powerful, beneficial properties of its own. ALCAR has shown protective effects in brain,[1051] myocardial[1052] and tissue ischemia,[1053] positive effects on aspects of aging (especially in the brain)[1054-1056] and its ability to lower cholesterol levels that rise as a result of age.[1057]

Systemic administration of ALCAR in a dose-dependent manner stimulates acetylcholine (ACh) release in the striatum and hippocampus of freely moving rats, suggesting that the increase in ACh release is the result of ALCAR activation of a physiological mechanism in cholinergic neurons.[1058]

The findings of one study confirmed the multiple effects of acetyl-L-carnitine in brain, and suggest that its administration can have a positive effect on age-related changes in the dopaminergic system.[1059] In this study, long-term acetyl-L-carnitine treatment had significant effects on age-related changes in striatal dopamine receptors and brain amino acid levels. Another study found that ALCAR, when administered intracerebrally at fairly high concentrations, can affect the level and the release not only of such neurotransmitters as acetylcholine and dopamine, but also of amino acids.[1060]

Other studies have documented the neuroprotective effects of acetyl-L-carnitine (ALCAR), its effects on metabolites involved in energy and phospholipid metabolism, and the possible therapeutic effects on neurodegenerative diseases such as Alzheimer's.[1061] The results of one study suggest that treatment with ALCAR is responsible for a reduction in brain glycolytic flow and for enhancing the utilization of alternative energy sources, such as lipid substrates or ketone bodies.[1062]

Studies have also shown that ALCAR has antioxidant actions that decrease free radical-mediated, site-specific protein oxidation implicated in the pathophysiology of ischemia/reperfusion brain injury. The results of one study indicate that brain protein oxidation does occur in a clinically relevant model of complete global cerebral ischemia and reperfusion, and that oxidation is inhibited under treatment conditions that improve neurological outcome.[1063]

ALCAR has been considered of potential use in senile dementia of the Alzheimer type because of its ability to serve as a precursor for acetylcholine.[1064] However, pharmacological studies with ALCAR in animals have demonstrated its facility to maximize energy production and promote cellular membrane stability, particularly its ability to restore membranal changes that are age related.

Since recent investigations have implicated abnormal energy processing, leading to cell death and severity-dependent membrane disruption in the pathology of Alzheimer's disease,[1065] the beneficial effects associated with ALCAR administration in Alzheimer patients may be due not only to its cholinergic properties, but also to its ability to support physiological cellular functioning at the mitochondrial level. This hypothetical mechanism of action is discussed in one study with respect to compelling supportive animal studies and recent observations of a significant decrease of carnitine acetyltransferase (the catalyst of L-carnitine acylation to acetyl-L-carnitine) in autopsied Alzheimer brains.[1066]

ALCAR has a protective effect in brain,[1067-1069] myocardial,[1070] and tissue ischemia. In one study it was found in animals that L-acetylcarnitine markedly enhances functional muscle reinnervation, which in this study was unaffected by L-carnitine.[1071] In another study by the same principal author, L-acetylcarnitine was shown to markedly favor the process of reinnervation of the oculomotor nerve sectioned at the intracranial level in guinea pigs.[1072] Acetyl-L-carnitine produces a significant increase in the survival time-course of adult rat sensory neurons maintained in primary cultures up to 40 days and thus might be involved in reducing neuronal loss observed in nervous system aging.[1073]

Aging results in a decrease of carnitine content in muscle of mice and humans.[1074] Analyses of muscle samples of healthy humans of different ages showed a drastic reduction of carnitine and acetylcarnitine in the older subjects, with a strong reverse correlation between age and carnitine levels. Acetylcarnitine lowers free and esterified cholesterol and arachidonic acid levels in the plasma often seen with aging.[1075] As well, it is possible that acetylcarnitine has antidepressant effects.[1076,1077]

A study set up to examine the effects of L-carnitine and acetyl-L-carnitine in rats and mice with experimental alloxan diabetes found that acetyl-L-carnitine may be more effective against diabetes in increasing glucose tolerance, restoring the impaired response of glucagon to glucose, and showing glycogen-sparing action than is L-carnitine.[1078]

Besides the above effects, ALCAR has several other properties that are of interest to athletes. With increasing work intensity the level of carnitine in muscle decreases and that of acetylcarnitine increases.[1079-1081] The results of these studies indicate that acetylcarnitine is a major metabolite formed during intense muscular effort and that carnitine functions in the regulation of the intramitochondrial acetyl-CoA/CoA ratio by buffering excess production of acetyl units. Modulating the rise in intramitochondrial acetyl-CoA/CoA ratio relieves the inhibition of many intramitochondrial enzymes involving glucose and amino acid catabolism.[1082]

The use of ALCAR may have implications in the recovery from training and injuries in that it has beneficial effects on spontaneous and induced lipoperoxidation in rat skeletal muscle,[1083] and accelerates the disappearance of DNA single-strand breaks induced by oxygen radicals and alkylating agents.[1084]

As well, acetylcarnitine seems to have an effect on the hypothalamic-pituitary-testicular axis. Studies have shown that ALCAR (like the BCAA — see above) prevented the decrease in plasma testosterone levels after chronic exercise stress such as swimming,[1085] and that ALCAR stimulates testosterone production.[1086] It may also have a protective effect on selected body tissues, including skeletal muscle.[1087]

METHIONINE

Methionine and cysteine are the principal sources of sulfur in our diets. The body can make cysteine from methionine but not vice versa, so methionine is the dietary essential.

Methionine has many functions in the body and the metabolic consequences of methionine deficiency are many and varied. The multifunctional role of methionine includes its participation in methyl-group metabolism, the synthesis of carnitine, creatine, glutathione, nucleic acids, polyamines, and catecholamines, as well as serving as a substrate for protein synthesis.

Methionine deficiency has been shown to adversely affect serum cholesterol levels. In one study, very-low-density lipoprotein (VLDL) plus LDL susceptibility to peroxidation was higher in rats fed soy protein than in casein-fed rats, which could reflect in part the lack of sulfur amino acid availability, since methionine supplementation led to a partial recovery of lipoprotein resistance to peroxidation.[1088] These findings suggest that amino acid imbalance could be atherogenic by increasing circulating cholesterol and leading to a higher lipoprotein susceptibility to peroxidation.

Ethanol fed to rats alters methionine metabolism by decreasing the activity of methionine synthetase.[1089] This is the enzyme that converts homocysteine in the presence of vitamin B_{12} and N-5-methyltetrahydrofolate to methionine. Methionine may mitigate some of the harmful hepatic effects of alcohol.

A deficiency of choline and methionine produces hepatic steatosis similar to that seen with ethanol, and supplementation with these lipotropes can prevent ethanol-induced fatty liver.[1090] Dietary deficiency of methionine in rats results in a fatty liver which can be cured by restoring this amino acid to the diet, or alternatively by giving the choline which the body would normally form from it, or by giving betaine, another methyl donor.[1091]

Methionine, among its other roles, is also concerned with the important process of transmethylation and provides methyl groups (methyl donors) for the synthesis of choline, which contains three such groups in each molecule. The chief dietary sources of methyl groups appear to be methionine and betaine. Methionine gives up the terminal CH_3 group attached to its sulfur atom.

Methionine has a high intracellular turnover because it is involved in the initiation of peptide synthesis and in a variety of transmethylation and transsulfuration reactions.[1092,1093] Methionine may be the endogenous amino acid that is most limiting for maintenance of body protein and nitrogen balance and for effective reutilization of other amino acids.[1094,1095] Since methionine is a nutritionally indispensable amino acid, its continued availability in free amino acid tissue pools is important for maintaining an anabolic drive for protein synthesis[1096] under conditions of greater protein turnover.

Methionine deficiency has been shown to decrease protein synthesis while its reintroduction increases protein synthesis. In one study, small amounts of methionine, along with threonine, significantly reduced nitrogen excretion in rats fed a protein-free diet.[1097]

Much of the work involving the need for methionine in protein synthesis has been done with burn and trauma patients. Major trauma, including thermal injury of the skin, results in a profound loss of body nitrogen, altered rates of whole-body protein synthesis and breakdown, and increased nitrogen and amino acid requirements relative to those in normal, nonstressed individuals.[1098,1099] However, the *in vivo* mechanisms responsible for the altered nitrogen economy of the host and their relationship to the metabolism of specific nutritionally indispensable (essential) and dispensable (nonessential) amino acids are not fully defined.[1100]

The fluxes of the major components of the methionine cycle *in vivo* include transmethylation (Tm), homocysteine remethylation (Rm) (recycling of homocysteine), oxidation or transsulfuration (C), the disposal of methionine via nonoxidative pathways (assumed to be protein synthesis (S) and its appearance via protein breakdown (B)).

A recent study explored quantitative aspects of methionine metabolism in patients recovering from severe burn injury.[1101] In this study, radiolabeled methionine was given by continuous intravenous infusion to 12 adult patients. Each of the adults was studied in the fasted and in the fed state while receiving parenteral nutrition. Compared with findings obtained in other studies in healthy adults using a similar protocol,[1102,1103] the rates of transmethylation (Tm), homocysteine remethylation (Rm), and methionine oxidation (C) were all substantially increased in burn patients. From the relationships between these systems, it appears that there is a relative increase in the recycling of methionine carbon via Rm during the fasted state.

This increased recycling of methionine via Rm of homocysteine would promote the availability of S-adenosyl methionine, required in numerous Tm reactions within the body.[1104] Thus, because methionine is the major methyl-donor, and the increased rates of Rm and Tm indicate a high level of methyl group transfer and utilization in these patients, it seems likely that the synthesis rates of polyamines, choline, creatinine, and carnitine are increased.[1105-1107] In this context, the polyamines are involved in normal growth and cell proliferation, and a higher turnover of these amines might well be expected where there is active and extensive tissue repair.[1108]

Increased requirements of carnitine have also been claimed in traumatized patients,[1109] and the methylation of DNA is important for the production of acute-phase proteins and other proteins involved in renewal of tissues.[1110] Finally, the methionine-homocysteine cycle is also connected with the *de novo* synthesis of a wide range of dispensable amino acids, including glutamate, glycine, serine, and histidine.[1111] The increased activity of the methionine cycle therefore is probably causally linked to the enhanced metabolic requirements indicated above, and also, perhaps, to the higher rates of utilization and catabolism of these nutritionally dispensable amino acids and of histidine in traumatized patients.[1112]

For these reasons, the methionine cycle would appear to play an important metabolic role in response to burn injury. However, despite the increased activity of the cycle, it appears to be linked with a relative reduction in the fraction of homocysteine entering the transsulfuration pathway, leading to the formation of cysteine. Perhaps the need to maintain high rates of methyl transfer reactions is of greater priority than is the synthesis of cysteine. Optimum body function and maintenance of protein homeostasis therefore may require an exogenous supply of cysteine for these patients.

In summary, this investigation has shown that methionine kinetics are profoundly altered by burn injury and that the nutritional requirements for sulfur-containing amino acids are significantly increased. This increase is, in part, caused by or associated with enhanced activity of methyl transfer reactions within the body. This leads to increased rates of homocysteine formation and the question arises whether an exogenous supply of cysteine might further reduce the degradation of homocysteine via the transsulfuration pathway and potentially promote whole-body protein synthesis and the maintenance of sulfur amino acid homeostasis in these patients.

Clearly, additional tracer studies are needed to explore the metabolic and nutritional importance of methionine-cysteine interrelationships in burn and trauma patients and, for our purposes, in athletes secondary to intense and prolonged exercise.

Methionine is also essential for the formation of creatine.

CREATINE MONOHYDRATE

Creatine is an amino acid derivative that is obtained from food (especially red meat — 2 lb of steak has about 4 g of creatine) and is also formed in the liver from the amino acids arginine, glycine, and methionine. Creatine is then taken up by skeletal muscle where it forms phosphocreatine, the high-energy phosphate compound. In humans, over 95% of the total creatine content is located in skeletal muscle, of which approximately a third is in its free form. The remainder is present in a phosphorylated form.

Phosphocreatine serves as a backup source of energy for ATP, the immediate source of energy for muscular contraction. The amount of phosphocreatine in skeletal muscle partially determines the length of time that maximum muscle work can be done. Once the phosphocreatine is gone, ATP must be regenerated through the metabolism of substrates such as glycogen, glucose, fatty acids, ketones, and amino acids.

While the building blocks of ATP can be recycled, creatine cannot due to the reactivity of the phosphoguanidine group in which the carboxyl group displaces the phosphate. The resultant cyclic compound is creatinine, which is excreted in the urine. A dramatic increase in muscle use as in high-intensity training for bodybuilding results in an increase in creatine phosphate breakdown, an increase in creatinine excretion, and an increased synthesis of creatine from the AAs arginine, glycine, and methionine.

Creatine, Phosphocreatine, and Creatinine Metabolism

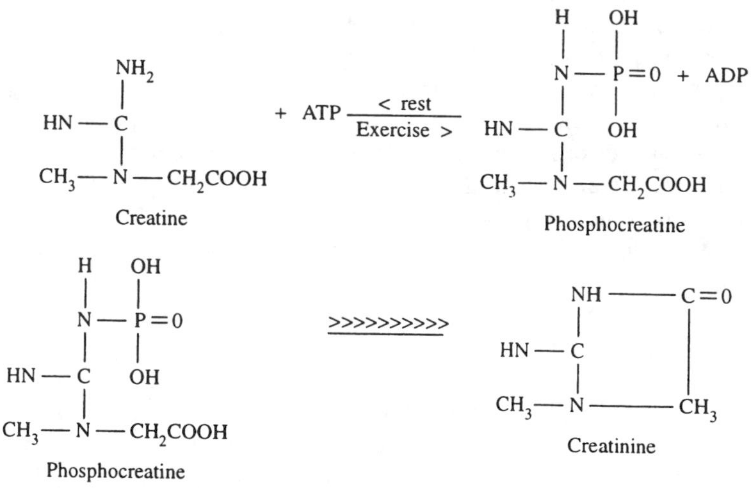

NH_2 | HN — C | CH_3 — N — CH_2COOH (Creatine) + ATP $\underset{\text{Exercise} >}{\overset{< \text{rest}}{\rightleftharpoons}}$ H, OH | N — P=O + ADP | HN — C, OH | CH_3 — N — CH_2COOH (Phosphocreatine)

Creatine

Phosphocreatine

H, OH | N — P=O | HN — C, OH | CH_3 — N — CH_2COOH >>>>>>>>>> NH —— C=O | HN — C | CH_3 — N —— CH_3

Phosphocreatine

Creatinine

It's believed that of the many causes of fatigue, one of the more important is the decrease in phosphocreatine in muscle. In the past, creatine supplements have been used by some athletes to try to increase phosphocreatine in muscle and thus increase the intensity and the length of muscular contraction during short-term, high-intensity work. Lately, use of creatine monohydrate (CM) has risen dramatically, as have the advertised claims for it.

The observation that increased muscular activity leads to muscle hypertrophy is well known and many studies have attempted to identify the biochemical and physiological mechanisms by which this occurs. Some of these studies looked into the possibility that creatine may be the chemical signal coupling increased muscular activity and increased contractile mass. In the past, two muscle models have been used in experimental tests of this hypothesis: differentiating skeletal muscle cells in culture and the fetal mouse heart in organ culture. Using these culture models, it is possible to alter the intracellular creatine concentration and to measure the effect of increased creatine concentrations on the rates of synthesis and accumulation of both muscle-specific and nonspecific proteins. The results show that muscle-specific protein synthesis in both skeletal and cardiac muscle is selectively stimulated by creatine.[1113]

CREATINE SUPPLEMENTATION

A century ago, studies with creatine feeding concluded that some of the ingested creatine was retained in the body.[1114] Recent research has shown that oral creatine supplements not only increase creatine content in muscle (the increase is greatest in exercised muscles)[1115] but delays fatigue,[1116] improves recovery (by increasing the rate of phosphocreatine resynthesis in muscle),[1117] and increases muscle torque during repeated bouts of maximal voluntary exercise.[1118]

Other studies have shown that oral creatine supplements increase both power output and the total amount of short-term work,[1119] and enhance single and repeated short sprint performance.[1120] Creatine may also independently result in increased body mass,[1121] although much of this increase seen in the first few weeks may be due to increased water retention.

A recent study investigated the effect of carbohydrate (CHO) ingestion on skeletal muscle creatine (Cr) accumulation during Cr supplementation in humans.[1122] Creatine supplementation had no effect on serum insulin concentration, but Cr and CHO ingestion dramatically elevated insulin concentration. These findings demonstrate that CHO ingestion substantially augments muscle Cr accumulation during Cr feeding in humans, which appears to be insulin mediated.

The results of an unpublished study (presented May 30, 1997 at the American College of Sports Medicine Annual Meeting), indicate that ingestion of creatine with glucose, taurine and electrolytes during training promotes greater gains in upper extremity lifting volume and sprint capacity as compared to glucose, taurine and electrolytes ingestion alone.[591]

Another recent study concluded that in competitive rowers, a 5-day period of creatine supplementation was effective in raising whole-body creatine stores, the magnitude of which provided a positive though statistically nonsignificant relationship with a 1000-m rowing performance.[1123] This study investigated the change in a 1000-m simulated rowing performance in 2 matched groups of 19 competitive rowers following a 5-day period of supplementation with placebo (CON group) or creatine at a dose equivalent to 0.25 g creatine monohydrate per kilogram of body mass (BM) (EXP group). Creatine uptake was calculated from the difference between the amount fed and the amount recovered in urine during each 24-h period of supplementation. After supplementation with placebo, the CON group showed no change in 1000-m rowing performance; of these subjects, 7 decreased and 10 increased their performance times. By contrast, 16 of the 19 subjects in the EXP group improved their performance times. The mean improvement in rowing performance for the EXP group was just over 1%.

The results of another study suggest improvements in performance secondary to creatine monohydrate use were mediated via improved ATP resynthesis as a consequence of increased PCr availability in type II fibers.[1124] In this study 9 male subjects performed 2 bouts of 30-s maximal isokinetic cycling, before and after ingestion of 20 g creatine monohydrate (Cr) per day for 5 days. Cr ingestion produced a 23.1 ± 4.7 mmol/kg dry matter increase in the muscle total creatine (TCr) concentration. Total work production during bouts 1 and 2 increased by 4% and the cumulative increases in both peak and total work production over the 2 exercise bouts were positively correlated with the increase in muscle TCr. Cumulative loss of ATP was 30.7 ± 12.2% after Cr ingestion, despite the increase in work production. Resting phosphocreatine (PCr) increased in type I and II fibers. Changes in PCr prior to exercise bouts 1 and 2 in type II fibers were positively correlated with changes in PCr degradation during exercise in this fiber type and changes in total work production.

On the other hand, some studies have not shown any ergogenic effects from creatine supplementation.[1125] A recent study concluded that a 4-day period of Cr supplementation failed to significantly raise resting muscle creatine, or that multiple sprint performance was not enhanced by increases in resting muscle creatine.[1126] In this study the influence of oral creatine monohydrate supplementation on repeated 10-s-cycle ergometer sprint performance was examined and 17 recreationally active males participated in the 16-day experiment. All subjects initially completed a VO_2 peak test and were then administered glucose (4 × 10 g/d) in a single-blind fashion for 4 days, after which they completed the first series of multiple sprints (7 × 10 s). For the following four days, diets were supplemented with either Cr (4 × 70 $mg.kg^{-1}$ body mass per day mixed with 5 g glucose) or glucose (4 × 10 g/d); supplementation during this phase was double-blind. Subjects then repeated the multiple sprint and VO_2 peak tests. Measures of peak power output (PPO), mean power output (MPO), end-power output (EPO), and percent power decline were recorded during the sprints. Analysis of variance revealed that 4 days of Cr supplementation did not influence multiple sprint performance, plasma lactate, blood pH, and excess postsprint oxygen consumption. Furthermore, VO_2 peak was unchanged following Cr supplementation.

There are reproducible and consistent data showing that CM supplementation increases lean body mass and strength. By increasing the PC in muscle, more energy is available for contraction, decreasing the need for anaerobic and aerobic mechanisms (such as hepatic gluconeogenesis and oxidation of AA) as well as possibly increasing the available intracellular energy, leading to an increase in protein synthesis and a decrease in protein catabolism. Under normal conditions muscle contraction places such a demand on ATP and PC that there is insufficient amounts available for active protein synthesis at the same time that muscle contractions are occurring.

One caveat — don't use caffeine if you use creatine monohydrate. A new study has shown that the use of caffeine negates the ergogenic effects of creatine monohydrate. This may explain why creatine supplementation doesn't seem to work for some athletes.[1127]

PHENYLALANINE

Phenylalanine is the major precursor of tyrosine. While the body can convert phenylalanine to tyrosine, it cannot convert tyrosine to phenylalanine. Tyrosine is the parent compound for the manufacture of the hormones norepinephrine and epinephrine by the adrenal medulla and thyroxine and triiodothyronine by the thyroid gland. Also, the pigment melanin which occurs in the skin, hair, and choroid lining of the eye forms from the enzymatic conversion of tyrosine.

Those individuals not able to convert phenylalanine to tyrosine due to a hereditary lack of phenylalanine hydroxylase, suffer from the inborn error of metabolism known as phenylketonuria.

THREONINE

Threonine is generally low in vegetarians (see above). Lack of threonine in high-protein diets may compromise protein synthesis (see above).

TRYPTOPHAN

Serotonin, an important neurotransmitter of the brain, forms from tryptophan. The plasma tryptophan ratio has been shown to determine brain tryptophan levels and, thereby, to affect the synthesis and release of the neurotransmitter serotonin.

In a review on the effects of tryptophan on serotonin[1128] the authors summarize evidence showing that: (1) the synthesis of serotonin in the brain depends directly on the amount of tryptophan available to it from the circulation; (2) tryptophan uptake into brain depends on the blood levels not only of tryptophan, but also of other aromatic and branched-chain amino acids that compete with tryptophan for a common transport carrier into brain; and (3) dietary factors that influence the blood levels of tryptophan and these other amino acids can modify tryptophan uptake into brain, and consequently the rate of serotonin formation. Additionally, data are reviewed that attempt to show that appetite for protein and/or carbohydrates is dependent on the relationship between food intake, plasma amino acid pattern, brain tryptophan uptake, and serotonin synthesis.

As we have seen, the essential amino acid tryptophan is the precursor for serotonin, which is in turn an intermediary product in the synthesis of melatonin.[1129,1130] A dose-dependent rise of circulating melatonin has been observed after L-tryptophan infusions.[1131] Studies have also shown that reduced plasma tryptophan levels, and presumably brain serotonin concentrations, decrease nocturnal melatonin secretion in humans.[1132,1133]

Niacin is the generic term for nicotinic acid (pyridine-3-carboxylic acid) and derivatives that exhibit the nutritional activity of nicotinic acid. In one sense, niacin is not a vitamin, since it can be formed from the essential amino acid tryptophan. In the human, an average of about 1 mg of niacin is formed from 60 mg of dietary tryptophan.

L-Tryptophan has a small but significant effect on growth hormone secretion[1134] and may significantly increase athletic performance. In 1988 Segura and Ventura[1135] reported that 1.2 g of L-tryptophan supplementation, because of its effect on the endogenous opioid systems and pain tolerance, increased total exercise time by 49.4% when the subjects were running at 80% of maximal oxygen uptake (VO_2max). A more recent study failed to repeat these results and found that oral L-tryptophan supplementation does not enhance running performance.[1136]

In the more recent study, 49 well-trained male runners aged 18 to 44 participated in a randomized double-blind placebo study. Each subject underwent four trials on the treadmill. The first two served as a learning experience, including measurement of VO_2max and anaerobic threshold. During the last two trials the subjects ran until exhaustion at a speed corresponding to 100% of their $V^{\circ}VO_2max$ — first in an initial trial and then after receiving a total of 1.2 g L-tryptophan or a placebo over a 24-h period prior to the run. No significant difference between the improvements in the L-tryptophan and placebo group could be demonstrated.

The use of L-tryptophan increased dramatically in the 1980s, mainly because it is useful in treating insomnia and PMS.[1137,1138] Athletes also use it to increase their growth hormone levels (see above). The free form of L-tryptophan, because of its possible association with eosinophilia-myalgia syndrome (EMS), is no longer available in North America and athletes have been warned not to use it.[1139]

The L-tryptophan scare began in late 1989, when FDA officials ordered products containing large doses of the amino acid health supplement off the shelves, citing a link with EMS.[1140,1141] In March, 1990 the FDA recalled all products containing any dosage of the supplement after several cases of the disease were reported in people who had taken relatively small amounts of L-tryptophan. By the time the product was recalled, more than 1500 cases of EMS had been reported in the U.S., with 21 deaths confirmed.[1142-1144]

EMS is a painful and occasionally life-threatening condition associated with ingestion of the nutritional supplement L-tryptophan.[1145-1149] The syndrome is characterized by eosinophilia and generalized severe myalgias, and a variety of neurologic, psychiatric, cutaneous, and pulmonary features, with significant long term sequelae.[1150-1152] The chronic, often worsening pattern of illness seen in EMS suggests an ongoing pathogenetic mechanism.[1153]

The exact cause of EMS has not as yet been identified,[1154] although contaminants formed during the process of purifying L-tryptophan are suspected and may have been isolated.[1155-1157] However, the continuing occurrence of EMS, in light of the ban on the sale of the free form of L-tryptophan and its availability only by prescription, brings causal interpretations of earlier studies into question.[1158] As well, a case has been described in someone who developed EMS in 1986 without the ingestion of any nutritional supplements.[1159]

The authors of a recent review examined the methodology of the epidemiological studies of the association between L-tryptophan and EMS and evaluated the validity of the conclusions from these studies.[1160] They found that the studies showing a L-tryptophan-EMS association had important methodological inadequacies. Subsequent studies of a brand of L-tryptophan also contained errors in design, which may have produced biased results and call the conclusions into question. The authors concluded that the cause of eosinophilia-myalgia syndrome remains unknown.

Chapter 8

CONDITIONALLY ESSENTIAL AMINO ACIDS

INTRODUCTION

Several amino acids are considered conditionally essential as they are rate limiting for protein synthesis under certain conditions. Individual amino acids are often described as conditionally essential, based on requirements for optimal growth and maintenance of a positive nitrogen balance. While in extreme circumstances, such as in the absence of certain nonessential amino acids from the diet and the presence of limited amounts of essential amino acids from which to synthesize the nonessential amino acids, any of the amino acids might be considered conditionally essential including arginine, citrulline, ornithine, proline, cysteine, tyrosine, histidine, taurine etc.[1161-1165] However, practically, only seven other amino acids can be considered essential under certain conditions.

Amino acids can be considered to be conditionally essential (dispensable) based on the body's inability to actually synthesize them from other amino acids under certain conditions. By this criterion, the following seven amino acids are conditionally essential in humans:

Arginine
Cysteine, Cystine
Glutamine
Histidine
Proline
Taurine
Tyrosine

ARGININE

Arginine, normally a nonessential amino acid in humans (but essential in some other species such as the rat), is considered essential under certain conditions.[1166] Several studies have pointed to the essential nature of arginine in a variety of catabolic conditions including surgery and trauma and in conditions where growth is accelerated.[1167-1169]

Arginine has a significant role in nitrogen detoxification and has been shown to be beneficial in various diseases including liver and other diseases in which ammonia levels are extremely high.[1170] In the urea cycle, ammonia is converted to urea and is subsequently excreted in the urine (see above).

Arginine also has effects on the immune system, on cancer, and on stressful situations such as surgery, burns and infection.[1171-1175] Impaired host immunity is associated with neoplasia, protein calorie malnutrition, and the administration of immunosuppressive drugs. Arginine appears to enhance immune function in both animals and humans. Peripheral blood lymphocytes from healthy human males have demonstrated *in vitro* an increased activity of natural killer cells and lymphokine-activated killer cells with increasing concentrations of arginine.[1176]

It is well accepted that protein calorie malnutrition impairs host immunity, with particularly detrimental effects on the T-cell system, resulting in increased opportunistic infection and increased morbidity and mortality in hospitalized patients. Arginine has been demonstrated to be essential to the traumatized host and may have tissue-specific properties which influence components of the immune system. Thus, arginine may be of value in clinical situations where the immune system is compromised. In a series of experiments in normal animals, arginine was demonstrated to enhance cellular immune mechanisms, in particular, T-cell function.[1177] It also has a marked immunopreserving effect in the face of immunosuppression induced by protein malnutrition and increases in tumor burden.

In postoperative surgical patients, arginine supplementation results in enhanced T-lymphocyte response and augmented T-helper cell numbers, with a rapid return to normal of T-cell function postoperatively compared with control patients. These data suggest that arginine supplementation may enhance or preserve immune function in high-risk surgical patients and theoretically improve the host's capacity to resist infection.[1178] Because of its effects on the immune system, arginine might be useful for enhancing the anabolic effects of exercise by improving training and recovery, immunologic responses, and modulating any immunologic depression secondary to intense exercise.

Supplemental parenteral or enteral arginine has been shown to stimulate secretion of growth hormone, insulin, and prolactin in humans.[1179-1183] Several supplement studies have shown both arginine and ornithine promote growth hormone and insulin secretion with anabolic effects in postoperative patients.[1184] In one study an oral administration of arginine resulted in an anabolic state mediated by insulin.[1185] Changes included decreases in serum leucine and isoleucine concentrations, reductions in serum glucose and free fatty acid contents, and a rapid increase in serum insulin level.

Arginine, along with lysine, has recently been shown to be effective orally in increasing GH levels.[1185a] In this study, 16 men completed 4 trials at random as follows: (Trial A) performance of a single bout of resistance exercise preceded by placebo ingestion (vitamin C); (Trial B) ingestion of 1,500 mg L-arginine and 1,500 mg L-lysine, immediately followed by exercise as in Trial A; (Trial C) ingestion of amino acids as in Trial B and no exercise; (Trial D) placebo ingestion and no exercise. GH concentrations were higher at 30, 60, and 90 min during the exercise trials (A and B) compared with the resting trials (C and D). However, no differences were noted in GH between the exercise trials. GH was significantly elevated during resting conditions 60 min after amino acid ingestion compared with the placebo trial. The authors concluded that ingestion of 1,500 mg arginine and 1,500 mg lysine immediately before resistance exercise does not alter exercise-induced changes in GH in young men. However, when the same amino acid mixture is ingested under basal conditions, the acute secretion of GH is increased.

Because arginine potentiates the release of several pituitary hormones, it can be hypothesized that the beneficial effects of pharmacological doses of the amino acid on protein synthesis, wound healing, and immune function may be mediated via a pituitary messenger such as growth hormone.

Arginine is also a precursor of creatine phosphate, one of the most important sources of cellular energy. One study has shown that muscle creatine content was significantly increased by arginine supplementation (along with glycine).[1186] In this study, supplementing a 25% casein-based diet with arginine and glycine significantly improved apparent nitrogen retention both in untraumatized as well as in traumatized rats.

Dietary intervention with L-arginine has resulted in amelioration of a number of experimental kidney diseases, such as those caused by subtotal nephrectomy, diabetic nephropathy, cyclosporin A administration, salt-sensitive hypertension, ureteral obstruction, puromycin aminonucleoside nephrosis, kidney hypertrophy due to high-protein feeding, glomerular thrombosis due to administration of lipopolysaccharide, and cytokine-mediated renal disease.[1187] A recent review has addressed the current evidence for these beneficial effects and describes the basis for the concept of L-arginine deficiency (absolute or relative) in certain settings in which supplementation of the diet with this amino acid may be beneficial.[1188]

In this review, the authors point out the important metabolic contributions arginine makes, not only to protein synthesis in cells and tissues, but also to the synthesis of urea, nitric oxide, creatine, creatinine, orotic acid, and agmatine, and its influence in hormonal release and the synthesis of pyrimidine bases. This places L-arginine and its precursors and its metabolites at the center of the interaction of different metabolic pathways and interorgan communication. Thus L-arginine participates in changing the internal environment in different but simultaneous ways ranging from disposal of protein metabolic waste, muscle metabolism, vascular regulation, immune system function, and neurotransmission, to RNA synthesis and hormone-mediated regulation of the internal milieu.

Recent research has shown that arginine is involved in nitric oxide production.[1189,1190] Few discoveries have had as comprehensive an impact on the understanding of cellular physiology as the production of nitric oxide (NO) from the terminal guanido amino group of L-arginine through nitric oxide synthases. Because of the sheer volume of data presently coming forth on the physiology and pathophysiology of NO, a full review is beyond the scope of this book.

How changes in the concentration of L-arginine influence the initiation, development, and resolution of the processes affected by nitric oxide is largely unknown. So far, it seems that increased ingestion of this amino acid reverses the changes in vascular reactivity and reduces intimal thickness in atherosclerosis, and may also reduce blood pressure and the excessive proliferation of smooth-muscle cells in hypertension.[1191]

NO functions as a regulator of blood pressure, as a powerful cytocide released by white blood cells to kill bacteria and tumor cells, and as a messenger molecule in the brain; it is involved with, among other things, memory and thought processes,[1192] regulation of inflammation and the immune system,[1193] and in many other processes in the body.[1194]

In normal rats, inhibition of the nitric oxide pathway results in systemic hypertension and decreased glomerular filtration rate and effective renal plasma flow. If the inhibition of this pathway is sustained, then glomerulosclerosis and death from uremia follow.[1195]

A recent study in rabbits has shown that L-arginine, the precursor of endothelium-derived relaxing factor (EDRF), decreases atherosclerosis in hypercholesterolemic animals.[1196] Similar results have been reported in studies done on humans when examining the effects of arginine on coronary artery disease.[1197]

Recently it has been shown that the L-arginine-nitric oxide pathway is responsible for the relaxation of the corpus cavernosum and thus the development of penile erections in humans, and is probably the final common mediator of penile erection.[1198,1199] Another recent study has shown that although dihydrotestosterone is the active androgen in the prevention of erectile failure seen in castrated rats, this effect may be mediated, at least partially, by changes in nitric oxide synthase levels in the penis.[1200]

ARGININE AND THE ATHLETE

Arginine has several important biological effects including the ability to stimulate insulin and GH secretion, leading to anabolic and anticatabolic effects on skeletal muscle. As well, nitric oxide may be required for the protein synthesis (growth hormone-like) response of muscle to IGF-1, and thus may further enhance the anabolic effects of exercise.[1201] Another study has found a role for nitric oxide on the neurochemical mechanisms elicited by corticosterone.[1202]

Although most studies on the effects of arginine administer it parenterally, arginine is also effective orally. The liver possesses high arginase activity as an intrinsic part of urea synthesis and would consume most of the portal supply of dietary arginine. The gut reduces this possibility by converting dietary arginine to citrulline, which effectively bypasses the liver and is resynthesized to arginine in the kidney.

Anabolic steroids have been shown to induce changes in behavior of the nitric oxide dilator system.[1203] Arginine treatment also prevents the development of hypertension in animals prone to this disease and also causes a rapid reduction in systolic and diastolic pressures when infused into healthy humans and patients with essential hypertension.[1204] It's possible that hypertension[1205] and hypercholesterolemia,[1206] both side effects of chronic anabolic steroid abuse, are also associated with abnormalities in the nitric oxide pathway. Arginine may offer some corrective or protective effects in those athletes using drugs.

Arginine has potent modulating effects on the immune system. Several studies have found that arginine, either alone or combined with omega-3 fatty acids and ribonucleic acid, improves immunologic responses, helps to overcome immunologic depression, accelerates recovery, and reduces infection.[1207-1210] As noted above, the suppression of the immune system can be counterproductive for athletes.

Arginine thus has significant anabolic and anticatabolic effects that if harnessed would be useful in increasing lean body mass and strength. Studies have shown the effects of arginine on strength and lean body mass.[1211]

In one study, 22 adult males participated in a 5-week progressive strength training program. Half the subjects received the amino acids L-arginine and L-ornithine and the other half were given a placebo.[1212] The study used a double-blind protocol so that the subjects as well as the investigators had no knowledge of which substances were being administered. Dosages amounted to 2 g or 1 g each of L-arginine and L-ornithine, or 600 mg of calcium, and 1 g of vitamin C as placebos. These supplements were taken orally for a total of 25 administrations.

Following the short-term strength program using progressively higher intensities, tests were taken for total strength, lean body mass, and urinary hydroxyproline (UH). The results showed that subjects who were taking the arginine-ornithine combination scored significantly higher in total strength and lean body mass, and significantly lower in UH, than subjects on placebos. It was concluded that arginine and ornithine taken in prescribed doses can, in conjunction with a high-intensity strength training program, increase total strength and lean body mass in a relatively short period of time. Arginine and ornithine also aid in recovery from chronic stress by quelling tissue breakdown, as evidenced by lower urinary hydroxyproline levels.

Thus, there is direct evidence that oral supplementation with amino acids (arginine and ornithine) leads to enhanced muscle mass and strength in conjunction with resistance training.

L-CYSTEINE

L-Cysteine is utilized for protein synthesis, glutathione synthesis, and taurine production.

Cysteine and methionine are the principal sources of sulfur in the diet. Sulfur is necessary for the formation of coenzyme A and taurine in the body. Methionine can convert to cysteine, but not vice versa, so that methionine is the dietary essential. Methionine also converts to S-adenosylmethionine, an active methylating (CH_3) agent in the formation of compounds such as epinephrine, acetylcholine, and creatine.

Cysteine is essential for the formation of skin and hair. It contributes to strong connective tissue and tissue antioxidant actions, aids in the healing process, stimulates white blood cell activity, and helps diminish pain from inflammation.

Cystine is formed when two molecules of cysteine are reduced and linked by an –S–S– bond. It is present in the keratin of hair and in insulin, in each of which it forms about 12% of the whole protein molecule.

Connective tissue growth factor (CTGF) is a cysteine-rich peptide that exhibits platelet-derived growth factor (PDGF)-like biological and immunological activities. Because of the high-level selective induction of CTGF by TGF-beta, it appears that CTGF is a major autocrine growth factor produced by TGF-beta-treated human skin fibroblasts.[1213] Similar regulatory mechanisms appear to function *in vivo* during wound repair where there is a coordinate expression of TGF-beta 1 before CTGF in regenerating tissue, suggesting a cascade process for control of tissue regeneration and repair.[1214]

CYSTEINE AND N-ACETYLCYSTEINE

N-acetyl-L-cysteine (or NAC) is the N-acetyl derivative of L-cysteine (a nonessential amino acid). As with other amino acids, only L-isomers are biologically active. The main difference between dietary supplements of NAC and cysteine is stability. Supplements of cysteine, but not NAC, are readily oxidized (inactivated) in the gastrointestinal tract, and can lead to toxic side effects.[1215] NAC is thus the preferred form for oral use.[1216]

Aside from protein synthesis, cysteine/NAC is an essential component of glutathione (L-gamma-glutamyl-L-cysteinylglycine — one of the main cellular antioxidants). NAC and cysteine also act as potent antioxidants, both by themselves[1217] or in concert with glutathione and other antioxidants.[1218]

Cysteine serves as a component of coenzyme A which is involved in carbohydrate and fat metabolism. Cysteine is also a precursor of taurine. Numerous studies have shown the clinical use of NAC supplements in chronic[1219] but apparently not acute[1220] pulmonary problems. NAC is marketed in European countries for use in chronic pulmonary diseases.

NAC has been shown to have hepatoprotective effects against various toxic liver compounds such as alcohol, acetaminophen, carbon tetrachloride, and drugs used in cancer chemotherapy.[1221] Much of the protective effects are due to NAC's antioxidant properties and its ability to increase cellular levels of glutathione.

As well, NAC and other reducing agents have been shown to be useful for the treatment of AIDS and the wasting seen in AIDS patients, since they have been shown to decrease viral replication and to inhibit the action of inflammatory cytokines.[1222,1223]

NAC, because of its potent antioxidant properties, may prove useful in decreasing the oxidative stress seen with exercise.[1224] Recent human studies performed by Dr. Lester Packer of the University of California at Berkeley, and presented at the 1996 American College of Nutrition meeting in San Francisco, found that supplementation with NAC improved exercise performance times and also reduced oxidative stress by preserving glutathione levels during exercise. This finding is pending publication, but is extremely important because it provides evidence of positive effects of amino acid supplementation on human exercise performance and recovery. If this response were to continue for an adequate time period, then enhanced results from resistance training (faster increase in muscle mass and strength) could be expected.

GLUTAMINE

Glutamine, a neutral amino acid, is the most abundant amino acid in human muscle and plasma and is found in relatively high levels in many human tissues. Glutamine constitutes over 50% of the total amino acid pool, making it the most highly concentrated amino acid in the plasma. Whole-blood concentration of glutamine is higher than any other amino acid concentration.[1225] About 80% of the free amino acids of the body reside within the intracellular compartment of skeletal muscle cells. Of this pool, glutamine constitutes over 60% of the total intramuscular amino acids.

Glutamine plays fundamental physiological roles as a precursor of hepatic ureagenesis and renal ammoniagenesis (see above); in the maintenance of the acid-base balance during acidosis; as a nitrogen precursor for the synthesis of nucleotides; as cellular fuel in certain tissues such as muscle, intestine, skin, and in the immune system; and as a direct regulator of protein synthesis and degradation.[1226-1230]

From a review of the extensive literature on glutamine it would appear that the release and utilization of glutamine is a response to physiological and pathological stressors. In respect to glutamine, it also seems that all forms of stress including trauma, surgery, burns, infections, fasting, malnutrition, and exercise deplete muscles of glutamine.[1231-1234] During catabolic stress, reductions up to 50% have been documented.[1235]

This drop in glutamine occurs in spite of the effect of stress hormones in increasing the production of glutamine secondary to muscle catabolism and *de novo* synthesis. In these cases the production of glutamine cannot keep up to the demand. As well, because of the use of other amino acids (especially the BCAAs) to produce glutamine, and the relative need for glutamine by other tissues, less glutamine and other amino acids are available for protein synthesis.

In times of stress, protein synthesis takes a back seat to other events that are more important in terms of survival. The utilization of glutamine by the gut and immune system takes precedence over protein synthesis. When the body is subjected to stress, although glutamine is the most depleted amino acid as well as the last one to be replenished, little of this glutamine serves for the synthesis of structural or contractile protein. The increase in glutamine turnover rate seen in these various conditions likely represents an adaptative mechanism to the stressor for preservation of immune and visceral function.

Glutamine concentrations decrease and tissue glutamine metabolism increases markedly in many catabolic, stressful disease states, and whole-body exchange rates of glutamine can exceed the body's total stores of glutamine by severalfold each day. Under stressful conditions there is a constant requirement for *de novo* synthesis of glutamine to match the rate of utilization. In healthy skeletal muscle, intracellular glutamine concentrations can reach more than 33 times the extracellular concentrations.[1236] The maximal synthesis rate of glutamine in human skeletal muscle (about 50 mmol/h) has been shown to be higher than that of any other amino acid.[1237]

Thus while nonessential under normal conditions,[1238] during periods of stress (e.g., intense exercise, sepsis, and conditions generating an acid load) the demand for glutamine can exceed its supply; hence, its classification as a conditionally essential amino acid.[1239] This position has been supported by recent studies that have shown trophic effects of glutamine-supplemented diets on the growth of specific tissues and on total body nitrogen balance.[1240]

GLUTAMINE METABOLISM

Glutamine homeostasis is dependent upon the net balance between release and utilization of glutamine by the various organs and tissues of the body.[1241] The simultaneous sampling of arterial and venous blood across various organs can help to classify them as either predominantly releasing or taking up glutamine.

The two principal intracellular enzymes of glutamine metabolism are glutaminase, which catalyzes glutamine hydrolysis to glutamate and ammonia, and reversibly, glutamine synthetase, which catalyzes glutamine synthesis from ammonia and glutamate.[1242] Tissues differ markedly in the direction of the reaction, determining whether a tissue or organ is a net consumer or producer of glutamine.

The major organs and tissues of glutamine synthesis in the body have been identified as primarily the skeletal muscle, but also the lungs, liver, brain, and possibly the adipose tissue. Glutamine utilization is high in cells of the intestine and in cells of the immune system (lymphocytes and macrophages), both for the synthesis of DNA and RNA and for provision of energy in these cells.[1243-1246]

Skeletal muscle is the principal site of glutamine production and provides the majority of glutamine required by other tissues.[1247] Skeletal muscle is capable of increasing the rate of release and synthesis of glutamine in response to increased demand from other organs and tissues of the body.

ANABOLIC AND ANTICATABOLIC EFFECTS OF GLUTAMINE

Glutamine plays an important role in protein metabolism by acting as a labile store of nitrogen mobilized from the periphery in times of stress, such as in sepsis and following surgery. Also this amino acid plays a direct role in the maintenance of protein balance in muscle.[1248-1250] Thus glutamine acts as a regulator of protein synthesis, increasing protein synthesis and decreasing protein degradation in skeletal muscle — both actions being dependent on the size of the intracellular glutamine pool.[1251-1256]

Glutamine is also a readily available store of protein and nitrogen for utilization by the liver,[1257,1258] and is selectively extracted from muscle tissue to become incorporated into the activity of gluconeogenesis (carbohydrate/sugar formation) by the liver.[1259] Glutamine, in addition to alanine, is the major interorgan nitrogen carrier,[1260] and both are released by muscle under the influence of glucocorticoids.[1261,1262] Further, some 90% of the nitrogen derived from branched-chain amino acid catabolism is released as glutamine.[1263] This amino acid is utilized extensively by the intestine, and there is a positive digestive balance only with high-protein diets.[1264]

The intramuscular glutamine concentration is decreased in various catabolic conditions including injury, surgery, uncontrolled diabetes, sepsis, burns, and high-intensity exercise. Indeed, one of the most typical features of the body's response to trauma appears to be a 50% reduction in the muscle glutamine content. It has been shown that an increase in muscle glutamine release and a corresponding rise in plasma glutamine levels occurs during intensive isometric exercise.[1265]

There appears to be a link between the size of the glutamine pool in muscle and the rate of protein synthesis by muscle.[1266,1267] A diminished supply of intramuscular free glutamine concentration,[1268] and especially intracellular glutamine concentration,[1269-1271] has been theorized to contribute to the significant degree of proteolysis observed in the acute-phase response in wasting. Animal studies suggest that glutamine supplements can prevent or reverse the atrophy of the small intestine that occurs during total parenteral nutrition,[1272-1274] and decrease structural damage in the epithelium of the small intestine during the systemic response to trauma and surgery.[1275,1276] Similarly, improvements in the immune function of injured animals have been noted.[1277,1278]

Many of the studies documenting the anabolic and anticatabolic effects of glutamine in humans have been done on trauma or surgically stressed patients. Glutamine added to commercially available parenteral amino acid solutions and enteral diets leads to a significant improvement in nitrogen balance and immune function, and has an anabolic effect on intestinal mucosa.[1279-1291]

Addition of glutamine to total parenteral nutrition after elective abdominal surgery has been shown to spare free glutamine in muscle, counteract the fall in muscle protein synthesis, and improve nitrogen balance.[1292] Either glutamine or its analogues (ornithine-alpha-ketoglutarate, alpha-ketoglutarate, or alanylglutamine), counteract the postoperative fall of muscle free glutamine and of muscle protein synthesis.[1293,1294] Furthermore, statistical correlations can be shown between the changes of muscle glutamine and muscle protein synthesis and the postoperative nitrogen losses.[1295]

GLUTAMINE REGULATION OF GLUCONEOGENESIS

Glutamine is a potent regulator of not only protein but of fatty acid and glycogen metabolism. To test the hypothesis that glutamine may act as a physiological regulator of gluconeogenesis, the authors of a recent study infused 16 normal postabsorptive volunteers with glutamine estimated to approximate its appearance in plasma after a protein meal and assessed changes in production of glucose from glutamine, systemic glucose appearance and disposal, and uptake and release of glucose, glutamine, and alanine by forearm skeletal muscle.[1295a] Although infusion of glutamine increased plasma glutamine concentration and turnover only threefold, formation of glucose from glutamine increased sevenfold. Formation of glucose from alanine was also stimulated in the absence of a change in plasma alanine concentration. Furthermore, glutamine infusion decreased its own *de novo* synthesis while increasing that of alanine. Systemic glucose appearance, systemic glucose disposal, and forearm balance of glucose and alanine were not altered. Because the stimulatory effects of glutamine on gluconeogenesis occurred in the absence of changes in plasma insulin and glucagon levels, these results provide evidence that, in humans, glutamine may act both as a substrate and as a regulator of gluconeogenesis as well as a modulator of its own metabolism.

As well, as we have seen above, there is evidence that glutamine may act as a regulator of protein, free fatty acid, and glycogen metabolism during and after exercise.

GLUTAMINE AND CORTISOL

Hypercortisolemia has been shown to increase glutamine flux in a dose-dependent fashion through an increase in protein breakdown and in *de novo* synthesis.[1296] Under stress the increase in glucocorticoid synthesis and release activates muscle catabolism[1297] and intracellular amino acid (mainly BCAA) oxidation. Both these processes result in increased glutamine formation and release of glutamine into the general circulation for the use of other tissues, mainly the GI tract and the immune system.[1298-1300]

Glucocorticoids that increase in catabolic states have been reported to mediate such changes[1301-1306] by:

1. Increasing glutamine efflux from skeletal muscle in rats and humans
2. Increasing glutamine synthetase activity and mRNA expression
3. Decreasing intramuscular glutamine stores
4. Changing glutamine transporter kinetics such that glutamine efflux could still occur maximally at lowered intramuscular glutamine levels

Together, these effects ensure that skeletal muscle glutamine release and synthesis would be adequate to supply the glutamine needed during catabolic states. However, the possibility remains that these changes may still be insufficient to balance an increased rate of utilization by other organs.

Studies have shown that glutamine supplementation may decrease the effect of increased cortisol levels secondary to physical and psychological stressors and can even prevent the decline in protein synthesis and muscle wasting associated with repeated glucocorticoid treatment. In one study it was shown that glutamine infusion was effective therapy in counteracting glucocorticoid-induced muscle atrophy.[1307] The authors of this study felt that atrophy attenuation appears related to maintaining muscle glutamine levels, which in turn may limit the glucocorticoid-mediated downregulation of protein synthesis.

The authors cited studies indicating that during conditions of muscle atrophy associated with excess circulating glucocorticoids, muscle protein synthesis is markedly depressed, intramuscular glutamine concentration is decreased, glutamine synthetase activity is elevated, and skeletal muscle releases glutamine at a high rate.

The authors also remarked that a number of investigations have provided evidence that glutamine supplementation can prevent muscle glutamine loss in patients undergoing surgical trauma, and that decreases in the concentration and size distribution of ribosomes and reduction in nitrogen balance were attenuated in those subjects receiving glutamine: "On the basis that muscle glutamine depletion is related to the atrophy process, the provision of additional glutamine could serve as effective therapy altering the course of muscle wasting from glucocorticoids."

In the study, cortisol-treated rats were infused with either saline or glutamine. Glutamine infusion attenuated the decline of glutamine concentration in the plantaris muscle and prevented >70% of the total muscle mass losses due to the glucocorticoid injections. Glutamine prevented 50% of the cortisol-induced decline in myosin heavy chain (a contractile protein in muscle) synthesis. It was concluded that glutamine infusion is effective therapy in counteracting glucocorticoid-induced muscle atrophy. The authors stated that atrophy attenuation appears related to maintaining muscle glutamine levels, which in turn may limit the glucocorticoid-mediated downregulation of myosin heavy chain synthesis.

In another study, dexamethasone, a synthetic glucocorticoid, was shown to cause striking receptor-mediated increases in both glutamine synthetase activity and the steady-state glutamine synthetase mRNA level.[1308] This effect was observed in rat skeletal muscle cells in culture, as well as in rat muscles *in vivo*. In this study glucocorticoid-mediated induction of glutamine synthetase was blocked by androgenic/anabolic steroids at high doses, suggesting that anabolic steroids might have an anticatabolic mode of action in enhancing skeletal muscle mass in athletes. Glutamine seems to have a similar effect on glutamine synthetase.

In a study set up to investigate how glutamine prevents skeletal muscle atrophy from glucocorticoids, the authors found that glutamine diminished glucocorticoid effects on glutamine synthetase (GS) enzyme activity.[1309] Because the gene encoding glutamine synthetase (GS) is glucocorticoid inducible, it represented an appropriate model for testing whether glucocorticoids and glutamine exert opposing actions on the expression of specific genes related to atrophy in muscle tissue. In this study, rats were administered hydrocortisone-21-acetate or the dosing vehicle (carboxymethyl cellulose) and were infused with saline (SAL) or glutamine (GLN) for 7 days. In saline-infused animals, glucocorticoid treatment produced 200 to 300% increases in plantaris, fast-twitch white, and fast-twitch red muscle GS enzyme activity and mRNA. In contrast, in all muscles/types studied, glutamine infusion diminished glucocorticoid effects on GS enzyme activity to 131 to 159% and on GS mRNA to 110 to 200% of the values in saline-treated controls.

Since elevated cortisol levels associated with some forms of stress and exercise can, through various pathways, decrease protein synthesis and increase protein catabolism, the use of glutamine may be a valuable anabolic agent under these conditions. For example, both overtraining and high-intensity exercise can increase cortisol production, and it may be that glutamine could have an anticatabolic effect by limiting the catabolic effects of this increased cortisol. Glutamine supplementation may attenuate the cortisol response to stress and decrease both skeletal muscle catabolism and the oxidation of amino acids that can in turn be used for protein synthesis both during exercise and recovery.[1310] If maintained over a period of time, glutamine supplementation would enhance the results of resistance training.

ANABOLIC EFFECTS OF GLUTAMINE

Besides anticatabolic effects, glutamine appears to have significant anabolic effects. The aim of a recent study was to determine whether the putative protein anabolic effect of glutamine (1) is mediated by increased protein synthesis or decreased protein breakdown, and (2) is specific to glutamine.[1311]

Seven healthy adults were administered 5-h intravenous infusions of L-leucine in the postabsorptive state while receiving in a randomized order an enteral infusion of saline on one day or L-glutamine on the other day. Seven additional subjects were studied using the same protocol except they received an isonitrogenous infusion of glycine. The rates of leucine appearance (RaLEU), an index of protein degradation, leucine oxidation (OxLEU), and nonoxidative leucine disposal (NOLD), an index of protein synthesis, were measured using the ^{14}C-specific activity of plasma alpha-ketoisocaproate and the excretion rate of $^{14}CO_2$ in breath.

During glutamine infusion, plasma glutamine concentration doubled, whereas RaLEU did not change, OxLEU decreased, and NOLD increased. During glycine infusion, plasma glycine increased 14-fold, but in contrast with glutamine, RaLEU, OxLEU, and NOLD all decreased. The authors concluded that glutamine enteral infusion may exert its protein anabolic effect by increasing protein synthesis, whereas an isonitrogenous amount of glycine merely decreases protein turnover with only a small anabolic effect resulting from a greater decrease in proteolysis than protein synthesis.

As we noted above, protein turnover and degradation have been directly linked with cellular hydration states, and an increase in hydration (and resultant increased cellular volume) is directly correlative to a powerful, positive anabolic signal for further protein synthesis. Conversely, cell dehydration (shrinkage) directly stimulates catabolism.[1312]

The effect of changes in cell volume on the rates of release of glutamine and alanine from muscle and on the concentrations of these amino acids in muscle were investigated in one study.[1313] The results of this study suggest that cell volume may play a role in the regulation of amino acid metabolism (and thus protein anabolism) in skeletal muscle.

Muscle cell hydration offers an explanation to the previously observed potent anabolic effects of certain hormones and nutrients. Amino acids, for example, have long been known to be essential for promoting muscle protein synthesis. Newer research shows that certain amino acids exert an osmotic effect in cells, in effect drawing water into the cell. This, in turn, initiates a signal that somehow turns on the anabolic machinery of the cell.

Of all amino acids examined for cellular hydration effects, glutamine appears to be one of the most important. The relationship between glutamine and cellular hydration may be fundamental to protein synthesis.[1314] Liver cells have been shown to increase in volume by as much at 12% within 2 min of glutamine infusion, and stay at their increased volumes for as long as glutamine is present.[1315] As long as glutamine content remains high in the cell, cell hydration and anabolic processes also remain elevated,[1316] and when glutamine leaves muscle the cells lose water and catabolic processes begin.[1317]

Glutamine cell efflux occurs under many conditions including any type of stress. Glutamine acts as a primary fuel for certain immune cells, which are activated under stress conditions. High-intensity exercise, while considered a beneficial form of stress, still exerts a glutamine- depleting effect on muscle.

As well as affecting cellular hydration, glutamine can also stimulate glycogen synthesis and thus increases energy available for cellular metabolism. In one study, alanine and glycine infusion decreased muscle glutamine content 18%, while the direct glutamine infusion increased muscle glutamine by 16%.[1318] Within 2 h after exercise, the glutamine infusion increased muscle glycogen more than the other two infusions. The researchers speculate that glutamine itself may be a direct precursor for muscle glycogen replenishment after exercise. As a comparison, medical studies show that to get best results from glutamine requires 20 to 40 g a day.

GLUTAMINE AND ATHLETIC PERFORMANCE

Although there are differences between exercising individuals and those who are traumatically or surgically stressed, glutamine supplementation in athletes may be beneficial in increasing the anabolic drive.

During resistance exercise, skeletal muscle cells are damaged in numerous ways. Mechanical and chemical (e.g., enzyme-mediated) factors can play a role in the etiology of this microtrauma, which ultimately must be repaired. Thus, in order to permit this tissue reparation glucocorticoids may be elevated, thereby contributing to the catabolism of myofibrillar proteins. Also, while other amino acids are being shunted into glutamine production, myofibrillar protein synthesis will fall, owing to the reduced availability of amino acids.

As well as the direct effects on protein synthesis and catabolism, some other functions of glutamine, such as its potential effects on growth hormone and testosterone and its antioxidant and hepatoprotective properties, are also of interest to athletes. The results of a recent study suggest that, after exercise, increased availability of glutamine promotes muscle glycogen accumulation by mechanisms possibly including diversion of glutamine carbon to glycogen.[1319] As well, it's been shown that glutamine is a major gluconeogenic precursor and vehicle for interorgan carbon transport in humans.[1320] These facts might be helpful in increasing training intensity and aiding in recovery from training sessions.

Glutamine is a precursor of glutathione and as such has antioxidant effects by increasing intracellular glutathione content.[1321] A study recently has shown that glutamine has a therapeutic effect, along with vitamin E, on hepatic dysfunction.[1322] In those athletes using drugs, glutamine may play a significant hepatoprotective role against the hepatotoxic effects of drugs such as the anabolic steroids.

Glutamine may be an important modulator of growth hormone, prolactin, and ACTH secretion in humans.[1323] A recent study found that an oral dose of only 2 g of glutamine significantly elevated growth hormone release, indicating that significant amounts of an orally administered glutamine load did reach the periphery.[1324] Larger glutamine loads, while further increasing plasma glutamine, provoke an accelerated glutamine clearance consistent with activation of hepatic glutamine removal. Calling into play the formidable hepatic mechanism for responding to a large increase in plasma glutamine may be counterproductive. On the other hand, smaller oral loads ≤ 1 g run the risk of being unable to significantly elevate circulating plasma glutamine.

The authors of this study feel that their results clearly show that an oral glutamine load approximating the dose range used in their study appears to attain a "window" of effectiveness in achieving the desired increase in systemic glutamine and GH release.

How an oral glutamine load might stimulate basal growth hormone secretion was not elucidated. However, glutamine initiates secondary amino acid fluxes that could affect growth hormone secretion. For example, conversion of glutamine to citrulline in the small intestine supports renal arginine synthesis, a known stimulus for growth hormone secretion. In addition, conversion of glutamine to glutamate provides a stimulus for directly activating somatotrophic growth hormone release. Thus, either one or both effectors might play a role in stimulating growth hormone secretion in response to oral glutamine load.

Glutamine, along with glutamate, has a role in increasing gonadotropin hormone-releasing hormone (GnRH) release and thus indirectly may increase testosterone secretion.[1325] As well, the effects of glutamine in skeletal muscle include the stimulation of protein synthesis which occurs in the absence or presence of insulin, the response being greater with insulin.[1326]

GLUTAMINE AND OVERTRAINING

Exercise has been shown to mitigate muscle atrophy secondary to glucocorticoids and to antagonize the hormonal actions on glutamine synthetase.[1327,1328] However, extreme exercise can increase serum cortisol and have anticatabolic effects.

Given the fundamental roles played by glutamine in supporting cellular and organ function it is not surprising to find multiorgan-dependent processes such as the immune and anti-inflammatory response to be dependent, in part, on glutamine.

Glutamine is utilized at a high rate by some cells of the immune system (including neutrophils, lymphocytes, and macrophages) and is essential for the viability and normal functioning of these cells.[1329-1332] After prolonged intense exercise the number of lymphocytes in the blood is reduced, the function of natural killer cells is suppressed and secretory immunity is impaired.[1333]

Experiments on lymphocytes *in vitro* showed that the proliferative response of these cells was dependent on the concentration of glutamine, and this suggests that a decrease in plasma glutamine concentration could be responsible, at least in part, for the reported impairment of immune function in various conditions.

Overtraining in athletes is associated with depressed plasma glutamine concentration and immune system malfunction as judged by changes in various components of the immune system including lymphocyte subsets, immunoglobulin levels, the mononuclear phagocytic system, polymorphonuclear leukocytes and cytokines, especially IL-1, IL-2, IL-6, and TNF.[1334-1337]

The immunosuppressive effects of intense exercise and overtraining can affect an athlete's performance and might reduce the immune system's ability to ward off disease.[1338] In fact, it has been shown that athletes have an increased frequency of upper respiratory infections.[1339] As well, it appears that those athletes who perform better reported more symptoms,[1340] and that more symptoms were reported in the week following a competition.

A recent study suggested that sustained physical activity could damage the glutamine release process so that it does not respond adequately to increased glutamine requirement by the immune system.[1341] The study compared blood glutamine levels in seven men who exercised at different intensities once a week with levels in five soldiers who exercised intensively twice a day for 10 days. When the 7 men exercised at the most intense level, the average glutamine level fell 560 µmol/l from 1244. Blood glutamine levels fell immediately in 4 of the soldiers and all 5 had significantly lower levels 11 days into the program.

The authors concluded that blood glutamine tests may serve as a valuable tool for determining whether or not athletes are overtraining, before health and performance suffer. The researchers speculated that glutamine supplementation may also be beneficial in the treatment of athletes affected by exercise-induced stress and overtraining.

Other studies have also shown that decreased plasma glutamine concentrations represent an objective, measurable parameter in severe exercise stress and overtraining, and can be used as a measure of recovery from exercise stress.[1342,1343]

In one study, glutamine supplementation in rats proved useful in mitigating the negative effects of exercise stress.[1344] Although the plasma glutamine concentration was significantly decreased in the control group immediately after a treadmill exercise, compared to rested rats, the plasma glutamine concentration of rats fed a glutamine-supplemented diet for three weeks was significantly higher than that of the control group in resting and was not significantly decreased even immediately after a treadmill exercise. Immune system parameters were also significantly improved in the glutamine-supplemented group even immediately after a treadmill exercise. The results of this study indicate that there was an increased uptake of glutamine in glutamine-supplemented diets and that this glutamine was utilized by immune cells as sources of fuel and nucleotides.

Another study looked at the effects of BCAA supplementation on the reduced plasma glutamine concentration seen in overtrained athletes and after long-term exercise.[1345] BCAAs were shown to prevent this decrease in the plasma glutamine level. The authors of this study concluded that the decrease in plasma glutamine concentration in overtraining and following long-term exercise may contribute to the immune deficiency reported in these conditions.

ORAL GLUTAMINE SUPPLEMENTATION

Much of both the dietary glutamine and the glutamine released from muscle is utilized by the mucosal cells of the small intestine.[1346] Glutamine has been suggested as a therapeutic tool in patients with a variety of gastrointestinal diseases and those requiring extensive intestinal operations.[1347]

Glutamine has a protective effect on the gastrointestinal system against several types of insults including radiation. In one study it was found that oral glutamine accelerated healing of the small intestine and improved outcome after whole abdominal radiation.[1348] In this study glutamine ingestion decreased the morbidity and mortality and diminished bloody diarrhea and the incidence of bowel perforation in irradiated rats. Glutamine has also been shown to exert important benefits in preventing gut-origin sepsis after trauma[1349] and beneficial effects in small-bowel transplants.[1350,1351]

Oral glutamine is used by the gut; ordinarily, very little of the oral glutamine makes it past mucosal cells of the small intestine[1352] unless relatively large amounts of glutamine are ingested at one time. Perhaps two thirds of the dietary glutamine is metabolized within mucosal cells, and the glutamine that is released from muscle and provided to the gut via the mesenteric arteries is also an important fuel for these cells.[1353,1354] Utilization of exogenous glutamine by the gut is not wasted, however, since the dietary glutamine is used instead of endogenous glutamine and thus there is less need to cannibalize skeletal muscle to obtain the necessary glutamine.

Studies have shown that oral glutamine increases plasma glutamine levels. In one study, plasma glutamine concentration of rats fed glutamine-supplemented diet for three weeks was significantly higher than that of control group in resting, and was not significantly decreased even immediately after a treadmill exercise.[1355] In rats not given supplemental glutamine, glutamine levels were dramatically lower after a treadmill exercise. In this same study a positive effect of glutamine on the immune system was seen.

It has been shown that metabolic acidosis associated with the catabolic state mobilizes muscle nitrogen and releases it into blood as glutamine targeted for renal consumption and base generation. Under these conditions, oral glutamine has been shown to spare endogenous supplies and decrease muscle catabolism.[1356]

A recent study found that oral glutamine supplementation, through support of host glutamine stores and glutathione production, may decrease tumor growth by enhancing natural killer (NK) cell activity.[1357] Also, glutamine is utilized in large concentrations by lymphocytes and macrophages of the immune system to fight infection.[1358,1359] These glutamine level changes are felt to be one of the most important changes seen in acute-phase reactions and are chronically depleted in long-term wasting disease. Additionally, the concentration of muscle glutamine in septic patients has been highly correlated to the survival rates in these patients, irrespective of the cause of wasting.[1360,1361] Glutamine has also been found to promote interleukin-2 (a growth factor in the immune system) production in rat lymphocytes.[1362]

Glutamine supplementation may also be useful in cachexia secondary to AIDS and cancer. Tissue wasting often occurs during human immunodeficiency virus infection and acquired immune deficiency syndrome. While weight loss in the human immunodeficiency virus-infected individual can be seen as an isolated symptom, catabolism during acquired immune deficiency syndrome is usually associated with complications such as diarrhea, malabsorption, fever, and secondary infection. Since glutamine is an amino acid central to many important metabolic pathways, glutamine depletion may explain the progression of tissue wasting during human immunodeficiency virus infection.[1363]

In one recent study, enteral glutamine administration induced:

1. A dose-dependent increase in the plasma glutamine level
2. A rise in the plasma level and appearance rate of alanine and in plasma levels of glutamate, citrulline, aspartate, and urea
3. A decline in plasma free fatty acid and glycerol levels[1364]

Other anticatabolic and anabolic amino acids may exert their effects through glutamine. For example, the BCAAs may exert their anticatabolic effects by preserving glutamine.[1365] It is now established that skeletal muscle cells are active in the catabolism of BCAAs and in the subsequent synthesis and release of glutamine, which serves as a metabolic substrate for various cell types.[1366] In fact, 90% of the nitrogen derived from BCAAs is released as glutamine.[1367]

In the postabsorptive state, the main source of glutamine is from muscle, where the branched-chain amino acids, including leucine, supply the nitrogen for glutamine formation.[1368] Studies have shown that the carbon chains of BCAAs entering the citric acid cycle in muscle are not used for oxidation or for alanine synthesis, but are converted exclusively to glutamine.[1369]

GLUTAMINE IN SUPPLEMENTS

Since the total daily glutamine production in humans averages 50 to 120 g,[1370] small amounts of glutamine in the form of supplements are unlikely to have any effect. Although glutamine intake can be increased through the use of whole foods, the calorie content would be prohibitive since many of the foods high in glutamine (such as almonds, soybeans, and peanuts) are also high in calories. Thus the use of supplements containing large amounts of this amino acid without the calories is much preferred. However, determining the glutamine content of some of the supplements on the market is not straightforward.

Although the amino acid profile listed on many protein supplements does not include the glutamine content, the glutamic acid content is usually listed. The reason is that the acid hydrolysis stage of the analysis converts the glutamine into glutamic acid, releasing ammonia. Thus the glutamic acid level actually represents the combined levels of glutamine and glutamic acid.

Although one can figure out the amount of glutamine by the amount of ammonia released during the acid hydrolysis, this is not usually done. Instead, by taking a percentage of the glutamic acid listed one can get a rough idea of how much glutamine is in a protein supplement. In the case of proteins of animal origin, approximately 50% of the glutamic acid content will represent glutamine. For plant proteins, however, that figure can be as high as 80%.

SUMMARY

In summary, the reduction of skeletal muscle protein synthesis is associated with a decrease of muscle free glutamine proportional to the muscle protein catabolism. Protein catabolic states are accompanied by an increased rate of glycolysis, and subsequently an increased nonoxidative disposal of pyruvate, derived from alanine. This process reduces the availability of intracellular nitrogen for glutamine synthesis, thereby causing a depletion of the intracellular glutamine pool which, in turn, suppresses protein synthesis.

Glutamine supplementation may offer a number of advantages to athletes. Overall, the use of exogenous glutamine would spare intramuscular glutamine and result in decreased proteolysis and potentially increased levels of muscle protein. Gastrointestinal and immune functions would be maximized and the morbidity secondary to overtraining would be improved. Glutamine can efficiently release growth hormone and perhaps upregulate other anabolic hormones. All these factors strongly suggest that glutamine supplementation may play a major role in enhancing the effects of resistance training.

ALPHA-KETOGLUTARATE

Alpha-ketoglutarate (AKG) is a product of glutamine catabolism as well as a precursor to glutamine synthesis. The amino acid glutamine, in addition to arginine, histidine, and proline, are all degraded by conversion to glutamate which, in turn, is oxidized to AKG by glutamate dehydrogenase. Conversely, AKG is also a precursor to glutamine, for in a similar series of steps (but in reverse order), catalyzed by an entirely different set of enzymes, AKG is converted to glutamate which is then converted to glutamine. Glutamine synthetase, the enzyme which catalyzes the formation of glutamine, is activated by AKG.

There is evidence that alpha-ketoglutarate preserves muscle mass and acts as an efficient anticatabolic compound.[1371,1372] Addition of alpha-ketoglutarate to postoperative total parenteral nutrition prevented the decrease in muscle protein synthesis and free glutamine that usually occurs after surgery.[1373] One study has found that an alpha-ketoglutarate-pyridoxine complex may have some beneficial effects on human maximal aerobic and anaerobic performance.[1374]

Thus, by ingesting AKG in sufficient quantities the demand for muscle glutamine might ultimately be spared to some degree, thereby allowing muscle protein synthesis to proceed unhindered (e.g., such as during the muscle hypertrophic response which follows a resistance training workout), and reducing the catabolism of muscle tissue.

Studies have shown that:

1. AKG reduces the decline in muscle free glutamine that is associated with reductions in protein synthesis.[1375]
2. The use of AKG, instead of glutamine, prevents the decline in protein anabolism observed following surgery.[1376]

AKG seems to exert anticatabolic effects by preserving muscle glutamine,[1377] as does ornithine-alpha-ketoglutarate or OKG (see below for more on OKG). These results are not surprising in that the carbon skeleton of BCAAs can be used to synthesize glutamine after the transamination reaction of BCAAs, and ketoglutarate is the immediate carbon donor for glutamine synthesis. The utilization of arginine and ornithine as carbon sources for glutamine synthesis is also a possibility.

HISTIDINE

This amino acid is conditionally essential (see above). The removal of the COOH group of histidine by the enzyme histidine decarboxylase converts it to histamine, an important physiological substance which is normally freely present in the intestine and (in bound form) in basophil granules in cells of the reticuloendothelial system. Histamine is a powerful blood vessel dilator, and is involved in allergic reactions such as urticaria and inflammation. Also, histamine stimulates the secretion of both pepsin and hydrochloric acid by the stomach.

Histidine (His) is elevated in plasma and brain during protein deficiency as well as in several pathological conditions, leading to the possibility of a direct effect on central nervous system (CNS) function. In a recent study,[960] groups of weanling rats were fed diets containing graded levels of casein or a single indispensable amino acid (IAA: Leu, Val, Ile, Phe, Trp, Thr, Met, or Lys) in order to produce nutritionally deficient states. Body weight gains and food intakes were recorded daily for 2 weeks. Whole brain and serum samples were obtained and analyzed for amino acid (AA) content. The only consistent pattern observed in AA profiles which could be correlated with food intake was an increase in brain His concentrations. Limiting dietary casein or IAA elevated brain His above controls 2.5- and 1.5-fold, respectively.

Food intake was generally depressed by 50% at brain His concentrations above 105 nmol/g. Since His is the precursor of the depressant neurotransmitter histamine (HA), systemic increases may be significant in that HA could be a possible cause of the anorexia observed in protein and IAA deficiency.

CARNOSINE

Carnosine (beta-alanyl-L-histidine) and carcinine (beta-alanylhistamine) are natural imidazole-containing compounds found in the nonprotein fraction of mammalian tissues. Carnosine, a naturally occurring histidine-containing dipeptide in mammalian tissues, with antioxidant properties, is related metabolically to histidine and histamine, and has immunopotentiating properties *in vivo*[961] and may be useful for the treatment of immunodeficiency states.[962-964] Both compounds are capable of inhibiting the catalysis of linoleic acid and phosphatidylcholine liposomal peroxidation and are able to scavenge free radicals.[965] They are thus physiological antioxidants[966-970] able to efficiently protect the lipid phase of biological membranes and aqueous environments and may be effective as an anti-inflammatory drug and a prominent tool in wound healing.[971]

BUFFERING EFFECTS OF CARNOSINE

Intense exercise always involves an anaerobic component and thus results in significant reductions in ATP, a buildup of tissue lactic acid, and an increase in tissue acidity.[972] Although the acidity can normally be buffered by the body, under high stress conditions the buildup is too fast for the body to cope with. With increasing acidity comes premature muscle fatigue.

A buildup of lactic acid and hydrogen ions (H^+) in the skeletal muscle occurs whenever oxygenation is not sufficient to meet the needs of muscle. This relative hypoxia does not allow the full aerobic metabolism of glucose to water and carbon dioxide. Thus, ATP can not be generated in adequate amounts, and the skeletal muscle tires and becomes less efficient in contracting. In addition, there are large accumulations of anaerobic end products (due in part to the combined reactions of glycolysis and ATP hydrolysis[973]) which lower intracellular pH. Intracellular pH decrements of sufficient magnitude have been shown to inhibit athletic performances because of the inhibition of the enzymatic and contractile machinery.

Chronic metabolic acidosis has been shown to stimulate protein degradation. One study evaluated the effects of chronic metabolic acidosis on nitrogen balance and protein synthesis and found that chronic metabolic acidosis causes negative nitrogen balance and decreases albumin synthesis in humans.[974] Since in this study plasma concentrations of IGF-1, free T4, and T3 were significantly lower during acidosis, the effect on albumin synthesis may be mediated, at least in part, by a suppression of these hormones.

Metabolic fatigue is a characteristic muscle response to intense exercise that has outstripped the rate of ATP replacement. The accumulation of metabolic by-products, namely hydrogen ions and diprotonated phosphate, interferes with actin-myosin interaction, effectively preserving muscle ATP levels by preventing further ATP hydrolysis.[975] Intracellular acidosis, while an important factor in muscle fatigue, is not the only component to cause fatigue. There is evidence that there are components of fatigue that are not due to intracellular acidosis.[976] Another component of fatigue (which in many cases may be the major component), seems to be a change of state in one or more of the steps of the excitation-contraction coupling process.[977] Reversal of this state is sensitive to external pH, which suggests that this component is accessible from outside of the cell. Other components of fatigue are due to substrate depletion, electrical events and/or excitation-contraction coupling,[978,979] and changes in intercellular and extracellular calcium and potassium.[980-982]

There are two ways of biochemically approaching the problem that fatigue poses to athletes. One hypothetical way is to increase the level of ATP in the tissues, either by exogenous administration of ATP, or by increasing endogenous production of the energy-rich compounds (see section on creatine monohydrate). Second, one can try to reduce the effect intracellular acidosis has on the muscle directly, by buffering the H^+ ions and lactic acid with certain alkaline compounds, and thus decrease the local and the systemic acidosis.

H^+ ions are generated rapidly when muscles are maximally activated. This results in an intracellular proton load that comes from both lactic acid dissociation and anaerobic ATP production, and interferes with muscle contraction.

Lactic acid is produced during skeletal muscle exertion even when there is adequate oxygen available. The effect of this local lactic acid buildup in adequately oxygenated muscle has not been fully investigated. There is evidence, however, that acidosis in humans is a catabolic factor stimulating protein degradation and amino acid oxidation[983] and that utilization of buffering compounds does in fact have an enhancing effect in athletic events where relative tissue hypoxia is a factor in performance.[984]

The intracellular buffers that are capable of contributing to this enhanced buffering capacity are inorganic phosphate (although some studies have shown that phosphate loading did not enhance performance[985]), protein-bound histidine residues, the dipeptide carnosine, bicarbonate, and creatine phosphate.

Skeletal muscle is susceptible to oxidative deterioration due to a combination of lipid oxidation catalysts and membrane lipid systems that are high in unsaturated fatty acids. To prevent or delay oxidation reactions, several endogenous antioxidant systems are found in muscle tissue. These include alpha-tocopherol, histidine-containing dipeptides, and antioxidant enzymes such as glutathione peroxidase, superoxide dismutase, and catalase.[986] Histidine-containing dipeptides such as carnosine are present in high concentrations in most skeletal muscles.[987,988] These dipeptides have been shown to be actively synthesized by muscle cells and not merely deposited in skeletal muscles.[989,990]

In the blood, bicarbonate is the main buffer, with phosphate as one of the many other buffering agents. In muscle tissue, phosphate and carnosine together provide approximately 90% of the buffering capacity. Bicarbonate only plays a minor role. Studies have shown that maximal oxygen uptake (the best indicator of aerobic capacity) was increased by phosphate supplements.[991]

There have been numerous studies on the effects of alkalinizers such as bicarbonate on athletic performance. The general consensus is that bicarbonate loading and other alkalinizers have in some circumstances a positive effect on athletic performance.[992-995]

PROLINE AND HYDROXYPROLINE

These amino acids consist essentially of a pyrrole ring and are prevalent in collagen and other proteins of connective tissue. This same ring structure is found in the porphyrins, which are used to make hemoglobin, and the cytochromes.

In a study looking at changes in serum amino acid concentrations during prolonged endurance running, serum levels of both alanine and proline decreased gradually as exercise continued.[1380] In this study, serum free fatty acid (FFA) concentration was significantly higher at the end of exercise compared to the resting value. The increase in serum FFA concentration and the decreases in the concentrations in serum of alanine and proline were found to be highly correlated.

While the drop in alanine is to be expected because of its role in gluconeogenesis, it's interesting to see the drop in proline. The reason for this drop is not yet clear. It is known that in some cases long-term physical exercise enhances the uptake of ^{3}H-proline by lining cells along the bone trabecules.[1381] This uptake of proline may decrease serum levels in long-term exercise.

Skeletal muscle is able to oxidize several amino acids and amino acid metabolites and derivatives, including BCAA, alpha-ketoglutarate, glutamate, and proline.[1382] In one study, postabsorptive proline flux, oxidation, and endogenous biosynthesis were determined in five severely burned intensive-care-unit patients and in six healthy, young-adult control subjects.[1383] Burn patients, compared with normal individuals, demonstrated a doubling in proline and leucine flux, a threefold enhancement of proline oxidation, a trend toward decreased proline synthesis, and a 37% reduction in plasma proline concentrations. Further, the injured group, unlike the control group, was in a distinct negative body proline balance, as proline oxidation greatly exceeded endogenous proline biosynthesis. In another study intracellular proline concentrations were reduced by 33% following severe injury.[1384]

These studies indicate that significant proline deficits may evolve during the postabsorptive period in severely traumatized patients and the authors suggested that an exogenous supply of proline might benefit the nitrogen economy of the traumatized patient. Proline has been shown to be beneficial for optimal wound repair in traumatized rats.[1385]

A recent study has postulated that proline may be a conditionally essential AA during lactation[1386] and for premature neonates.[1387] Another study looked at the effects of removing proline from the diet on plasma leucine and proline kinetics.[1388] After a 1-week control period, during which young adult men received a diet containing a complete L-amino acid mixture, 7 subjects were given a diet devoid of proline for 4 weeks (group 1); 6 received a diet devoid of proline, arginine, aspartate, glutamate, and serine (group 2); and 7 continued with the complete diet (group 3). At the end of the control and 4-week periods subjects were given a continuous (3 h fast, 5 h fed) intravenous infusion of labeled L-leucine and L-proline.

Plasma proline was reduced significantly in groups 1 and 2, especially during the fed state, after the 4-week diet periods. Small but statistically significant reductions occurred in nonoxidative leucine disappearance and leucine appearance during the fasted state in group 2. Proline fluxes decreased by approximately 50% in fasted and fed states in groups 1 and 2. Mean *de novo* proline synthesis during the fasted state declined markedly after 4 weeks in groups 1 and 2.

A study examined plasma proline concentration flux, oxidation, and endogenous biosynthesis in 5 healthy young men given 3 isocaloric, isonitrogenous diets for 1 week — a complete egg-pattern amino acid diet (diet 1), an amino acid mixture devoid of proline (diet 2), and a diet composed solely of indispensable amino acids (diet 3).[1389] Plasma proline concentrations declined by 22% on diet 2 and by 29% on diet 3. The authors concluded that the metabolic significance of the reduction of plasma proline concentrations requires elucidation.

During exercise, the amino groups used in the synthesis of alanine and glutamine appeared to be derived from the catabolism of other amino acids, specifically leucine, isoleucine, valine, aspartate, glutamate, asparagine, arginine, and proline.[1390]

Overall, dietary proline deficiency may impair protein synthesis under certain conditions. The effect of proline deficiency or supplementation on the anabolic effects of exercise has not as yet been adequately studied, but appears to be important.

TAURINE

Unlike glutamine, taurine is not incorporated into muscle proteins. Taurine, a derivative of the transsulfuration pathway originating with methionine, is the second most abundant free amino acid in muscle after glutamine. Taurine may be involved in eliciting important cell-volumizing effects through the control of ionic flux,[1455] and its effect on osmoregulation,[1456] thereby influencing anabolic processes.

As a conditionally essential nutrient, taurine has several important properties, including antioxidant effects, that make it useful in preventive medical applications.[1457] For example, taurine may have a protective effect in joints by decreasing the degradation of hyaluronic acid.[1458] Taurine also has antihypertensive activity. The increase in serum taurine could contribute, at least in part through the reduction in plasma norepinephrine level, to the antihypertensive effect of exercise.[1459]

The results of one study indicate that taurine is an effective stimulator of GH secretion in rats, and that the mechanism of this action involves the opioid peptidergic system in the hypothalamus.[1460]

A recent study examined the effects of taurine (2-aminoethanesulfonic acid) on isometric force development using skinned muscle fiber preparations.[1461] In atrial and ventricular pig heart muscles, as well as in fibers of slow abdominal extensor muscle of crayfish, an increase of submaximal isometric force was observed in Ca^{2+}-activated skinned fiber preparations at physiological concentrations of taurine. The maximal isometric force remained unaffected in all preparations. It is assumed that taurine increases the Ca^{2+} sensitivity of the force-generating myofilaments in mammalian hearts and crustacean slow skeletal muscle fibers.

In a recent review Timbrell et al.[1462] listed some features of taurine as follows:

- Various *in vivo* data suggest that taurine has a variety of protective functions and a deficiency leads to pathological changes.
- Depletion of taurine in rats increases susceptibility to liver damage from carbon tetrachloride.
- Susceptibility to a variety of hepatotoxicants correlates with the estimated hepatic taurine level.
- *In vitro* data suggest that taurine can protect cells against toxic damage.
- Taurine protects isolated hepatocytes against carbon tetrachloride, hydrazine, and 1,4-naphthoquinone, but not against allyl alcohol, alpha-naphthylisothiocyanate (ANIT), or diaminodiphenyl methane (DAPM) cytotoxicity.
- The mechanisms of protection are unclear but may include modulation of calcium levels, osmoregulation, and membrane stabilization.

TYROSINE

Tyrosine, a nonessential amino acid since it can be produced from phenylalanine in the body, is essential for the production of catecholamine neurotransmitters including: dopamine, dihydroxyphenylalanine (DOPA), norepinephrine, and epinephrine. Variations in neurotransmitter concentrations have been shown to result in a variety of physiological and psychological changes. For example, reductions in brain catecholamines have been found in association with depression and memory deficits.

Animal studies have shown that norepinephrine agonists reduce age-related declines in memory. In a recent study, tyrosine (100 and 200 mg/kg of body weight were used 15 min prior to challenge) significantly improved memory-dependent performance.[1378] Tyrosine has been found to minimize or reverse stress-induced performance decrement by increasing depleted pools of brain norepinephrine.[1379]

Tyrosine is the precursor for the hormones thyroxine and triiodothyronine from the thyroid gland and growth hormone from the pituitary. Also, the pigment melanin, which occurs in the skin and retina of the eye, forms from the enzymatic conversion of tyrosine.

Chapter 9

NONESSENTIAL OR DISPENSABLE AMINO ACIDS

INTRODUCTION

Dispensable amino acids, also called nonessential amino acids, can be synthesized by the body from other amino acids. The following eight amino acids can be considered to be nonessential in humans based on the body's ability to actually synthesize them from other amino acids under almost all conditions although, as discussed above, there is likely no amino acid which is nonessential since limiting amounts of the precursors of these amino acids in a diet that doesn't contain adequate amounts of these amino acids, will limit the body's ability to synthesize them.

Alanine*
Asparagine*
Aspartic Acid
Citrulline*
Glutamic Acid
Glycine
Ornithine
Serine

*Discussed elsewhere in this book.

ASPARTIC ACID

During an exercise of a high intensity, such as resistance training, ammonia is produced in large quantities and has been suggested to play a role in fatigue. The origin of ammonia under these conditions is generally believed to be the catabolism of adenine nucleotides. This results from an imbalance between the rate of ATP (adenosine triphosphate) utilization and its resynthesis within the contracting muscle cells.

As high concentrations of ammonia are toxic, the ammonia produced is converted to urea, a less toxic waste product synthesized in the liver by the enzymes of the urea cycle. Following this, it is secreted into the blood and taken up by the kidneys to be excreted in the urine. Aspartate, an amino acid involved in what is considered to be the rate-limiting step of the urea cycle, is widely available in vitamin and health food stores. Supplementation with aspartate has been theorized to enhance high-intensity exercise performance by increasing the speed of this reaction.

However, supplementation with aspartic acid or aspartate has not consistently been shown to have any anabolic or ergogenic effects although some increase in endurance capacity because of effects on ammonia metabolism has been found in some studies.[1391] Another study found that 7 days of oral arginine aspartate administration (250 mg/kg/d, or 25 g/d for a 100-kg bodybuilder) resulted in increases in sleep-related GH release in 5 normal human subjects.[1392] Administering 100 mg/kg/d failed to produce any significant effects.

A recent study has looked into the effects of aspartate supplementation on ammonia concentration during resistance training.[1393] In it, 12 men, ages 18 to 30 years, participated in 2 testing sessions separated by 7 days. A randomized, counterbalanced, double-blind protocol was followed in administering two compounds: (1) potassium-magnesium aspartate (orally, 150 mg/kg), and (2) vitamin C (orally, 150 mg/kg). One third of the calculated dose was ingested 5, 4, and 3 h prior to working out. Vitamin C was chosen as a placebo as it has no known effects on ammonia production or clearance.

Each exercise involved a warm-up set of 8 repetitions with 50% of the 1RM followed by 5 sets of 8 repetitions with 70% of the 1RM for the bench press and 3 sets of 8 repetitions with 70% of the 1RM for the incline press, behind-the-neck press, supine triceps extension, and biceps curl. A 2-min rest was permitted between sets. Then 2 min after completing the resistance training workout, each subject performed repetitions of the bench press to failure with 65% of the 1RM in order to assess the difference in physical performance between aspartate and vitamin C trials.

Following statistical analysis, it was found that there was no significant difference in ammonia concentration or bench press performance between aspartate and vitamin C trials. The researchers proposed several theories to explain the lack of an ergogenic effect with aspartate supplementation:

1. The ammonia levels produced during the workout may not have been great enough to challenge the urea cycle. Saturating the cycle with additional aspartate, they remarked, would therefore not have increased ammonia clearance.
2. If the subjects were consuming a high-protein diet (an issue which was not investigated in this study), the urea cycle may have been saturated with aspartate already.
3. Resting muscle fibers (i.e., present in the lower-body musculature) may have acted as a reservoir for ammonia during the exercise period, reducing the load placed on the liver for ammonia removal. Their involvement as buffers in the purine nucleotide cycle, the urea cycle, in exercise, and other functions are covered elsewhere in this book.

D-Aspartic acid (D-Asp) is an endogenous amino acid which occurs in many marine and terrestrial animals. In fetal and young rats this amino acid occurs prevalently in nervous tissue, whereas at sexual maturity it occurs in endocrine glands, mostly in the pituitary and testes. In a recent study set up to see if a relationship exists between the presence of D-Asp and hormonal activity[1394] the following results were obtained:

1. Both D-Asp and testosterone are synthesized in rat testes in two periods of the animal's life: before birth at about the 17th day after fertilization, and after birth, at sexual maturity.
2. Immunocytochemical studies have demonstrated that this enantiomer is localized in Leydig and Sertoli cells.
3. *In vivo* experiments, consisting of i.p. injection of D-Asp to adult male rats, demonstrated that this amino acid accumulates in pituitary and testis (after 5 h, the accumulation was of 12- and 4-fold over basal values, respectively); simultaneously, luteinizing hormone, testosterone, and progesterone significantly increased in the blood.
4. Finally, *in vitro* experiments consisting of the incubation of D-Asp with isolated testes also demonstrated that this amino acid induces the synthesis of testosterone.

These results suggest that free D-Asp is involved in the steroidogenesis. While there are no studies substantiating this effect in humans, there is a possibility that a connection exists and that this connection will be discovered in the near future. For example, most of the studies finding an ergogenic effect of aspartate in animals and humans utilized DL-aspartate, which is 50% D-Asp. Perhaps the benefits seen were related to the D-Asp rather than the L-Asp.[1395]

GLUTAMIC ACID

Glutamic acid is one of the most common amino acids found in nature. It occurs both in proteins and in its free form (i.e., unattached to other amino acids) in a variety of foods. Glutamic acid is the predominant amino acid in wheat protein (gliadin). Glutamate is the salt form of glutamic acid. The most common glutamate salt is monosodium glutamate (MSG), a widely used food additive and flavor enhancer.

As similar as glutamine and glutamate may sound and appear chemically, their roles in the body are radically different. Glutamate is important in brain metabolism as a major precursor for gamma-aminobutyric acid (GABA), an inhibitory neurotransmitter. Glutamate also participates in transamination processes and easily loses its amino group to keto acids giving rise to other amino acids (e.g., alanine from the transamination of pyruvate). Glutamate is a direct precursor of glutamine, proline, ornithine, arginine, and indirectly for glutathione. Glutamate is also a potential source of energy and plays an important role in the metabolism of ammonia (see above under Skeletal Muscle Catabolism).

Oral and intravenous glutamate supplementation (as MSG), has reduced plasma ammonium levels in humans with hepatic failure,[1396] showing that glutamate supplements have biological effects in humans. One study administered 9 g of MSG intravenously to 6 healthy male volunteers, followed by exercise to exhaustion on a cycle ergometer.[1397] Compared to saline infusion, MSG halved exercise-induced ammonia levels, but caused nausea in most subjects. Since MSG is known to be more toxic than glutamic acid or glutamate dipeptides (such as arginine glutamate), these findings are worthy of further study to determine whether glutamate supplementation would affect exercise performance.

ORNITHINE

Ornithine has many similarities with its parent amino acid arginine. Both are dibasic amino acids, both are involved in the urea cycle, and both have effects on insulin, glucagon, and growth hormone secretion and release. Unlike arginine, however, ornithine is not used for protein synthesis.

Ornithine may help increase growth hormone secretion in high doses.[1398] In one study, 12 bodybuilders were given 3 different doses of ornithine on successive weekends. Half of the bodybuilders responded to the highest dose (170 mg/kg) with significant increases in GH. Ornithine had no effect on serum insulin levels.

As explained earlier, ornithine is involved in the urea cycle and thus may have some effect in reducing exercise induced increased ammonia levels, and thus possibly decreasing fatigue.[1399] Ornithine is also involved in polyamine synthesis. Polyamines are important regulators of cell growth (see above).

ORNITHINE-ALPHA-KETOGLUTARATE

Ornithine-alpha-ketoglutarate (OKG) is a salt formed of two molecules of ornithine and one molecule of alpha-ketoglutarate. OKG appears to have anabolic properties which are greater than when the individual factors are given separately. A recent study has shown that the combination of ornithine and alpha-ketoglutarate modifies AA metabolism in a way not observed when they are administered separately.[1400] In addition, the study also indicated that the OKG-mediated increase in insulin levels probably does not appear to result from a direct action of ornithine on pancreatic secretion. Another study has shown that in the immediate postoperative period, total parenteral nutrition supplemented with OKG countered the decline in the muscle free glutamine, but supplementation with the BCAAs did not.[1401]

OKG has been successfully used, or has the potential to be used, by the enteral and parenteral route in burn, traumatized, cancer, and surgical patients, and in chronically malnourished subjects.[1402-1404] According to the metabolic situation, OKG treatment decreases muscle protein catabolism and/or increases synthesis. In addition, OKG promotes wound healing. In children receiving home intravenous nutrition, large doses of OKG have produced improvement in growth.[1405]

OKG is used as a fuel source and is oxidized by the citric acid cycle, thereby sparing glucose and raising liver glycogen content. It can be used to make BCAAs or BCKAs, as well as glutamate and glutamine; thus, OKG is valuable in the removal (detoxification) of ammonia. OKG also acts as a precursor for gluconeogenesis. It can be transformed into BCAAs or BCKAs, glutamate, and glutamine. As well, OKG seems to exert anticatabolic effects by preserving muscle glutamine.[1406,1407]

In a study on rats, the authors looked at the effect of enterally administered OKG on muscular amino acid content, eicosanoid release, and polymorphonuclear leukocyte responsiveness after induction of burn injury in rats.[1408] They concluded that OKG administered to rats with burn injuries displays immunomodulatory properties that can enhance host-defense mechanisms in animals that are affected by a severe injury.

Thus numerous clinical and laboratory trials have demonstrated the anabolic effects of supplementary OKG (it increases nitrogen retention and increases lean body mass) in patients recovering from burns, trauma, or other conditions associated with abnormal muscle catabolism.

Recently, OKG has been observed to dramatically increase the blood levels of insulin-like growth factor-1 — one of the more important anabolic growth factors,[1409] and to have important immunomodulatory effects.[1410]

OKG is largely used in clinical nutrition for its anabolic effects. However, its mechanism of action is not fully understood although the secretion of anabolic hormones (insulin, human growth hormone) and the synthesis of metabolites (glutamine, polyamines, arginine, ketoacids) may be involved.[1411,1412] Since OKG significantly improves the muscle glutamine pool[1413] and has recently been shown to enhance the amounts of arginine and glutamine in skeletal muscle,[1414] glutamine and arginine likely play a role in its action. As well, there is likely a link between the polyamine biosynthesis pathway and the anabolic effect of OKG.[1415]

Results from one study[1416] suggest that (1) the anticatabolic/anabolic action of OKG (in burn patients) is not mediated by insulin or hGH, and (2) OKG probably induces an increase in glucose tolerance in burn patients, in whom there is a state of insulin resistance.

In an attempt to determine if the action of ornithine alpha-ketoglutarate is due to its alpha-ketoglutarate moiety (as a glutamine precursor), the authors of a recent study looked at the effects of alpha-ketoglutarate administered to rats as ornithine alpha-ketoglutarate, or in combination with arginine salt (arginine alpha-ketoglutarate), as the two closely related amino acids have similar metabolic behavior.[1416a]

The results of the study demonstrated, for the first time, the following: (1) the action of ornithine alpha-ketoglutarate as a glutamine precursor cannot solely be ascribed to alpha-ketoglutarate since arginine alpha-ketoglutarate combinations did not exhibit this effect to the same extent; and (2) the action of ornithine alpha-ketoglutarate is not due to its nitrogen content since isonitrogenous arginine alpha-ketoglutarate did not reproduce the effects of ornithine alpha-ketoglutarate.

Another recent study has shown that OKG is effective orally and that the bolus mode of OKG administration appeared to be associated with higher metabolite production compared with continuous infusion in burn patients, especially for glutamine and arginine.[1416b]

SERINE

Serine is widely used for synthesizing various proteins in the body and is an important glucogenic substrates in high-protein diets.[1417] Serine is also an integral component of the phospholipid phosphatidylserine (PS) and regulates both the formation of PS and the rate of decarboxylation of phosphatidylserine to phosphatidylethanolamine.[1418]

Phospholipids are fats similar to triacylglycerols (triglycerides) in that they are constructed from a glycerol backbone but have two fatty acids attached by ester bonds instead of three fatty acids. Instead of a third fatty acid, phospholipids have a negatively charged phosphate group coupled with a polar alcohol. Examples are phosphatidylcholine, containing choline, and similarly phosphatidylinositol with inositol, phosphatidylserine with serine, and phosphatidylethanolamine with ethanolamine. Phosphatidylserine (PS) is a natural fat-like substance found in cell membranes.

Cerebral cortex neuronal membrane phospholipids are composed of phosphatidylcholine, phophatidylethanolamine, phosphatidylserine, and phosphatidylinositol. While the membrane receptor and secondary messenger characteristics of phosphatidylinositol and its metabolites have been extensively investigated,[1419-1421] the functions of other phospholipids are less certain.

Phosphatidylcholine is known to confer a stabilizing influence within the neuronal membrane.[1422] The carboxyl groups of phosphatidylserine function as ion-exchange sites[1423] while both phosphatidylserine and phosphatidylethanolamine have an important influence on the distribution of protein molecules in the membrane.[1424] The degree of unsaturation present in neuronal phospholipid fatty acids can mediate the activities of membrane-bound enzymes.[1425,1426]

There is clustering of phosphatidylserine, phosphatidylethanolamine, and phosphatidylcholine head groups into membrane areas known as domains. The phosphatidylserine and phosphatidylethanolamine domains are critically important for neurotransmitter function. It has long been recognized that there are structural similarities between phosphoserine, which is the hydrophilic moiety of phosphatidylserine, and the major central nervous system activatory neurotransmitter glutamate (or aspartate) and the polar phosphoethanolamine of phosphatidylethanolamine, which resembles the inhibitory amino acid neurotransmitter gamma-aminobutyric acid (GABA). The phospholipids phosphatidylethanolamine and phosphatidylserine are known to exchange polar head groups directly *in vivo* and may also be interconverted in a simple irreversible decarboxylation reaction similar to that which neutralizes the effect of glutamate by its conversion to GABA.[1427] Although there is no direct evidence that phosphatidylserine functions in tandem with glutamate, it is known that L-AP4 (L-2-amino-4-phosphonobutanoic acid), a phosphorus-containing molecule structurally similar to phosphoserine, is a proven L-glutamate agonist at presynaptic terminals and retinal bipolar receptors.[1428-1430] It may be that phosphatidylserine and phosphatidylethanolamine have a neurotransmitter function that could be independent or work in parallel with the glutamate-GABA system.

PS administrations may be useful for treating the neurochemical and behavioral changes that occur with aging and for improving learning and memory.[1431-1435] Studies have shown that PS is produced less with age, and appears to beneficially affect brain function through interacting with brain neurotransmitters. In one study, PS induced consistent improvement of depressive symptoms, memory, and behavior in a group of ten elderly women with depressive disorders.[1436] Thus because of the potential role of PS in neuroendocrine-immune communications,[1437] PS is one of the agents proposed for the treatment of various disorders including Alzheimer's disease.[1438,1439]

PS is a necessary cofactor for protein kinase C (PKC) activation, and changes in the synthesis of PS have been shown to participate in the mechanism(s) involved in the transmembrane signaling of interleukin 1 (IL-1). In one study involving both *in vitro* and *in vivo* treatments with PS, the authors found that:[1440]

1. *In vivo* treatment of aging animals with the specific phospholipid PS is able to reverse the physiological decline of the humoral immune response induced by the ageing process.

2. Pharmacological depression of humoral immune response induced by a treatment of adult animals with dexamethasone was similarly reversed by a chronic treatment with PS.
3. Treatment of young rats with PS reversed the pharmacologically associated depression of specific antibody production.
4. The *in vitro* effects of the phospholipid on human PBMC and rat splenocytes suggests that PS is implicated in T-cell activation through its action on IL-2 receptors.

PS has recently been advertised and marketed as an ergogenic aid because of its anti-catabolic and anticortisol effects. PS readily penetrates the blood brain-barrier and may work by being incorporated into brain cell membranes and consequently altering the corticotrophin-releasing factor responses to cell receptor binding, which in turn prevents the associated stress hormone cascade.

Two studies done in Italy showed that PS given either systemically[1441] or orally,[1442] blunted the ACTH and cortisol response to exercise. In the 1992 study, 800 mg/d of PS for 10 days significantly blunted the ACTH and cortisol responses to physical exercise without affecting the rise in plasma growth hormone. Because of its effects in decreasing exercise-induced increases in serum cortisol, PS may increase the anabolic response to exercise although more research needs to be done to see if the decrease in cortisol translates into increased protein synthesis and lean body mass gains. As well, the effects of PS on training soreness, stiffness, and injuries potentially secondary to the cortisol reduction must be evaluated.

GLYCINE

Glycine, the simplest of the amino acids, can be derived by the loss of one carbon atom from serine and is used for the formation of other amino acids. While a nonessential or dispensable amino acid, during periods of rapid growth the demand for glycine may be increased. Glycine participates in the synthesis of purines, porphyrins, creatine, and glyoxylic acid. Glyoxylic acid is of interest because its oxidation yields oxalic acid, of which there is increased formation in the genetic disorder oxaluria. Furthermore, glycine conjugates with a variety of substances thus allowing their excretion in the bile or urine.

Glycine is an important constituent of collagen. Nearly one third of the amino acid residues in collagen are glycine (explaining the high glycine content of gelatin, which is denatured collagen), and another 15 to 30% of its residues are proline and 4-hydroxyproline (a compound released in increased quantities following resistance training).

Collagen, an extracellular protein that is organized into insoluble fibers of great tensile strength, occurs in all animals and is the most abundant protein of vertebrates. Collagen is found in virtually every tissue in the human body and is the major stress-bearing component of connective tissues such as bone, teeth, cartilage, tendon, ligament, and the fibrous matrices of skin and blood vessels.

Collagen and skeletal muscle are quantitatively important reservoirs for glycine. In the transurethral resection syndrome, when glycine is supplied in potentially toxic amounts (irrigation is done with a glycine-containing solution), the concentrations of glycine in plasma and muscle were equal within an hour of the operation, and at 4 h, the abnormally high glycine concentration persisted in muscle, though it had decreased rapidly in plasma.[1443]

Glycine used with arginine has been shown to increase endogenous creatine levels by increasing creatine synthesis.[1444-1446] A number of studies using glycine for the alleviation of fatigue and as a possible treatment for muscular dystrophy, myasthenia gravis, and other diseases were done in the 1930s and 1940s but the results were minimal.[1447]

Glycine is one of seven amino acids thought to have inhibitory neurotransmitter or neurotransmitter precursor function.[1448,1449] The others are GABA, taurine, serine, threonine, phenylalanine, and tyrosine and are used directly by certain neurons without change. Glutamic acid, aspartic acid, and glycine play roles as excitatory neurotransmitters, but exert a neurodegenerative effect in case of excessive release.[1450]

Glycine has also been shown to increase GH secretion in a dose-dependent manner. In one study the authors found that oral administration of 6.75 g of glycine to 19 human subjects increased growth hormone levels significantly for 3 h, peaking at 3 to 4 times baseline at 2 h.[1451]

In another study, different doses (4, 8, or 12 g) of glycine were intravenously infused over 15 or 30 min in normal subjects.[1452] Serum levels of GH (growth hormone) and prolactin were measured before and after the infusion, and also blood sugar levels were determined. The dose of 4 or 8 g glycine induced a significant increase in serum GH; however, a more pronounced and significant increase in serum GH levels was observed after infusion at a dose of 12 g glycine.

Because of the GH response, one might expect significant effects of glycine supplementation on protein synthesis. The result of a recent study, however, has shown that an isonitrogenous amount of glycine merely decreases protein turnover with only a small anabolic effect resulting from a greater decrease in proteolysis than protein synthesis.[1453] No studies have been done on the effects of oral glycine on GH levels and protein synthesis in athletes.

Glycine, as well as the other gluconeogenic amino acids (alanine, glutamine, threonine, serine, methionine, tyrosine, and lysine), are elevated in brief starvation and on low-protein diets.[1454] Brief starvation is associated with an increase in gluconeogenesis, suggesting increased release of amino acids from muscle (see above under Gluconeogenesis).

Chapter 10

NATURALLY ANABOLIC

INTRODUCTION

Both competitive and recreational athletes make use of a vast arsenal of drugs to improve their performance and appearance, and to combat some of the side effects of other drugs. Besides the well-publicized anabolic steroids, several classes of compounds are used in an attempt to increase muscle mass and strength and improve performance:

- Anabolic steroids and testosterone
- Stimulants
  - Adrenalin
  - Adrenergic compounds
  - Amphetamines and amphetamine derivatives
  - Arcalion
  - Caffeine
  - Cocaine
  - Heptaminol
  - Nicotine
  - Piracetam
  - Sydnocarb
- Narcotic analgesics — including agonists, partial agonists, and antagonists
- Growth factors and peptides
  - Growth hormone
  - Growth hormone-releasing hormone (GHRH)
  - Growth hormone stimulators such as arginine, ornithine, clonidine, L-dopa, etc.
  - Insulin-like growth factor-1 (IGF-1)
  - Epithelial growth factor (EGF)
  - Galanin
- Compounds that increase endogenous androgen levels
  - Human chorionic gonadotropin (HCG)
  - Menotropins (Pergonal)
  - Gonadorelin (Factrel)
  - Antiestrogens (clomiphene, cyclofenil, tamoxifen)
- Other hormones
  - Insulin and insulinotropic drugs (glyburide, metformin)
  - Thyroid hormone (T4, T3, tiratricol)
  - Hypothalamic and pituitary releasing hormones such as TRH, TSH, ACTH
  - ADH or Vasopressin
  - Pitocin
  - Erythropoietin (EPO)
  - Dehydroepiandrosterone (DHEA)
  - Melatonin
- Compounds to block the anticatabolic effects of cortisol
  - Aminogluthetimide
  - Mifepristone (RU486)
  - Mitotane
  - Trilostane
- Anti-inflammatory compounds
  - Corticosteroids
  - Nonsteroidal anti-inflammatory drugs (NSAIDs)
  - Dimethylsulfoxide (DMSO)
  - Veterinary cartilage-based compounds

Miscellaneous compounds with putative anabolic or ergogenic effects
- Beta 2 adrenergic agonists such as clenbuterol, cimaterol, salbutamol, and fenoterol
- Cyproheptadine
- Gamma-hydroxybutyrate (GHB)
- Pentoxifylline (Trental)
- Perchlorate
- Selegiline (deprenyl)
- Yohimbine
- Zeranol (Ralgro)

Miscellaneous compounds used in an attempt to enhance performance
- Alcohol
- Beta-blockers
- Calcium channel blockers
- Cyclobenzaprine
- Diuretics
- Local anesthetics
- Marijuana

This list is just the tip of the iceberg; in fact, it might be difficult to find a substance with which some aspiring athlete has not experimented.

Drugs work. They improve muscle mass, strength, and athletic performance. But for many reasons drug use by athletes is a serious problem. Not only are there moral and health ramifications to the use of performance-enhancing drugs by athletes, but for substances such as the illicit drugs, the amphetamines, anabolic steroids and growth hormone we also have to consider the legal consequences of their use. Anabolic steroids and growth hormone, drugs used mainly by athletes, have recently been classified as controlled substances in North America and other places.

In addition to the legal ramifications of anabolic steroid and growth hormone use, there are the health risks inherent in how these compounds are obtained and used. The main source for these drugs, and information on how to use them, is the black market, where counterfeit and tainted products and misinformation are the rule.

In light of the legal, moral, and health ramifications of drug use by athletes, it makes sense to dissuade the athlete from using performance-enhancing drugs. However, asking athletes to stop using drugs is not enough. We also have to offer the athlete a viable alternative to drug use. We believe that nutritional supplements, in conjunction with enlightened training and diet, is this alternative.

In this section we will present ways to maximize the anabolic effects of diet, exercise, and nutritional supplements (especially protein and amino acids), and offer a viable alternative to drug use by athletes. The information below will be useful not only for the elite athlete, but for anyone wishing to maximize their athletic prowess and maintain a vigorous, healthy body.

MAXIMIZING LEAN BODY MASS AND ATHLETIC PERFORMANCE WITHOUT DRUGS

HORMONAL MANIPULATION

In order to maximize gains it's important to maximize the anabolic environment by controlling the anabolic and catabolic hormones through the manipulation of training, diet, and nutritional supplements.

Although there are vast numbers of variables to consider when attempting to increase the anabolic and decrease the catabolic effects of exercise, a good starting point is the eight hormones that are intimately involved in muscle metabolism (see below). By manipulating the various endogenous anabolic and catabolic influences, we should, to some extent, be able to maximize the anabolic effects of exercise and minimize the catabolic ones.

With enough care and detail, it may be possible to maximize the effect of the endogenous hormones so that the use of exogenous hormones and compounds (such as anabolic steroids, growth hormone, and clenbuterol) would be superfluous and perhaps even counterproductive (since the use of exogenous drugs would disrupt the endogenous hormonal levels).

The eight main hormones to consider when attempting to maximize the body's natural anabolic drive are:

Testosterone
Growth hormone
IGF-1 (insulin-like growth factor-1)
Insulin
Thyroid
Cortisol
Glucagon
Catecholamines

While we still have a lot to learn about the various hormonal responses to changes in diet, training, and lifestyle, we do know enough to put together this information into a comprehensive system of eating, training, and nutritional supplementation. By manipulating our diet, exercise, and lifestyle, we can increase insulin, GH, and IGF-1 and testosterone levels, and decrease cortisol levels and other anticatabolic factors at specific times so as to maximize increases in lean body mass.

It's important to either create an anabolic hormonal cascade or to make proper use of natural fluctuations and spikes in the endogenous anabolic hormones. The end result is an anabolic and anticatabolic effect both in and around the time of training, in the critical posttraining period, and at other times of the day.

It's difficult, however, to get the hormones and nutrients synchronized so that they can work together synergistically. For example, the problem with natural growth hormone spikes is that they almost always occur in the postabsorptive phase where exogenous nutrients are in short supply and are not available to muscle cells. The main actions of GH under postabsorptive conditions is thus anticatabolic. That is, GH decreases muscle protein catabolism but has little anabolic action since there is relatively little influx of amino acids into the cells. As well, at these times there is very little insulin effect because there's no stimulus for insulin release.

Ideally, all the anabolic and anticatabolic effects of the various hormones should be maximized (through a synergistic action of testosterone, insulin, GH, IGF-1 and thyroid), and the catabolic effects of cortisol minimized at a time when the availability of nutrients is maximal. Creating this ideal environment for muscle growth requires both knowledge and dedication.

This is one of the main reasons that going natural, unless one is precise as to the timing of training, meals and supplements, can be so discouraging. When drugs are used this is not a problem. For example, the use of anabolic steroids and testosterone esters gives you a constant high level of testosterone with no dips or low-level intervals; then by using exogenous GH and insulin one can elevate all three anabolic hormones at the same time, when in fact this is not usually seen in those who don't use drugs since there are feedback loops regulating their actions.

For example, a recent study suggests the presence of a peripheral negative feedback loop that allows IGF-1 to limit locally the response of extrahepatic tissues to circulating GH.[1466] Add to this mix a large and ready supply of amino acids and other nutrients and you have a recipe for maximal muscle growth, albeit drug induced.

The idea behind the targeting of supplements (along with appropriate training and diet) is to do all this naturally. However, unlike the use of drugs, one has to be precise in the implementation of supplements and know exactly what one is doing in order to create and make maximum use of any possible synergism between elevated levels of endogenous testosterone, GH, insulin, and IGF-1, and decreased levels of cortisol.

Amino acid supplements can be very useful in manipulating protein synthesis. For example, as we've seen above, the use of the amino acid glutamine has been shown to prevent the cortisol-induced destruction of muscle contractile proteins. As well, glutamine has been shown to increase both growth hormone and insulin secretion. The judicious use of glutamine could give us both anabolic and anticatabolic effects.

All athletes could benefit from this manipulation, especially those involved in sports where strength and lean body mass are of primary importance for athletic success.[1467] The following steps make up a comprehensive natural system to maximize muscle mass and strength and enhance athletic performance.

STEP NUMBER ONE — LIFESTYLE CHANGES

Keeping testosterone and other anabolic hormones (such as GH and IGF-1) levels high, decreasing basal levels of cortisone, and increasing the testosterone/cortisol ratio are important in order to maximize strength, muscle mass and athletic performance. An athlete's lifestyle should be optimized so as to eliminate any factors that can adversely affect the endogenous hormones.

Many studies have highlighted factors (including the use of illicit drugs and alcohol) that can adversely affect the anabolic and catabolic hormones and the testosterone/cortisol ratio.

The use of illicit drugs as well as alcohol and nicotine are common among both professional and amateur athletes.[1468] A recent study examined the use of recreational and illicit drugs and alcohol in Canadian university athletes.[1469] The authors estimated the proportion of Canadian university athletes using social and/or ergogenic drugs through survey methods. Using a stratified random sampling procedure, 754 student athletes were surveyed in eight different sports from eight universities across Canada. Results showed that 17.7 percent of athletes have used major pain medications over the past twelve months, 3 percent reported use of weight loss products, 0.9 percent reported anabolic steroid use, 16.6 percent reported use of smokeless tobacco products, 94.1 percent reported use of alcohol, 65.2 percent reported use of caffeine products, 0.7 percent reported use of amphetamines, 1.0 percent reported use of barbiturates, 19.8 percent reported use of marijuana or hashish, 5.9 percent reported use of psychedelics and 0.8 percent reported use of cocaine/crack.

A recent study looked at the effects of alcohol on GH and testosterone in peripubertal rats.[1470] The authors measured serum levels of GH and testosterone were measured at 1.5, 3, 6, and 24 h after a single injection of either saline or ethanol. The authors found that acute alcohol use decreases both serum testosterone and growth hormone.

Several other studies have shown the testosterone lowering effects of an unhealthy lifestyle and the abuse of alcohol and other licit and illicit drugs. Studies have shown that sleep deprivation adversely affects testicular function leading to lower serum levels of testosterone.[1471] Decreased testosterone levels and secretion rates are observed under stressful conditions (anesthesia, anxiety, hangover, exhaustion, undernutrition, overtraining) as well as with increased serum cortisol levels and ACTH stimulation. Drugs such as alcohol,[1472-1475] marijuana,[1582,1583] narcotics,[1584,1585] and cocaine[1586,1587] have adverse effects on serum testosterone levels.

The repeated use of cocaine and amphetamines has been shown to enhance the activity of the hypothalamo-pituitary-adrenal axis and lead to a decrease in the hypothalamo-pituitary-gonadal axis activity.[1588,1589] The overall result of chronic use of these stimulants is counterproductive for athletes, leading to a decrease in serum testosterone, an increase in serum cortisol, and a decrease in the testosterone/cortisol ratio.

Alcohol has been shown to affect the circadian rhythms of LH, testosterone and its conversion to DHT, and to decrease the LH and testicular secretion in response to leutenizing hormone releasing hormone.[1590] One recent study looked at the combined effect of alcohol and physical exercise on serum testosterone, luteinizing hormone, and cortisol in males.[1591] The authors found that physical stress immediately before alcohol administration prolonged the depressant effect of alcohol on testosterone secretion.

While the acute and chronic use of alcohol has adverse effects on serum testosterone in men, such may not be the case in women. One study found that high doses of alcohol increases serum testosterone,[1592] while another found that daily alcohol intake appeared to be positively and independently correlated to both plasma total and free testosterone levels.[1593] Alcohol, however, has other ergolytic effects and overall adversely affects athletic performance in both men and women.

In 1982, based on an analysis of the research on alcohol and human performance, the American College of Sports Medicine issued a position statement decrying the use of alcohol in sports. Its two main conclusions were (1) the acute ingestion of alcohol can impair many psychomotor skills, including reaction time, balance, accuracy, hand-eye coordination, and complex coordination; and (2) alcohol will not improve, and may decrease strength, power, speed, local muscular endurance, and cardiovascular endurance.[1594]

Nicotine can also adversely affect performance. Another recent study was set up to examine the effects of long-term cigarette smoking on the levels of plasma testosterone, luteinizing hormone (LH) and follicle- stimulating hormone (FSH) in male adult rats and to examine morphological and histological changes in the testes.[1595] In this study rats were exposed to cigarette smoke generated by a smoking-machine and diluted with 90% air for 60 days (2 hours/day). Twelve rats were exposed to room air only under similar conditions as controls. The concentrations of plasma testosterone, LH and FSH were measured before and after exposure and the testes were examined histologically.

The results of this study showed that in rats exposed to smoke, testosterone levels decreased significantly, but there were no significant changes in testosterone in the control rats. The mean plasma LH and FSH levels of the two groups did not change significantly after exposure. In rats exposed to smoke, histological examination of the testes showed fewer Leydig cells and degeneration of the remaining cells. The authors concluded that the decrease in plasma testosterone levels induced by exposure to smoke was not associated with changes in plasma gonadotrophin levels but was likely related to the toxic effects of smoke on Leydig cells.

Many athletes expose themselves to nicotine by smoking or using smokeless tobacco. Nicotine can enter the body through the lungs by smoking, the buccal mucosa by way of smokeless tobacco (chewing tobacco and snuff) and nicotine gum, and transdermally by way of transdermal nicotine patches.

Smoking is the most common and least desirable way of taking nicotine. The effects and adverse effects of smoking are due to both nicotine and the over 2000 different chemical substances (including carbon monoxide) contained in tobacco smoke. Many of these substances act as irritants and carcinogenic agents and have also been shown to decrease the lungs ability to clean itself. The result can be severe lung disease and lung cancer.

Cigarette smoking can increase atherosclerosis and result in strokes, heart disease and sudden cardiac death.[1596] Smoking has an overall dysfunctional effect on the hypothalamic-pituitary-testicular axis, decreasing serum levels of androgens and impairing male reproduction.[1597,1598]

Perhaps even more important to the athlete is, as pointed out in the above study, cigarette smoking decreases plasma testosterone levels. Animal studies have shown that nicotine and cotinine, the major metabolite of nicotine, inhibit testicular steroidogenesis[1599,1600] and may act as a neuromodulator during sexual differentiation of the brain, demasculinizing the male progeny in rats. This effect is correlated with decreased testosterone levels during adulthood.[1601] Nicotine has been shown not only to effect basal testosterone levels but also human chorionic gonadotropin (HCG) induced testosterone secretion.[1602] As well, smoking and nicotine can increase circulating plasma concentrations of cortisol, in both smokers and non smokers (second hand smokers?).[1603-1605]

So with all these bad side effects why smoke? Because once you start it's hard to stop.

Nicotine, one of the most addictive drugs known, affects many body functions, influences the secretion of several hormones and stimulates the sympathetic and parasympathetic nervous system and adrenal glands. Small doses stimulate the autonomic nervous system and skeletal muscle neuromuscular junctions, and has effects similar to small doses of amphetamines. Larger doses act as a depressant at these sites. In addition, nicotine stimulates the central nervous system directly, desynchronizing cortical electrical activity and releasing vasopressin and beta-endorphins.

As if the addiction and all the side effects we've mentioned weren't enough the study below seems to indicate that smokers suffer more musculoskeletal pain than non smokers.[1606]

The present study was based on data from the Norwegian Health Survey 1985, a nationwide interview survey with members of a representative sample of households. Their sample comprised all adult respondents who had reported musculoskeletal pain. Smokers experienced more intense pain than nonsmokers. The association remained significant after adjusting for workplace factors, social network factors, alcohol consumption, and intake of cod liver oil as dietary supplement.

The message is simple. If maximizing lean muscle mass and strength is important to you then you should optimize your lifestyle including reducing stress, getting proper rest and keeping away from recreational drug use and the excessive use of alcohol and nicotine.

STEP NUMBER TWO — TRAINING WITHOUT OVERTRAINING

The next step is to make appropriate changes in training. Describing the right way to train would take another whole book. In short, however, to increase muscle mass, strength, and stamina (something all athletes strive for) one has to train in such a way that the anabolic and catabolic hormones are fine-tuned to give maximum results. Controlling anabolic and catabolic influences during training and recovery can maximize strength and muscle mass gains by most efficiently translating the response to exercise into increased protein synthesis and decreased protein catabolism.

That means having to train both hard and smart. To get ongoing consistent increases in muscle mass and strength, one needs to do enough exercise so that one's body must adapt to the new work load. For example, if the athlete is training with weights, in order to make any progress he or she will have to handle more weight and/or do more reps in a certain time interval. Unless one does enough work, the body is not going to grow because it doesn't need to adapt.

There's another side to this equation that's just as important. We now know that if the high-intensity training isn't there, then the athlete is not going to grow. However, if it is there but one cannot adapt to the training load, then one still won't grow. Successful adaptation to high-intensity exercise results in anabolic changes providing that the adaptive stress is high enough and forces adaptation to occur. Exercise stress that doesn't require any significant degree of adaptation will not result in a positive training effect.

The changes that occur in muscle protein metabolism are due to the duration, intensity, and type of exercise employed. For example, long-term heavy-resistance exercise leads to increases in muscle mass, while low-resistance endurance exercise causes little or no size changes but induces numerous subcellular changes that result in increased endurance capacity.

After exercise, adaptive protein synthesis starts. After endurance exercises the main locus of adaptive protein synthesis is in the mitochondrial proteins of oxidative or oxidative-glycolytic muscles, whereas after exercises for improved strength, adaptive protein synthesis will take place to the fullest extent in regard to the myofibrillar proteins of glycolytic fibers.

The molecular basis for muscle hypertrophy has been studied in animals through the use of various methods including surgical procedures, weights, or electrically stimulated contractions to produce chronic resistance or stretch on specific muscles. Muscle hypertrophy appears to require full extension of the muscle and resistance, while high levels of intensity and duration of the activity are not useful. These procedures produce rapid increases in muscle weight and protein content and corresponding increases in muscle RNA content and the rate of protein synthesis.

At the molecular level, these experimental models suggest that hypertrophy of skeletal muscle is dependent on stimulation of transcription to increase muscle protein synthesis. The regulatory controls and limits of this response remain unknown.

RECOVERY PHASE — PROTEIN SYNTHESIS AFTER EXERCISE

In the transition from high- to low-energy demands,recovery occurs. In this recovery period there occurs a restoration of energy resources, removal of metabolic waste material, and a return to normal levels of hydration, electrolytes, and tissue homeostatic levels.

In regard to metabolism, the recovery period means not only transition from high- to low-energy demands, but also restoration of energy reserves, abolishment of the accumulated metabolic intermediates, as well as normalization of water and ionic composition in body compartments. In the course of repletion of energy reserves the phenomenon of supercompensation has been found. This gives a peculiar feature to the delayed stage of the recovery period. Recovery period also means a change in protein metabolism opposite to that happening during exercise. The altered balance between anabolic and catabolic processes has to warrant an effective renewal of exhausted cellular structures and enzyme molecules as well as the opportunity for the increase in active structures and in the number of enzyme molecules.

The renewal of structural and enzymatic proteins in the muscular tissue can be completed only after the end of muscle activity. Accordingly, an elevated intensity of protein synthesis is considered to be common for the recovery period after exercise. The exercise-induced decrease of protein nitrogen is reversed after the cessation of contractile activity.

However, it would be an oversimplification to regard the postexercise recovery as a transition from exercise-induced overall catabolism to anabolism. The picture is more complicated.

During the first hours of postexercise recovery the rate of protein synthesis remains low in the skeletal muscle of humans and rats. During the recovery period the inhibition of protein synthesis in previously less active muscles and fibers makes it possible to concentrate the adaptive protein synthesis for structures that performed the highest load.

After exercise for improved strength, the main locus of adaptive protein synthesis is the myofibrillar proteins of fast-twitch glycolytic fibers. In men the action of a resistance training session (4 sets of 6 to 12 repetitions of the biceps curl, preacher curl, and concentration curl with a resistance equal to 80% 1RM) on protein synthesis in the biceps muscle was studied, using the opposite arm as a control.[1475a] Muscle protein synthesis was significantly elevated 4 h postexercise. The increased protein synthesis rate persisted for at least 24 h. The increase appeared to be due to changes in posttranscriptional events. The latter conclusion was founded on the unchanged RNA capacity (expressed as total RNA content relative to noncollagenous protein content) and elevated RNA activity (expressed as the amount of protein synthesized per unit time per unit RNA).

HORMONAL CHANGES WITH EXERCISE

Androgens such as testosterone (and trophic hormones such as luteinizing hormone [LH]) increase with intense exercise as long as the exercise is not exhausting. Thus, short, intense training sessions will give the best results and maximize lean body mass and strength. When exercise duration is too long, the level of testosterone decreases. Thus repetitive and prolonged heavy exercise results in overtraining and in decreased protein synthesis and increased muscle catabolism.

GH also increases with increasing intensity and duration of exercise. The degree of ATP regeneration, waste removal, and oxygen availability seem to dictate the GH response. We believe that the best marker of GH increase is the degree of ATP regeneration. Thus if ATP is not able to be regenerated maximally, then GH increases proportionally. It's important, therefore, to exercise in such a way that there is some anaerobic component present. Again, short, hard, intense training sessions would be most productive.

Overtraining is to be avoided since even though overtraining may result in elevated levels of GH and even testosterone during and shortly after exercise, it results in chronically lowered serum levels of both hormones. We thus need to strike a balance between GH and testosterone increases both during and between exercise sessions.

Conversely, cortisol (which induces the breakdown of cellular proteins) increases with increased duration of intense exercise. Cortisol induces the breakdown of cellular proteins, thereby liberating amino acids which can then undergo gluconeogenesis in the liver. Although cortisol and GH often rise simultaneously as testosterone decreases, there are ways of exercising so as to minimize cortisol and maximize GH and testosterone. An elevation in cortisol has been associated with decreased testosterone levels. Cortisol may act directly upon the testis to impair the biosynthesis of testosterone. Conversely, testosterone can decrease the catabolic effects of cortisol.

Insulin, an anabolic hormone, also should be brought into play. In order to increase insulin response during exercise, it's necessary to increase blood sugar levels or to use compounds such as certain amino acids that stimulate insulin secretion. Increasing serum glucose levels (either directly or through an increase in gluconeogenesis) may lead to decreasing levels of GH, but this is not necessarily the case. As discussed above, studies have shown that plasma glucose concentrations increase during exercise while GH is increasing. Therefore, although hypoglycemia is implicated in GH increase, this is not the mechanism of GH increase during exercise, and in fact serum glucose may not be a factor during exercise.

Weight-training sessions with shorter rest intervals also induce significant increases in serum IGF-1 concentrations both during exercise and for up to 90 min following exercise.

Ideally, in order to counteract some of the catabolic effects of exercise stress, it would be useful to limit extreme rises in corticosteroids (some elevation is necessary to prevent musculoskeletal fatigue, stiffness, and injuries) that would decrease serum testosterone levels, and to increase testosterone, GH, and insulin levels.

As we have seen, hormone responses are dependent on the intensity and duration of the training sessions and the level of physical fitness of the individual. Thus one of the bases for the improvement in muscle mass and strength is the successful adaptation to exercise which results in an overall increase in protein synthesis. The metabolic events both during and after exercise (both training and recovery periods) determine the degree of adaptation that occurs secondary to a training load.

Thus it's important to use a training program that is both specific to the changes desired and is of proper intensity and duration. Along with an adequate training program, assuming normal physiological (metabolic and hormonal) responses to this program, there must be a nutritional environment that can make maximal use of the exercise-induced metabolic and hormonal changes.

Although there is a variability in the hormonal response to exercise depending on the type of training, inter-individual variation, emotional states, environmental conditions, and nutrient availability (for example, protein, individual amino acids, and carbohydrate supply), a number of studies have shown that there are some common and predictable responses in some of the hormones.

Various studies have shown that growth hormone and testosterone levels may vary according to the type of resistance exercise. For example, when resistance is heavy and rest is long, as characterized by strength/power programs, little change is seen in circulating levels of growth hormone, but testosterone levels may rise if the amount of muscle tissue mass used in the exercise is great enough. Conversely, if resistance is moderately heavy and of sufficient duration and a short rest period is used, increases in growth hormone and testosterone can be expected.

The hormonal changes depend on the configuration of exercise stress and the subsequent alterations produced in the nerves and muscle. The amount of muscle mass stimulated, the rest between sets and exercises, and the resistance used are vital factors in eliciting hormonal increases.

High-intensity training that is not taken to exhaustion generally results in increases in GH and cortisol that continue in the recovery period, decreases in insulin, subtle increases in thyroid hormone, increase then a decrease in testosterone during training and a fluctuating level during recovery, increases in catecholamines during training, and a decrease in IGF-1.[1476,1477] The insulin level decline during exercise is an effect more evident in experienced athletes.[1478]

For athletes with a long training background and with a high training volume, the role of endogenous hormone optimization may be extremely important for strength development. During the most stressful training weeks, measurement of serum testosterone, GH, and cortisol may be of great importance for achieving maximum results.[1479-1481] Thus the monitoring of serum testosterone, GH, and cortisol might be a way of judging if an athlete is training maximally or overtraining. The drop in testosterone and/or GH levels, and a rise in cortisol levels, could be used as indicators of overtraining.

Since it's been shown that chronic high-intensity training actually lowers performance, periodizing your training helps prevent overtraining and makes your training more productive.[1482] The basic premise behind the periodization of training is that the body must be trained in a systematic step-like fashion, through various cycles or phases, towards ever-increasing performance levels.[1483-1485]

Making use of various kinds of training methods can enhance the anabolic response to exercise. For example, eccentric muscle actions (those in which a muscle generates force while lengthening) play an important role in the hypertrophic response to exercise and should be incorporated into the training of those athletes looking to increase muscle mass and strength.[1486]

MAXIMIZING THE ANABOLIC AND MINIMIZING THE CATABOLIC EFFECTS OF EXERCISE

Exercise is the most potent catabolic and anabolic agent known. Performed to excess, whether with resistance training or marathon running, exercise will result in an overall catabolic process that will result in loss of muscle and strength. In such cases we often find chronically lowered serum testosterone and elevated serum cortisol levels. Elevated cortisol levels decrease amino acid transport and protein synthesis, and increase muscle breakdown.

In order to maximize athletic performance, it's important to not only increase protein synthesis but to decrease protein degradation. Today there is a faddish interest in anticatabolic compounds and supplements. Anticatabolic really means much the same as protein sparing (a term that has been around for a number of years) as far as end results. Protein sparing is generally applied to certain measures that decrease muscle breakdown. For example, taking in adequate carbohydrates is known to have a protein-sparing effect.

There is some confusion, however, about exactly what the term anticatabolic means. Some people are using the term anticatabolic interchangeably with the term antiglucocorticoid. This can lead to misconceptions even though in many cases an anticatabolic effect may be mediated by decreasing the effect of glucocorticoids on muscle tissue. However, there are other factors and influences to consider when a certain substance or regimen produces an overall anticatabolic effect.

As well, the popular notion of cortisol being solely a catabolic hormone is not accurate. Too much cortisol can certainly be a problem, but cortisol is a necessary hormone and in athletes plays a role in decreasing muscle stiffness and inflammation. Without normal and even somewhat elevated cortisol levels we couldn't even exercise properly, so it wouldn't matter what training, diet, drugs, and nutritional supplement regimens we were following. In fact, in some sports short cycles of synthetic cortisol-like drugs are used to enhance both strength and endurance.

Protein balance is a function of intake relative to output (utilization and loss). Body proteins are in a constant state of flux, with both protein degradation and protein synthesis constantly going on. Normally, these two processes are equal with no net loss or net gain of protein taking place. Protein intake usually equals protein lost.

There are a number of ways to manipulate exercise and diet to maximize the overall anabolic effect of a substance or activity. For example, if a compound or activity increases both protein synthesis and protein breakdown (as many do) it might have a positive or negative anabolic effect. The overall effect is anabolic if the increase in protein synthesis is greater than the increase in protein breakdown, and catabolic if protein breakdown exceeds protein synthesis. It would also be useful to quantify the anabolic effect so we can tell which substances and procedures would be more effective than others for increasing muscle mass and strength.

On the other hand, a substance or activity may decrease both protein breakdown and synthesis. Again, the anabolic effect would depend on the degree that it does either one. If we examine clenbuterol we see that some studies show that while clenbuterol has potent anticatabolic properties, it also, to a lesser extent, suppresses protein synthesis.[1487] The overall effect, however, is anabolic since the net result of the decreased protein breakdown and decreased protein synthesis is an increase in muscle protein content.

There are many variables to consider when trying to determine the most anabolic diet and exercise regimen for athletes. Even for those well versed in the complex hormonal interactions that are involved in the anabolic-catabolic processes of the body, there are many areas that are confusing because of contradictions in the literature and the lack of specific studies.

While minimizing the effects of cortisol (at least the catabolic effect on muscle protein and not the anti-inflammatory effect) is important in the overall scheme of things, there are many other hormones and factors to consider that will influence the net result. And many of the variables act on more than one level. For example, an increase in endogenous testosterone can directly increase protein synthesis, and in part by mitigating the catabolic effect of the corticosteroids, lead to decreased protein degradation.

Decreasing catabolism by using appropriate methods and supplements can have dramatic effects on increasing protein synthesis and muscle mass. One of the ways to decrease the catabolic process is to decrease the excessive secretion or effects of the glucocorticoid hormones, the most important being cortisol. Cortisol, a catabolic hormone, can, if inappropriately elevated, be counterproductive for athletes who are trying to increase their muscle mass.

There are several ways to decrease the breakdown of muscle tissue both during and after exercise and thus provide potent anticatabolic effects. Substances that decrease catabolism can have anabolic effects on muscle. Many nutritional supplements, drugs, and even lifestyle changes can have anticatabolic effects. Increasing dietary carbohydrates and/or calories, increasing dietary protein, using branched chain amino acids, glutamine, alanine, and other amino acids, vitamin C, beta carotene and other antioxidant vitamins all have been shown to lessen muscle breakdown.

As we have seen, chronically elevated cortisol levels have a catabolic effect on muscle and decrease the effect of the anabolic hormones. Cortisol also increases fat mobilization and oxidation. This fat mobilization effect occurs several hours after initial cortisol release by the adrenals. If insulin is low, cortisol promotes increased ketone production from fat. Although ketones exert an anticatabolic effect on structural proteins, the effect is negated by cortisol's potent catabolic effects.

Thus decreasing or attenuating the rise in cortisol seen after exercise can give an added anabolic boost by decreasing muscle tissue breakdown and increasing AA influx and utilization by muscle cells.

STEP NUMBER THREE — MAXIMIZING DIET AND NUTRITION

We have seen that the nutritional needs of athletes are above those of the general public. The first source for the needed macro- and micronutrients should be from following a proper diet: one that will satisfy the needs of energy, water, protein, glucose, and most of the vitamins and minerals such as thiamine, riboflavin, niacin, iron, zinc, and chromium.[1488-1493] Varying the diet can also be productive. Several studies have shown that an appropriate diet, begun several days before a competition, can assist in loading the glycogen stores of muscle and improve performance.[1494,1495] At times, special dietary practices — such as carbohydrate loading offer a competitive advantage.[1496]

While hormones play an important role in the muscle hypertrophic response to resistance training,[1497] the hormonal response will not result in a maximal anabolic response without an optimal dietary intake of protein and other nutrients. Thus, the anabolic effects of training are dependent not only on the resulting immediate and delayed hormonal changes, but also on the presence of a systemic and cellular environment both during training and recovery that provides the nutrients needed to translate the training effect into increased protein synthesis. As well, the presence of certain nutrients around the training period and in the recovery period can accentuate the hormonal response of training and thus increase protein synthesis, further maximizing the anabolic response to training.

Dietary protein appears to stimulate muscle growth directly by increasing muscle RNA content and inhibiting proteolysis, as well as increasing insulin and free T3 levels. Studies have shown that the anabolic effect of intense training is enhanced by a diet high in protein. When intensity of effort is maximal and stimulates an adaptive response, protein needs increase in order to provide increased muscle mass.

The first rule in gaining muscle mass is to make sure to take in enough calories. You can't gain significant amounts of lean body mass by starving yourself. Your body will break down other tissues, including your muscle, to make up for the lack of dietary calories.

Amino acids will not be efficiently incorporated into protein without enough energy sources from other foods — first because of the energy consumed in heat loss during their metabolism, and second because incorporation of amino acids into peptides requires three high-energy phosphate bonds, thereby using 10 kcal/mol derived from hydrolysis of ATP. Any excess of dietary energy over basic needs thus improves the efficiency of dietary nitrogen utilization.

Thus there is a need to take in enough calories to match calorie output and goals. Trying to lose body fat and still gain or maintain muscle size can drop the calories some, but if they drop too much, some lean body mass will be lost. The trick to losing body fat and maintaining or even increasing muscle mass is to gradually drop the calories as one increases protein intake and supplement intake.

No matter what kind of diet is followed, whether low- or high-complex carbohydrate or how many calories are taken in, the diet needs to be high in protein. The consensus in the past has been that the Recommended Daily Allowance (RDA) figures we're all supposed to live by provide enough protein for the athlete.[1498] But in recent years a number of studies done with both strength and endurance athletes have clearly indicated that exercise increases the need for protein and amino acids, protein's building blocks. While those RDA levels might cut it for the couch potato, they're sadly lacking for the athlete.

Intense muscular activity increases protein catabolism (breakdown) and protein use as an energy source. The less protein available, the less muscle is going to be built. A high-protein diet protects the protein to be turned into muscle by, among other things, providing another energy source for use during exercise. The body will burn this protein instead of the protein inside the muscle cells.

In fact, studies have shown that the anabolic effects of intense training are increased by a high-protein diet. When intensity of effort is at its maximum and stimulates an adaptive, muscle-producing response, protein needs accelerate to provide for that increased muscle mass. It's also well known that a high-protein diet is necessary for anabolic steroids to have full effect.

It's our belief that once a certain threshold of work intensity is crossed, dietary protein becomes essential in maximizing the anabolic effects of exercise. Exercise performed under that threshold, however, may have little anabolic effect and may not require increased protein. As a result, while serious athletes can benefit from increased protein other athletes who don't undergo similar, rigorous training may not.

Whether or not one needs to supplement the diet with extra protein depends on one's goal. For those of us who don't have to worry about gaining some fat along with the muscle (traditionally, athletes in sports without weight classes or those in the heavyweight classes in sports that do, where mass is an advantage — for example in the shotput and in weight-lifting), high-caloric diets will usually supply all the protein needed provided plenty of meat, fish, eggs, and dairy products are included. With the increased caloric intake and including high-quality protein foods, the athlete will get extra protein at the dinner table without thinking about it.

Most athletes, however, need the economy of maximizing lean body mass and minimizing body fat. These athletes, both competitive and recreational, are on a moderate or at times a low caloric intake. In order to increase their protein intake, they need to plan their diets carefully and in many cases use protein supplements, since they can't calorically afford to eat food in the volume necessary to get enough protein.

On the average, we recommend a minimum of 1 g of high-quality protein per pound of body weight every day for any person involved in competitive or recreational sports who wants to maximize lean body mass but doesn't wish to gain weight or have excessive muscle hypertrophy. This would apply to athletes who wish to stay in a certain competitive weight class or those involved in endurance events.

However, for those athletes involved in strength events such as Olympic field and sprint events; those in football or hockey; or weight lifters, power lifters and bodybuilders; we recommend between 1.2 to 1.6 g of high-quality protein per pound of total body weight. That means that an athlete who weighs 200 lbs and wants to put on a maximum amount of muscle mass will have to take in as much as 320 g of protein daily. We know of several competitive weight lifters, power lifters, and bodybuilders who take in 2 to 3 g of high-quality protein per pound of body weight.

When trying to lose weight and/or body fat it's important to keep dietary protein levels high. That's because the body oxidizes more protein on a calorie-deficient diet than it would in a diet that has adequate calories. The larger the body muscle mass, the more transamination of amino acids occurs to fulfill energy needs. Thus for those wishing to lose weight but maintain or even increase lean body mass in specific skeletal muscles, I recommend at least 1.5 g of high-quality protein per pound of body weight. The reduction in calories needed to lose weight should be at the expense of the fats and carbohydrates, not protein.

UNUSUAL DIETARY PRACTICES

Although the above dietary guidelines will suffice for most athletes, those who are more advanced may find that experimenting with the content and composition of their diets may result in a greater anabolic response. In some cases, frequent and extreme changes in diet may result in adaptive responses that may lead to further increases in muscle mass and strength.

Considerable research has been done on the effects of varying the content and composition of diets on lean body mass and strength. Studies have shown that both underfeeding and overfeeding are accompanied by changes in the anabolic and catabolic hormones. They also show that it is the change from one state to another which causes dramatic changes in the hormones and that these changes attenuate once the body adjusts, or attempts to adjust, to the new state.

Thus any dramatic change in a diet (or anything else for that matter including exercise, lifestyle, nutritional supplements etc.) results in adaptive responses. For example, drastically cutting back on calories and protein intake can result in reductions in GH, IGF-1, insulin, and testosterone and significant skeletal muscle catabolism within just a few days. One study examining adaptations of leucine and glucose metabolism to 3 days of fasting in six healthy young men found that there is increased proteolysis and oxidation of leucine on short-term fasting.[1607] They found that leucine flux increased 31% and leucine oxidation increased 46% after 3 days of fasting compared with leucine flux and oxidation after an overnight fast. Glucose production rate declined 38% and resting metabolic rate decreased 8% during fasting. Plasma concentrations of testosterone, insulin, and triiodothyronine were reduced by fasting whereas plasma glucagon concentrations were increased.

On the other hand, other studies have shown that overfeeding results in an increase not only in fat but also in significant amounts of lean body mass and in the anabolic hormones. The increase in lean body mass is thought to be at least in part to increases in anabolic hormones including GH, IGF-1, and testosterone. One study assessed the hormonal status of adult female volunteers before and during a 3-week period of weight gain induced by mixed diet overfeeding.[1608] Forty-six percent of the 4.3 kg average weight gain experienced by these subjects consisted of lean body mass (LBM) and it is of interest that there were also increases in plasma IGF-1 and testosterone concentrations as well as insulin. The authors suggested that it was the combined anabolic effect of these three hormones that facilitated the increase in LBM. Of the other assays done, increases were recorded for urinary 17-ketosteroids, 17-hydroxysteroids, epinephrine, and creatinine, whereas there were no changes in serum cortisol or triiodothyronine (T3), or urine norepinephrine; serum thyroxine (T4) fell slightly.

In this study, there were progressive increases in LBM and the hormones IGF-1, testosterone and insulin during the first two weeks of overfeeding. However, during the final week hormone levels reached a plateau or even declined somewhat even though during that final week there was a further increase in LBM.

Thus it is possible that cycles of overfeeding and underfeeding, with mini cycles that manipulate the macronutrient composition of each feeding, may result in adaptive responses that would lead to increased muscle mass and strength, while at the same time limiting any increase in or perhaps even decreasing body fat.

There is one caveat, however. Excessive amounts of weight gain are likely counterproductive even though with this weight gain there is a gain in lean body mass. It appears that the increased lean body mass seen in the obese may not be as dense or as functional as normal muscle. Thus while gaining significant amounts of weight may result in an increase in lean body mass, the effects on lean tissue density are less clear. One study examined the effects of obesity and non-insulin-dependent diabetes mellitus (NIDDM) on lean-tissue composition and density.[1609] Cross-sectional computed tomography (CT) scans of the midthigh were obtained in 20 men of various weights. Obesity was associated with increases in thigh-adipose and lean-tissue volume and with reduced density of lean tissue. The increased lean tissue in obesity was due to a nonadipose tissue component with a density below the normal range of muscle, an effect compounded by NIDDM, whereas normal-density muscle volume was unchanged.

Once a certain amount of weight is gained, loss of the excess body fat, desirable for most athletes since for maximum efficiency their muscle mass to body weight ratio should be as high as possible, can be a problem. Ideally as much lean body mass should be retained while dieting down. Studies, however, have shown that significant amounts of lean body mass are lost in as little as a few days into a diet. Exercise alone has been shown to attenuate the loss in lean body mass and preserve muscle at least in the muscle being exercised.[1610] Muscle mass may be lost in those muscles that are not being adequately worked.

Also if LBM is lost during weight reduction, this loss of fat free mass should ideally be in the less dense (and likely less essential) FFM rather than the normal density and more functional FFM. Research has been focusing on the need to maintain FFM during weight loss because of its integral role in metabolic rate regulation, preservation of skeletal integrity and maintenance of functional capacity. It has been suggested that FFM loss should compose no more than 30% of total weight loss.[1611] Because skeletal muscle in the obese has been shown to consist of an increased amount of low density muscle tissue, impaired strength: size ratio, less capillarisation, decreased mitochondrial density, and consequently impaired work capacity, it may be necessary to stratify FFM into essential and less essential FFM categories.[1612] With this categorization, more specific quantification of FFM loss and maintenance can be made. While FFM influences several physiological functions, it may be that a minimal loss of FFM from the obese state is not only unavoidable, but actually desirable if the loss is in the form of less essential FFM.

It would seem that the degree of muscle mass retention while dieting is to some extent genetically determined. Thus variations in human energy expenditure and the response to various diets are partly due to an influence of the genotype. In one study the authors, using the techniques of genetic epidemiology, found that about 40% of the variance in resting metabolic rate, thermic effect of food, and energy cost of low-to-moderate intensity exercise (< or =3D 5 times the resting metabolic rate) is explained by inherited characteristics.[1613]

A significant genetic effect has also been reported for the level of habitual physical activity. The existence of a genotype-environment interaction has also been investigated. Thus, in response to chronic overfeeding, as well as negative energy balance, changes in the components of energy expenditure exhibit significant identical twin pair resemblance. Nutrient partitioning is emerging as a major determinant of the individual differences in metabolic rate responses to overfeeding or negative energy balance conditions. Taken as a whole, these observations consistently support the hypothesis that heredity plays a significant role in the various components of energy expenditure in humans.

In a study using identical twins plasma glucose, insulin, and glucagon levels were measured before and after long-term overfeeding (4.2 MJ/d during a 100-day period) in 24 lean adults (12 pairs of monozygotic twins).[1614] Fasting plasma glucose, insulin, and glucagon were significantly increased by overfeeding. Significant twin intrapair similarity was observed for fasting plasma glucagon before overfeeding and for the changes in fasting insulin and glucagon with overfeeding. The results of this study indicate that (1) in response to long-term overfeeding, both fasting insulin and glucagon are increased; (2) initial levels of glucose, insulin, and glucagon do not predict the gains in body weight and total body fat during overfeeding, but are related to changes in indicators of fat topography (fasting glucagon before overfeeding was positively correlated with the gains in abdominal visceral fat and in femoral fat); (3) the changes in total subcutaneous fat represent an important correlate of insulin changes with overfeeding; and (4) the genotype could be an important determinant of insulin and glucagon responses to a prolonged positive-energy-balance period. Interestingly in this study the changes with overfeeding in insulin area during a 75 gram oral glucose tolerance test were positively correlated with the changes in total subcutaneous fat, even after adjustment for total body fat gain.

There are significant and as yet not fully known changes in macronutrient balance during over- and underfeeding. Both the amount and composition of food eaten influence bodyweight regulation. For example, the authors of one study set out to determine whether and by what mechanism excess dietary fat leads to greater fat accumulation than does excess dietary carbohydrate.[1615] The authors overfed isoenergetic amounts (50% above energy requirements) of fat and carbohydrate (for 14 days each) to nine lean and seven obese men. A whole-room calorimeter was used to measure energy expenditure and nutrient oxidation on days 0, 1, 7, and 14 of each overfeeding period. From energy and nutrient balances (intake-expenditure) they estimated the amount and composition of energy stored. Carbohydrate overfeeding produced progressive increases in carbohydrate oxidation and total energy expenditure resulting in 75–85% of excess energy being stored. Alternatively, fat overfeeding had minimal effects on fat oxidation and total energy expenditure, leading to storage of 90–95% of excess energy.

The authors concluded that excess dietary fat leads to greater fat accumulation than does excess dietary carbohydrate, and the difference was greatest early in the overfeeding period. It would have been interesting to have measured the amount of lean body mass gain in each instance. In any case, it seems from this and other studies that fat oxidation is regulated primarily by carbohydrate intake rather than by fat intake.[1616]

It also appears that in light of available information, experimentation with various diets, for example switching between a high fat, high protein, low carbohydrate diet with a low fat, moderate protein, high carbohydrate diet on a weekly basis, might be beneficial in increasing muscle mass.[1617] Stabilization from a change in diet can take from a few to several days.

Another approach would be to switch between periods of overfeeding and underfeeding consisting of anywhere from five days to two weeks since according to the literature the body adapts to extreme dietary changes in that period of time. And even after macronutrient partitioning has stabilized, the effects of the dietary change may continue for one to several days more. Thus a period of diet induced obesity would be followed by a period of relative starvation. A study undertaken to examine whether diet-induced obesity alters the amount and/or composition of weight lost during starvation found that diet-induced obesity leads to preferential loss of body fat and conservation of lean mass during starvation.[1618] Thus increasing bodyweight dramatically and then dieting down to lose the extra bodyfat gained may produce an overall increased anabolic response with increased lean body mass and decreased body fat. Gaining and then losing weight in a cyclical may force the body to continually increase muscle mass.

However, while changes in diet composition and content may be productive, the best way to manipulate diet has yet to be determined. For example combining underfeeding and overfeeding with a low carbohydrate, high fat, high protein diet and a high carbohydrate moderate protein, low to moderate fat diet may be one of the best ways to force the body to adapt and grow. In fact, it's been shown that being on a higher fat/low card diet makes the insulin response to a high carbohydrate diet even greater than it normally would be.[1619,1620] Overcompensation occurs in glycogen, fat and protein storage when switching from underfeeding to overfeeding and when varying the content of the diet.

Describing in detail various diet principles, timing of the time periods in which to overeat and then to diet, and determining the composition of the foods in each phase is beyond the scope of this book and will be extensively covered in one of my upcoming book dealing with diet and nutrition for the competitive athlete.

STEP NUMBER FOUR — NUTRITIONAL SUPPLEMENTS

In adition to drugs, athletes also use a large variety of nutritional supplements to improve their performance and appearance. Some of the more common supplements used by athletes are:

Adenosine
Aloe
Alpha-ketoglutarate (either alone or complexed with pyridoxine [PAK] or ornithine [OKG])
Amino acids
Amino acid neurotransmitters (such as gamma-aminobutyric acid [GABA])
Antioxidant vitamins (vitamin A, beta carotene, vitamin C, vitamin E, selenium, zinc)
Antioxidants (from various plants, fruits, and vegetables)
Aspartic acid
ATP
Bee pollen
Betaine (trimethylglycine or TMG)
Boron
Branched-chain amino acids
Brewer's yeast
Boron
Caffeine
Calcium
Carnitine
Carnosine
Choline
Chondroprotective agents
Chromium (in the picolinate or other form)
Coenzyme Q10
Colostrum
Conjugated linoleic acid (CLA)
Creatine monohydrate
Creatine phosphate
Cyanocobalamin (vitamin B_{12})
Cyclofenil
Cytochrome C
Dehydroepiandrosterone (DHEA)
Desiccated liver
Dibencozide (cobamide)
Dimethylglycine (DMG)
Ecdysterone
Essential fatty acids
Ferulic acid
Folic acid
Gamma-linolenic acid (GLA)
Gamma-hydroxybutyrate (GHB)
Gamma oryzanol
Gelatin
Gerovital H3 and GH3 (procaine HCl)
Gerovital KH3 (a combination of procaine HCl, hematoporphyrin, and magnesium carbonate)
Ginseng
Glandular preparations (such as orchic)
Glutamine

Glutathione
Glycerol
Growth hormone stimulators (such as arginine, lysine, ornithine, and L-dopa)
Herbal preparations (such as Smilax Officinalis — advertised as an alternative to anabolic steroids)
Homeopathic mixtures (such as Musco-Mxt- another anabolic steroid substitute)
Hydroxycitrate (HCA)
Hydroxymethylbutyrate (HMB)
Inosine
Inositol
Iron
Ketoisocaproic acid (KIC)
Ketones
Lactate
Lecithin
Magnesium
Ma huang (containing *Ephedra*)
Medium chain triglycerides (MCT)
Minerals
Miura Puama
MSM (methylsulfonylmethane)
Mumie
N-Acetyl-L-cysteine
Neonatal pituitary extract
Neurofor
Octacosanol
Omega-3 fatty acids
Orotates
Oryzanols and ferulic acid
Pantocrine
Perchlorates
Phenylalanine
Phosphatidylserine
Phosphorus
Plant sterols (such as sitosterol and diosterol)
Potassium
Protein supplements (MET-Rx, Phosphagain)
Pyruvate
Ribose
Royal jelly
Rubranova
Silymarin
Sodium succinate
Superoxide dismutase (SOD) and catalase
Taurine
Tribestan
Tryptophan
Vanadyl sulfate
Vitamin B15 (pangamic acid)
Vitamins and minerals (oral and injectable)
Weight gain products (such as Gainer's Fuel and Mega Mass)
Wheat germ oil
Yohimbe
Zinc

While many athletes make extensive use of nutritional supplements, they usually have distorted ideas on their usefulness. In many cases the only information they have comes from the manufacturers, distributors, and retailers of these products. This information and the advertisements for these compounds are tainted by commercial bias and contain false and misleading information and claims.[1499]

The references sometimes used to substantiate their claims deal with disease or deficiency states and are not even remotely translatable to healthy athletes who do not have any significant disease or deficiencies. For example, a study used to validate the testosterone-raising effects of boron shows that boron raised testosterone levels in postmenopausal women.[1500] There is no evidence that boron does so in athletes, male or female, and indeed there is evidence that it does not[1501,1502] and that boron supplementation may even be harmful.[1503]

Even articles found in the various sports magazines, especially the bodybuilding magazines, that support the use of various compounds are often commercially biased. Either the authors have a financial edge to grind, or the magazine does, or both.

Many of these compounds are used in the hope that they will provide the benefits of anabolic steroids without the side effects and without the stigma of possible detection. Some of these compounds are advertised commercially in the many bodybuilding, power-lifting, and other sports magazines, as anabolic steroid substitutes — many claiming to be even more effective but with none of the side effects associated with anabolic steroids.

Nearly all the claims made by proponents of nutritional, herbal, homeopathic, and glandular products (almost always associated with a commercial bias) are unsubstantiated by scientific research. They may be safer than anabolic steroids but they are also relatively ineffective. However, there are commercially available supplements that can favorably affect athletic performance and increase lean body mass.

Supplements can do wonders for training including increasing anabolic drive and workload capacity and decreasing recovery time. In order to accomplish these things, however, one has to take the right supplements at the right time and in the right amounts. Unfortunately most people who use supplements don't use them properly and thus don't get any significant benefits. Largely due to mistrust and ignorance, supplements are not used with the same "seriousness" as drugs.

However, there are several supplements that if used at the right dosage, at the right time and with the right diet and training program can help athletes maximize their lean body mass and their athletic potential without the use of drugs. As a rule, the useful supplements will work to make training more productive than if the supplements weren't used.

Many supplements that have some anabolic potential usually do so by increasing an athlete's ability to train (for example by increasing endurance or by enhancing muscular contraction) by increasing the production of endogenous testosterone and/or growth hormone and/or decreasing cortisol secretion, or by directly influencing protein synthesis.

Under specific conditions many nutritional supplements can have some positive effects on lean body mass, strength, and endurance. The trick in using supplements is to know enough about them in order to use them effectively. Overall, maximizing the diet of an athlete is a fundamental factor in improving athletic performance.

One caveat. Nutritional supplements should not be used as a substitute for sound dietary planning. However, once a comprehensive diet and exercise program is started, then the proper use of specific supplements will lead to further gains. Targeting these supplements is the key to further improving gaining significant amounts of lean body mass and increasing athletic performance.

BENEFITS OF NUTRITIONAL SUPPLEMENTS

Supplements can help in attaining athletic goals by increasing the anabolic and decreasing the catabolic effects of exercise, increasing endurance and training capabilities, and decreasing recovery time.

Recovery from training is critical to improving muscle mass, strength, and athletic performance. Immediately after a training session, the body goes through the process of recovery. The sooner it recovers from a training session, the sooner it can further adapt to increasing training loads.

The athlete who doesn't fully recover from training can go into chronic overtraining; thus losing the appetite and actually losing muscle instead of gaining it, and lacking the energy and stamina for the next training session. Overall, instead of improving, ground will be lost.

Certain supplements can have a very strong effect on lowering recovery time and increasing muscle growth and strength. Supplements targeting recovery can also help handle additional stress during training.

The most useful commercially available supplements at present are listed below. The * indicates compounds that have been covered in detail above. Compounds denoted with a # are covered briefly in this chapter.

Acetyl-L-carnitine *
Alanine *
Alpha-ketoglutarate (AKG) *
Antioxidants (amino acid based) *
Antioxidants (vitamin and mineral) #
Arginine *
Branched-chain amino acids (BCAA) *
Calcium #
Carnitine *
Chromium #
Creatine monohydrate *
Di- and tripeptides *
Glutamine *
High quality whey protein hydrolysate *
Beta-hydroxy-beta-methylbutyrate (HMB) *
Iron #
Ketoisocaproic Acid (KIC) *
Magnesium #
N-Acetyl-L-cysteine *
Omega-3 fatty acids #
Ornithine-alpha-ketoglutarate (OKG) *
Potassium #
Vitamin C #
Zinc #

Other supplements that may be useful are:

Coenzyme Q-10 #
Conjugated linoleic acid (CLA) #
Glycerol #
Ketones *
Phosphatidylserine *
Pyruvate #

As well there are a number of drugs that are contained in certain nutritional supplements and foods that may also be useful such as:

Caffeine #
Ephedrine #

All of these nutritional supplements can be found in one or more offerings from various supplement companies. In many instances two or more of these supplements are found in meal replacement and compound mixtures (such as Phosphagain and MET-Rx) from several of the well-known and not so well-know companies such as Champion Nutrition, EAS, Twin Labs, Weider, etc.

VITAMINS AND MINERALS

In a recent review on the nutrition of children and adolescents engaged in high-level sports activities, the authors recommended mineral and vitamin supplementations. They feel that for minerals, perspiration losses may be associated with dietary deficiency, and possible vitamin deficiencies concern B_1, B_2, B_6, B_9, B_{12}, C, and D vitamins.[1504]

Vitamins and minerals, although widely used by athletes, and by the general population, are the subject of much controversy. They are useful in correcting specific deficiencies that interfere with maximal physical performance (such as thiamine, vitamin C, sodium, and especially iron[1505-1509]), and may be useful under certain conditions. For example, greater requirements for sodium, potassium, magnesium and iron may be present in athletes who train for prolonged periods of time in hot weather.[1510]

Certain vitamins and minerals have been shown to be important for athletic performance. For example, a recent study examined the effect of thiamine supplementation on exercise-induced fatigue.[1511] The authors concluded that thiamine supplementation significantly suppressed the increase in blood glucose in the normal thiamine group and significantly decreased the number of complaints shortly after exercise in the subjective fatigue assessment of 30 items. Vitamin B_6 is an essential cofactor necessary for the metabolism of protein and a useful supplement to take with any protein product. Usual dose for athletes is 25 mg daily.

Vitamin C

Vitamin C is essential to proper collagen synthesis, and this is evident in the vitamin C deficiency disease scurvy, in which the collagen fibers synthesized in the body cannot form fibers properly, resulting in lesions, blood vessel fragility, and poor wound healing.

Vitamin C has been shown to have some anticatabolic effects that likely involve decreasing exercise-induced cortisol but may also have some effects through its antioxidant action. Conversely, some of the anticatabolic effects of antioxidants may be mediated through a decrease in cortisol.

Antioxidants may be of some use in training-induced muscle ischemia and injury. Research shows that exercise can adversely affect muscle tissue by increasing the formation of free radicals. These free radicals can then lead to muscle fatigue, inflammation, and muscular damage.[1512] During normal conditions free radicals are generated at a low rate and neutralized by antioxidant enzymes in the liver and skeletal muscle and other systems. Unfortunately, the increase in free radicals caused by exercise accompanies a simultaneous decrease in the supply of antioxidants to handle them. Vitamin E, for instance, can be severely decreased by training, thus depleting muscle of its major antioxidant force.[1513]

A recent study examined the potential protective effect of pretreatment with corticosteroids or antioxidants (ascorbic acid or allopurinol) in rabbits with reperfusion-induced damage to skeletal muscle after ischemia.[1514] In this study 4 h of limb ischemia induced by a pneumatic tourniquet, followed by reperfusion for 1 h, caused a considerable amount of ultrastructural damage to the anterior tibialis muscles accompanied by a rise in circulating creatine kinase activity. Pretreatment with depomedrone by a single 8-mg bolus injection led to a preservation of the anterior tibialis structure on both light and electron microscopy. High-dose continuous intravenous infusion with ascorbic acid (80 mg/h) throughout the period of ischemia and reperfusion also preserved skeletal muscle structure, although allopurinol in various doses had no protective effect.

These data are fully compatible with a mechanism of ischemia/reperfusion-induced injury to skeletal muscle involving generation of oxygen radicals and neutrophil sequestration and activation. They also indicate that damage to human skeletal muscle caused by prolonged use of a tourniquet is likely to be reduced by simple pharmacological interventions.

Coenzyme Q10 (Ubiquinone-10)

Coenzyme Q10 acts as an electron carrier of the respiratory chain in mitochondria. It has also been shown that the reduced form of coenzyme Q10 is an important physiological lipid-soluble antioxidant and scavenges free radicals generated chemically within liposomal membranes.[1515,1516] It has also been shown that vitamin E and ubiquinone increase physical working capacity of experimental animals.[1517]

Generation of free radicals and subsequent lipid peroxidation have been proposed to contribute to delayed tissue damage. One study has found that ascorbate and ubiquinol levels were decreased after trauma.[1518] In this study, changes in tissue levels of ubiquinol, but not ascorbate, reflected the degree of trauma. The authors suggest that ubiquinol levels may provide a useful marker of the oxidative component of the secondary injury response.

Zinc

Zinc deficiency in humans is widespread[1519] and athletes may be particularly prone to lower plasma zinc levels.[1520] Zinc is a constituent of more than a hundred fundamentally important enzymes, so zinc deficiency has many negative effects on almost every body function.[1521] As well, zinc deficiency can adversely affect the reproductive hormones and as such impair athletic efforts.[1522]

Zinc deficiency adversely affects protein synthesis. In one study the effects of zinc deficiency in rats on the levels of free amino acid in urine, plasma, and skin extract were investigated.[1523] Zinc deficiency adversely affected skin protein synthesis. Especially where a deficiency may be present, supplemental zinc has resulted in an increase in the secretion of growth hormone, IGF-1,[1524] and testosterone,[1525] and raises plasma testosterone and sperm count.[1526,1527]

ZINC AND PROTEIN SYNTHESIS

In one study published this year it was found that zinc stimulates protein synthesis in the femoral-metaphyseal tissues of normal and skeletally unloaded rats.[1527a] Skeletal unloading was designed using the model of hindlimb suspension in rats. Animals were fed for 2 or 4 days during the unloading. [3H]Leucine was added to the reaction mixture containing the 5500 g supernatant fraction of the homogenate prepared from the femoral-metaphyseal tissues. In vitro protein synthesis was significantly decreased in the bone tissues from the rats which had undergone unloading for 2 or 4 days. When the metaphyseal tissues were cultured for 24 h in the presence of zinc sulfate (10(-5) M) or beta-alanyl-L-histidinato zinc (AHZ, 10(-5) M), zinc compounds clearly stimulated protein synthesis in the metaphyseal tissues from the 4-d unloaded rats. The zinc effect was also seen in the metaphyseal tissues from normal rats. The addition of zinc sulfate (10(-5) M) or AHZ (10(-7) to 10(-5) M) into the reaction mixture containing the 5500 g supernatant fraction of metaphyseal homogenate from normal or unloaded rats produced a significant increase in protein synthesis. This increase was clearly inhibited in the presence of cycloheximide. The present result demonstrates that protein synthesis is impaired in the femoral-metaphyseal tissues of rats with skeletal unloading, and that this impairment is clearly restored by zinc supplementation.

Zinc also affects immune function. In a study set up to examine the effect of zinc (Zn) supplementation on exercise-induced changes in immune function, five male runners were randomly assigned in a double-blind crossover design to take a supplement (S; 25 mg of Zn and 1.5 mg of copper) or placebo (P) twice daily for 6 days.[1527b] On morning 4 of each phase, 1 h after taking S or P, subjects ran on a treadmill at 70 to 75% of maximal oxygen uptake until exhaustion (approximately 2 h). Blood samples were obtained before (Pre), immediately after (Post), and 1 (Rec1) and 2 (Rec2) days after the run. [3H]thymidine incorporation by mitogen-treated mononuclear cell cultures was significantly lower Post than Pre, Rec1, or Rec2 for both S and P. Respiratory burst activity of isolated neutrophils was enhanced after exercise with P but not with Thus supplemental Zn blocked the exercise-induced increase in reactive oxygen species. This antioxidant effect of Zn may benefit individuals exposed to chronic physical stress.

Magnesium

Magnesium supplementation has been shown to increase protein synthesis and strength.[1528] In another study, the authors felt that insulin sensitivity can be improved by reduction of excessive body weight, regular physical activity and, possibly, by correcting a subclinical magnesium deficiency.[1529]

Calcium

Calcium permits the contractile filaments of the muscle cell — actin filaments and myosin filaments — to associate and produce the force that generates movement. When the nerve cell innervating a muscle cell signals that cell to contract, calcium is released from the sarcoplasmic reticulum into the region of the contractile filaments, thereby permitting contraction to occur. In one study, calcium was shown to be effective in prolonging time of onset of fatigue in striated muscle.[1530]

Chromium

It has been shown through various studies that chromium is an essential element involved in carbohydrate and lipid metabolism. Since the need for chromium increases with exercise,[1531] and modern refined foods are low in chromium, there may be a need for incorporating chromium-rich food into the diets of athletes.[1532]

Insufficient dietary chromium has been linked to maturity-onset diabetes and cardiovascular diseases, with supplemental chromium resulting in improvements of risk factors associated with these diseases.[1533]

Potassium

Potassium is one of the essential dietary minerals. While most diets supply an adequate amount of potassium, athletes may have increased needs since it is one of the electrolytes lost in sweat. While it is important for athletes to replace the increased electrolytes lost due to sweating, it is especially important to replace potassium.

Even mild potassium deficiency can lead to fatigue and decreased performance,[1534] while a significant deficiency can lead to cardiac problems. Muscular fatigue is manifested by a decline in force- or power-generating capacity and may be prominent in both submaximal and maximal contractions. Disturbances in muscle electrolytes play an important role in the development of muscular fatigue. Unfortunately, surprisingly little research has been carried out to investigate the effects of exogenous potassium on training intensity and muscle hypertrophy.

Studies with isolated animal muscle fibers have shown that potassium may help alleviate muscle fatigue. KCl^- or caffeine-induced release of Ca^{2+} from intracellular stores has been shown to decrease fatigue by reversing long-lasting interference in excitation-contraction coupling.[1535]

Since some studies have implicated the decline of the intracellular to extracellular potassium gradient, and extracellular K^+ accumulation during activity is an essential factor of muscle fatigue,[1536] it might be argued that excessive potassium accumulation at the surface of the muscle cell might increase fatigue. A recent study investigated the role of K^+ in muscle fatigue by testing whether an increased extracellular K^+ concentration in unfatigued muscle fibers caused a decrease in force similar to the decrease observed during fatigue.[1537] The authors concluded that exogenous potassium does not cause accumulation of K^+ at the surface of the sarcolemma that is sufficiently large to suppress force development during fatigue.

It has been shown that potassium deficiency can result in lower GH and IGF-1 levels and that potassium replacement restores these levels. The problem appears to be at the pituitary level rather than the muscular level since the use of GHRH did not correct serum levels.[1538] As well, a recent study has shown that potassium deficiency inhibits protein synthesis.[1539]

OMEGA-3 FATTY ACIDS

Omega-3 fatty acids are long chain polyunsaturated fatty acids that havc biological functions because they are converted to a number of active substances in the body such as prostaglandins and leukotrienes and are involved in a number of metabolic events. Linolenic acid is an essential fatty acid since it cannot be synthesized in the body. Other omega-3 fatty acids can, however, be synthesized from linolenic acid.

Omega-3 fatty acids, eicosapentaenoic acid (EPA) and docosahexaenoic acid (DHA), are found in fish oils. Studies have shown that fish oils, because of their vasodilation, anti-aggregation, anti-inflammatory, and plasma lipid-lowering effects may be useful in a wide variety of diseases,[1540] including certain inflammatory, degenerative, and autoimmune diseases,[1541-1543] and may be effective in the prevention of coronary heart disease[1544] and headaches.[1545]

As well, fish oil may, through perhaps more than one mechanism, have anticatabolic properties. By extrapolating from burn injury studies, there is the possibility of modifying the catabolic processes secondary to training through the use of fish oil.[1546,1547] There is the possibility that fish oil may modulate PGE_2-mediated muscle proteolysis. Studies have shown that thc mechanism of interleukin-1 (IL-1)-induced muscle proteolysis involves PGE_2 synthesis.[1548] Thus it is likely that omega-3 fatty acids from fish oil competitively inhibit the PGE_2 synthesis,[1549,1550] resulting in less muscle proteolysis. Furthermore, it has been shown that fish oil feeding in healthy volunteers can reduce the *in vitro* production of IL-1 and tumor necrosis factor by macrophages.[1551] Thus, the reduction of IL-1 level may represent another mechanism by which fish oil moderates muscle proteolysis.

Omega-3 fatty acids may increase growth hormone secretion since they are involved in the formation of prostaglandin E1, which in turn is involved in GH release.[1552]

CONJUGATED LINOLENIC ACID (CLA)

Conjugated linoleic acid (CLA) is a mixture of positional and geometric isomers of linoleic acid (LA) found preferentially in dairy products and meat. CLA is present in cheese, milk and yogurt which have undergone heat treatment, and also in beef and venison. Supplementation with 4 oz of cheddar cheese daily was found to increase the ratio of CLA to LA by 130%.

CLA has been shown to have properties above and beyond those of linoleic acid. It has shown potential as a powerful anticarcinogen[1553,1554] and exhibits potent antioxidant activity.[1555] Recent studies have suggested that CLA may be cytotoxic to human cancer cells *in vivo*.[1556]

Of equal importance for those wishing to maximize lean body mass, is the possible anticatabolic effects of CLA.[1557,1558]

GLYCEROL

The products of the hydrolysis of triglycerides, the storage form of fat, are fatty acids and glycerol (also called glycerine or glycerin). The free fatty acids are transported to muscle in a loose combination with plasma albumin where they are released and taken up and oxidized. Glycerol is not used directly as a substrate but undergoes gluconeogenesis in the liver. Glycerol is metabolized to pyruvate, which in itself may be a useful ergogenic aid (see below), and two pyruvate molecules are used to make up a glucose molecule. This process produces glucose and helps restock liver glycogen stores which, in turn, provides glucose as a fuel for the central nervous system and for muscle metabolism.

As well, a recent study has shown that glycerol competitively inhibited gluconeogenesis from amino acids.[1559] In this way glycerol may have important anticatabolic properties because of its protein-sparing action.

Both training and the high-fat/low-carb diet increase the capacity of skeletal muscles to use fat as an energy source. An increase in fat metabolism during prolonged exercise has a glycogen-sparing effect and as such improves endurance capacity. Thus, with diet and training lipolysis may provide more energy during heavy-resistance exercise of relatively short duration than in a normal high-carb diet.

Glycerol taken 45 min prior to exercise has been shown to decrease fatigue and to decrease glucose oxidation when compared to glucose ingestion.[1560] Orally administered glycerin also has an effect on insulin secretion, especially when it reaches the highest blood levels 60 to 90 min after ingestion.[1561]

Besides the above effects, glycerol may also have some beneficial effects on athletic performance due to its osmotic action. Recent research has shown that when a glycerol and water mix is used as a hydration beverage before training or competition, performance improves. Thus glycerol-induced hyperhydration, by delaying the adverse effects of dehydration, reduces the thermal burden of exercise.[1562]

PYRUVATE

Pyruvate, along with lactate, glycerol, and the amino acids glutamine and alanine, are the major gluconeogenic precursors, and as nutritional supplements have both anabolic and anticatabolic effects (see above). Calcium pyruvate (calcium salt of pyruvic acid) is now commercially available as a nutritional supplement. Benefits may include antioxidant and nitric oxide effects,[1563,1564] increased endurance,[1565-1567] and increased weight and fat loss.[1568,1569]

Several patents have been registered outlining methods of using pyruvate and dihydroxyacetone for a variety of problems and diseases including obesity, diabetes, heart disease, alcoholic fatty liver, and for inhibiting the generation of free radicals.[1570]

CAFFEINE AND EPHEDRINE

A number of studies have shown that caffeine may favorably affect long-term endurance performance[1571] but research results concerning high-intensity, short-term exercise have been a bit mixed.[1572] Still, it seems very likely from an analysis of the biochemical effects of caffeine that it has a beneficial effect on short-term fatigue and muscle fiber in high-intensity, short-term exercise like weight lifting.[1573,1574]

Ephedrine has mild amphetamine-like CNS effects and is used by athletes to enhance training and performance. Aspirin is widely used by athletes for several reasons. It is a common mild pain killer, has anti-inflammatory properties, and has some thermogenic effects.

The combination of caffeine, ephedrine, and aspirin is commonly used as a thermogenic cocktail.[1575,1576] This cocktail promotes lipolysis while decreasing muscle breakdown — the result is an increased ratio of lean body mass to fat. A recent study measured the effects of ephedrine (75 to 150 mg), caffeine (150 mg), and aspirin (300 mg) on weight loss in 24 human volunteers.[1577] The combination proved effective in increasing weight loss after 8 weeks of treatment — those using the compound averaged 3.2 kg vs. 1.3 kg for the placebo group.

ANTI-CORTISOL SUPPLEMENTS

Any type of stress, including high-level exercise, physical or emotional trauma, infections, and surgery translates into hypothalamic and pituitary changes that result in increased cortisol secretion.

Exercise itself, while increasing cortisol, has compensatory anticatabolic effects. Short, intense training sessions tend to result in more moderate cortisol secretion. In addition, well-conditioned athletes show less cortisol secretion during exercise compared to their out-of-shape peers. One measure of overtraining is the testosterone/cortisol ratio. Elevated cortisol in relation to testosterone is considered indicative of overtraining. Taken from another angle, when training properly, testosterone will rise while cortisol remains stable.

Vitamin C has been shown to have some anticatabolic effects that likely involve decreasing exercise-induced cortisol but may also have some effects through its antioxidant action. Conversely, some of the anticatabolic effects of antioxidants may be mediated through a decrease in cortisol. A gram or so of vitamin C, along with some vitamin E (400 IU), beta-carotene (20,000 IU), zinc (50 mg), and selenium (50 μg) before workouts might be useful.

A new supplement has recently been marketed that may decrease exercise-induced cortisol increase. Studies have shown that phosphatidylserine blunts the ACTH and cortisol response to exercise (see above). Although more research needs to be done to see if the decrease in cortisol translates into increased gains, PS may be of benefit and could be included in the supplement stack — 1 to 2 g could be used prior to each training session. One caveat, there may be an increase in training soreness, stiffness, and injuries secondary to the cortisol reduction. The benefits-to-risk ratio should be considered when using these compounds.

AMINO ACID AND PROTEIN SUPPLEMENTATION

As we have noted above, increased blood amino acid levels secondary to a high-protein meal have been shown to cause insulin and growth hormone levels to rise. Increasing these hormones as well as increasing amino acid levels, but at the same time decreasing muscle catabolism, leads to an enhanced anabolic response. As well, studies have shown that branched-chain amino acid ingestion modifies the hormonal milieu.

There is also some information that amino acids, primarily methionine, and the dipeptides methionine-glutamine and tryptophan-isoleucine, have a profound anabolic effect on increasing protein synthesis for reparative and muscle wound healing and on protein synthesis. The amino acid and two dipeptides could override or block the increase in glucocorticoid levels found in diabetic patients.

As well, protein taken after training may increase both insulin and growth hormone, and thus have anabolic effects. Increased amino acid availability has been shown to directly influence protein synthesis, especially within a few hours after physical exercise. The rate of protein synthesis, protein catabolism, and amino acid transport is normally increased after exercise and depends on amino acid availability. If there is an increase in the availability of amino acids during this postexercise time interval or window, then the catabolic processes are more than offset by the increased anabolic processes, resulting in an overall increase in cellular contractile protein. Thus it is vital to increase the absorption of amino acids as quickly as possible after exercise.

WHEN AND HOW TO TAKE THEM AND HOW MUCH TO TAKE

Because we're all different and have disparate needs, it's necessary to fine-tune our supplement intake. Like everything else in life whatever one is doing or taking must be adapted so that it works best. There's both a science and an art to taking supplements. The science involves knowing what the supplements do and how they might be a benefit under certain conditions and provide possible dosages and times that will theoretically maximize their effects. The art involves finding out just what works and in customizing these supplements to the athlete's own needs and metabolism.

The bottom line is to try out potentially useful supplements and determine if the benefits are worth the cost. That means experimenting with various combinations of supplements under different conditions, keeping such variables as diet and training relatively constant so the effects of the supplements themselves can be determined. It's not possible to find out what's working and not working if everything is changed at the same time. For example, dramatically changing one's diet and training routine won't tell much about some new supplement that is being tried out. There are just too many changes taking place to allow one to figure out what is doing what.

Various studies have shown that certain supplements can have anabolic and anticatabolic effects. For example, studies have shown that the use of branched-chain amino acids (BCAAs) before training increases insulin secretion and decreases the drop in testosterone both during and after exercise.

Athletes who use a complete amino acid mixture or hydrolysate or even a whole protein supplement prior to working out still run into declining testosterone levels as they train and after the workout. However, the use of BCAAs prior to training counteracts this. Unfortunately the use of BCAAs blunts the growth hormone response during training and decreases the formation of IGF-1. While the blunting of GH and IGF-1 might have catabolic effects, the relatively increased levels of testosterone would likely overshadow this effect. Nonetheless, if GH and IGF-1 could be made to increase along with testosterone and insulin then the overall anabolic effect of exercise could be maximized.

So what's an athlete to do in order to get all the hormones working together? Well, first of all an athlete could use an amino acid and protein stack as follows — now while this stack is not written in stone, it will work.

First of all increase the daily dietary protein intake to between 1.2 and 1.6 g of protein per 1 lb of bodyweight. Train in the morning or don't eat a meal within a few hours prior to working out. Especially don't take in any carbohydrates. We don't want a grossly elevated insulin level to decrease the use of free fatty acids as energy substrates while training. Also, unopposed high insulin levels have an adverse effect on training-induced elevations of GH and IGF-1 levels.

It seems that during morning workouts, more fat is metabolized than at any other time of the day. As well, the amount of protein oxidized decreases rather than increases when exercise is done in the postabsorptive state.

Although during sleep our bodies seem more efficient at decreasing protein catabolism and decreasing hunger. Nocturnal rises in prolactin, thyroid-stimulating hormone, free fatty acids and leptin could have an effect in suppressing muscle catabolism and appetite during the night while sleeping.[1578] However, because of the lack of food intake athletes will still go through a significant catabolic phase after the first three to four hours of sleep.

Between a half hour and an hour prior to training, take in 5 g of glutamine, 5 g of alanine, 5 g of leucine, and 5 g of arginine, either in powdered form or mixed with water or a noncaloric drink. As well, with these amino acids take in an antioxidant mixture containing 400 IU vitamin E, 1500 mg vitamin C, 50 μg of selenium, 20,000 IU beta-carotene, 50 μg chromium, and 50 mg zinc.

The use of other antioxidants such as glutathione, NAC, etc. and the use of magnesium, potassium, folic acid, and calcium can also be considered either prior to workouts or spaced out in two or three doses daily.

Taking too many supplements prior to working out may cause some GI upset and may thus be somewhat counterproductive so use the amino acids and the chromium and vitamin C first and introduce any other supplements as tolerated.

Right after training, before doing anything else, take in about 20 g of protein in the form of both free AA, and a protein hydrolysate that has an abundance of di- and tripeptides. Don't take in any whole foods since digestion, absorption, and thus increased amino acid plasma levels take too long. As well, don't take in any carbohydrates at this time since carbs slow down the absorption of the protein and can decrease GH levels. The use of the full-spectrum, free-form amino acids along with a well-hydrolyzed protein supplement will get needed AA into the system the quickest and will increase insulin to some extent without affecting the elevated GH levels. Along with the 20 g of this protein take 5 g of glutamine and 5 g of lysine to further increase insulin, GH, and testosterone levels and to counteract the immune-suppressant effects of intense exercise.

As we have seen above, there is evidence that glutamine may act as a regulator of protein, free fatty acid, and glycogen metabolism during and after exercise.About 1/2 hour later — say after showering and dressing — take in 20 to 40 g of protein in the form of free AA and a hydrolysate containing mostly free AA, di- and tripeptides along with some carbohydrates. The use of carbohydrates after exercise has been shown to increase postexercise insulin and growth hormone levels.[1579] How many grams of carbs to take depends on the diet. On a low-carbohydrate diet limit the carbs to about 15 g mostly simple high glycemic carbs and use about 40 to 50 g of protein. For those on a moderate to high complex carb low-fat diet use between 100–150 g of a combination of simple and complex carbs (depending on body weight — roughly 1.5 g per kg of body weight) along with about 30 g of AA and protein hydrolysate.

A few hours later eat a moderately sized meal. The composition of the meal will depend on whether one is following the high complex carb diet or low carbohydrate diet.

Since there is an increase in protein synthesis for up to 36 h after exercise, it's important to keep the body in as much of an anabolic state as possible over this time period. Thus, decreasing the amount of time spent in a postabsorptive state is of primary importance. Perhaps the ideal routine is taking in the right combination of foods continuously. Studies in rats have shown that in certain animals under certain conditions, around-the-clock feedings are best for rapid growth.[1579] Studies have yet to be done on humans to see if continuous feeding infers an anabolic advantage.

To be practical, however, intermittent feedings no more than 3 hours apart would seem to decrease the postabsorptive catabolic response. Depending on one's needs and time constraints, taking some well-hydrolyzed whey protein along with 5 g of glutamine between high-protein meals might work best.

Unfortunately, we can't keep the body from going into a postabsorptive state while we're sleeping; although, during sleep our bodies seem more efficient at decreasing protein catabolism and decreasing hunger. Nocturnal rises in prolactin, thyroid-stimulating hormone, free fatty acids, and lectin could have an effect in suppressing muscle catabolism and appetite during the night while sleeping.[1578] However, because of the lack of food intake athletes will still go through a significant catabolic phase after the first three to four hours of sleep.

There are ways, however, of minimizing the late phase catabolic response of sleep. Ideally, regular feedings would prevent or attenuate the catabolic effects seen at night. Although no studies have been done in normal humans to see what effect regular feeding would have, studies in animals have shown that for maximal protein synthesis round-the-clock feedings are best.[1580]

Practically, the most effective way to attenuate the catabolic response seen with sleep is to eat a small to medium sized high-protein, high to moderate fat, low-carbohydrate meal an hour or so before bed. With this meal I take about 15 g of fresh oils consisting of 7 g of fish oil (such as salmon oil), 1 g of GLA (say in the form of evening primrose oil), and 7 g of flaxseed oil.

Then right before bed take some well-hydrolyzed whey protein and 5 g of glutamine. This combination will likely keep the body in an anabolic phase for at least the first 4 h of sleep. In order to abort any catabolic phase as soon as possible, first thing in the morning take a protein fix and then have breakfast at your usual time.

Of course if one naturally wakes up once or twice a night, this is the perfect time to take 20 to 30 g of preprepared, easily digestible and palatable protein (for example a protein shake). This protein will prevent the postabsorptive catabolic state and in many cases will likely make it easier to fall back to sleep.

What about OKG, KIC, HMB, carnitine, vanadyl sulfate, ALCAR, creatine monohydrate, conjugated linoleic acid (CLA), glycerol, and a host of others nutritional compounds? I believe that these compounds should be reserved for specific training and competition phases especially when athletes are attempting to decrease body fat and maintain or increase lean body mass. Once your body has derived from the benefits of a high protein diet and the more basic protein and amino acid supplements discussed above, these extra supplements should give you that extra edge you need in the rigorous pre-competition training and during competitions.

For example, HMB, KIC and ALCAR would be useful prior to training, immediately after training, several hours after training and three times a day when not training. I would recommend about one grams of each at those times. OKG can also be used in a pre-training stack. Vanadyl sulfate, a compound which exerts insulin-like effects on glucose metabolism, is one of the few compounds widely used by athletes that I believe should not even be on the market.[1581] First of all it doesn't work,[1621] is potentially hepatotoxic[1622] and more importantly, a recent study has shown that it may actually inhibit protein synthesis. In this study, vanadate and pervanadate (both tyrosine phosphatase inhibitors) mimic insulin to stimulate glucose uptake but inhibit system A amino acid uptake.[1623]

Creatine monohydrate can be used 5 g 2 to 4 times a day on its own (you can take the powder straight, washing it down with some water) or with some simple carbs (either mixed into a drink or with some juice or carb drink to wash it down) to increase its absorption. The usual advice is to take 20 to 30 g a day for five days and then go on a maintenance dose of 10 to 15 grams per day. An as yet unpublished study has shown that the ergogenic effects of creatine monohydrate can likely be obtained by using only 5 to 10 grams daily without a loading phase. On the other hand some athletes believe that the loading phase should be repeated on a monthly basis so as to "prime" the system and force an increase in CP. More research is being carried out to determine whether other compounds such as glucose, taurine, glutamine, other amino acids, and certain electrolytes increase the absorption and utilization of CM, and lead to greater increases in intracellular CP.

The bottom line, just as with other supplements, is that you have to experiment with different doses to see what is the most cost effective dose for you. If CM is going to be useful, you should see some results during the first few weeks of supplementation.

CYCLING OF SUPPLEMENTS

Variety is the spice of life, otherwise you get used to the same old fare. Cycling your supplement stack, along with your training and diet, makes good sense. The proper cycling or periodization of supplements will save you money and also give you the greatest benefit from the supplements you do use when you most need them. By cycling your supplement stack you can keep the body from adapting to the supplements being used and therefore decreasing their effects. I usually recommend that supplements be used in three stages. Cycling supplements can be intertwined with cycling your training and diet.

Stage One — Detraining or rest phase. Diet, protein intake and training should be relaxed. Minimal supplementation with the use of a general purpose vitamin and mineral supplement, extra antioxidants, and perhaps some essential fatty acids in the form of flaxseed and fish oils.

Stage Two — Beginning training phase. Strength and mass building. Diet high in calories and high in protein. Supplements used before and after exercise and before bed include general vit/min, antioxidants, arginine, alanine, glutamine, leucine and hydrolyzed whey, and depending on your goals, the use of either a high-calorie weight gain product such as Mega Mass, medium calorie protein and meal replacement supplement such as MET-Rx, or a product like Phosphagain (for those who want to minimize body fat and maximize lean body mass). Two new EAS (Experimental and Applied Research) products on the market make ideal meal replacement or meal enhancement supplements. Myoplex Plus Deluxe powder that can be mixed as a drink and the very handy Myoplex Plus Deluxe Bar. Certainly the best tasting and most nutritious "snack bar" on the market.

Stage Three — The precompetition and competition phase. Maximizing lean body mass and strength and decreasing body fat (except for those sports where weight is an advantage such as Sumo wrestling and heavyweight categories in weightlifting and powerlifting).

Decreased caloric intake (the same or increased caloric intake where increased levels of body fat and muscle mass can be an advantage), increased protein intake, the use of the same supplements as in stage two but with the addition of more hydrolyzed whey protein and full spectrum amino acid products (since the use of whole protein foods would overly increase calories) and the use creatine monohydrate, ALCAR, KIC, HMB, and ketones. As well the use of CLA, OKG, AKG, and other compounds might be beneficial. Two products from EAS fit the bill. Both Cytovol (a glutamine, taurine, alanine, AKG, potassium, calcium mix) and Betagen (creatine monohydrate plus HMB, with lesser amounts of potassium, glutamine and taurine) would be useful supplements in stage three.

Meal replacement products such as MET-Rx and Phosphagain and their clones (depending on content, price, and palatability) are useful in this phase as well.

In stage three compounds such as the ASA-caffeine-ephedrine mixture might be useful to decrease body fat while maintaining lean body mass.

SUMMARY

The supplement combinations suggested in this chapter will likely give good results since they make the best use of the latest research and knowledge. Other combinations may also have significant effects and can be tried in different cycles. Products such as CLA, phosphatidylserine, and various minerals may be more effective for some than others.

The use of nutritional supplements is both an art and a science. We can present the scientific end. However, because each individual has a unique makeup and thus different needs and goals, only that person can work out which supplements work best and when to use them.

It's important for athletes to determine the usefulness of the supplements by rationally evaluating any perceived ergogenic effects — keeping an open but critical mind as to the benefits they receive from using the supplement and determining if there is progress above and beyond that which they would ordinarily expect from their diet and training. Is there an objective increase in any measurable parameters such as stamina, strength, and lean body mass? And if there is an increase is it a result of the supplement or of increased training intensity and enthusiasm?

Despite the potential benefits of many of the nutritional supplements, especially protein and amino acids for increasing lean body mass and athletic performance, the use of nutritional supplements needs to be more systematically investigated. We need more empirical evidence to fine-tune the use of supplements in order to maximize the anabolic effects of exercise.

Unfortunately nutritional supplement companies, except for one, do not fund valid scientific studies on their products or other supplements. It would appear that most of these companies are more interested in profits than in arriving at some factual information about their products. However, the people today are demanding to know more and are accepting of results obtained through valid research. In the end this kind of research can only benefit the companies that conduct them by increasing the credibility and usefulness of certain nutritional supplements, and thus increasing their sales and profits.

The one exception is Experimental and Applied Research (EAS). This company is involved in funding dozens of studies by well known scientists in the field of nutritional supplement research. And their products reflect the results of their research. The preparations sold by EAS often take the guesswork and bother of trying to make up a supplement stack on your own. The convenience of using their products, coupled with the research behind their products, makes their offerings very attractive to the athlete wanting to use cutting-edge nutritional supplements. More nutritional companies should follow EAS's lead and fund research on nutritional supplements.

Chapter 11

SUMMARY

PROTEIN AND AMINO ACIDS AND MUSCLE HYPERTROPHY

We can maximize protein synthesis and minimize muscle catabolism by several means including:

1. Increase the available AA pool in muscle cells so that AAs are available for protein synthesis. Decreasing the oxidation of AAs in the pool during exercise would decrease the catabolic effect and increase the anabolic effects of exercise.
2. Spare structural and more important contractile protein catabolism by providing adequate substrates for oxidation so that muscle catabolism is not needed to provide these substrates.
3. Increase intracellular phosphocreatine (PC). The reason that this might increase skeletal muscle hypertrophy may be due to the fact that by increasing the PC in muscle, more energy is available for contraction, decreasing the need for anaerobic and aerobic mechanisms (such as hepatic gluconeogenesis and oxidation of AA) as well as possibly increasing the available intracellular energy, leading to an increase in protein synthesis and a decrease in protein catabolism. Under normal conditions muscle contraction places such a demand on ATP and PC that there are insufficient amounts available for active protein synthesis at the same time that muscle contractions are occurring.

For reasons given in this book, dietary protein supplementation and selectively increasing the intake of specific amino acids has profound effects on all three mechanisms. As well, protein and amino acid supplements can have important effects on many functions in the body including the antioxidant and immune systems.

Amino acid and protein supplements have been proven to favorably affect the secretion of anabolic hormones and growth factors and protein synthesis, and to decrease protein catabolism. If we were to look at only two of the many studies quoted in this book, we can see the powerful effects of protein and amino acid supplements. The studies by Chandler et al.[1464] and by Carli et al.[1465] show that supplementation both before and after training has profound anabolic effects.

Some protein and amino acid supplements, if used in proper dosages and at the right times, may have effects similar to those obtained through the use of exogenous anabolic drugs including anabolic steroids and growth hormone. At present, we can, based on current research and valid extrapolations, recommend nutritional alternatives to the use of potent and potentially harmful ergogenic drugs such as anabolic steroids, growth hormone, IGF-1, thyroid, and insulin.

SUMMARY AND CONCLUSIONS

In summary we have seen that:

1. Athletes need significantly higher protein intakes than normal sedentary people, and depending on the sport, may need specific protein and amino acid supplementation.
2. In order to keep the body in a positive anabolic state, protein must be consumed every 2 to 3 h. Otherwise catabolism of body protein occurs.

3. Certain amino acids have to be present in the dietary protein in specific amounts in order to have maximal protein synthesis and minimal protein catabolism.
4. The absence of adequate amounts of certain amino acids can result in decreased protein synthesis, even in the presence of a high-protein diet.
5. Certain whole food protein supplements offer distinct advantages over high-protein foods.
6. Certain amino acids and their metabolites, either alone or in specific combinations, in pharmacological doses and at specific times (for example before and after exercise) regulate protein syntheses and protein catabolism (either by their direct effects or their effects on the anabolic and catabolic hormones), and can result in increased lean body mass that cannot be duplicated through the use of a high-protein diet or specific foods.
7. The use of specific protein and amino acid supplements can have anabolic and anticatabolic effects (through their intrinsic activity and by stimulating anabolic and decreasing the effect of catabolic hormones) similar to those obtained through the use of exogenous anabolic drugs including anabolic steroids and growth hormone.
8. The use of pharmacological doses of certain supplements, such as creatine monohydrate, that are derived from amino acids, can result in an increased skeletal muscle hypertrophy that cannot be duplicated by the use of high protein or specific foods.
9. The use of protein and amino acid supplements can have important effects on many other functions in the body including the antioxidant and immune systems that affect protein synthesis and lean body mass.
10. Some amino acids in themselves trigger cellular reactions that initiate peptide formation and increase protein synthesis.
11. Oral ingestion of several amino acids in proper doses consistently and reproducibly elicits release of growth hormone and insulin in healthy athletes.
12. Ingestion of protein supplements or particular amino acids (e.g., arginine and ornithine) enhanced the results of resistance training by improving lean body mass (mostly muscle) and increasing strength as compared to control groups not using these supplements.

The information presented in this book shows that amino acid and protein supplements used properly are superior to high protein and other diets using whole food protein sources. The physiological and pharmacological effects that can be obtained by the use of protein and amino acid supplements cannot be duplicated through a high protein or other diet alone, no matter how meticulously that diet is prepared.

REFERENCES

1. Guyton & Hall. *Textbook of Medical Physiology,* 9th ed. W.B. Saunders 1996. page 877.
2. Chesley A, MacDougall JD, Tarnopolsky MA, et al. Changes in human muscle protein synthesis after resistance exercise. *J Appl Physiol* 1992; 73:1383-1388.
3. Metcoff J. Intracellular amino acid levels as predictors of protein synthesis. *J Am Coll Nutr* 1986; 5(2):107-20.
4. Haussinger D. The role of cellular hydration in the regulation of cell function. *Biochem J* 1996; 313(Pt 3):697-710.
5. Hamilton MT, Ward D, Watson PD. Effect of plasma osmolality on steady-state fluid shifts in perfused cat skeletal muscle. *Am J Physiol* 1993; 265(6 Pt 2):R1318-23.
6. Haussinger D, Roth E, Lang F, et al. Cellular hydration state: an important determinant of protein catabolism in health and disease. *Lancet* 1993; 341:1330-1332.
7. Haussinger D, Stoll B, Morimoto Y, Lang F, Gerok W. Anisoosmostic liver perfusion: redox shifts and modulation of alpha-ketoisocaproate and glycine metabolism. *Hoppe-Seyler Biol Chem* 1992; 373(8):723-34.
8. Haussinger D, Hallbrucker C, vom Dahl S, Decker S, Schweizer U, Lang F, Gerok W. Cell volume is a major determinant of proteolysis control in liver. *FEBS Lett* 1991; 283(1):70-2.
9. Lang F, Ritter M, Volkl H, Haussinger D. The biological significance of cell volume. *Renal Physiol Biochem* 1993; 16(1-2):48-65.
10. Vom Dahl S, Haussinger D. Nutritional state and the swelling-induced inhibition of proteolysis in perfused rat liver. *J Nutr* 1996; 126(2):395-402.
11. Fiers W. Tumor necrosis factor. Characterization at the molecular, cellular and in vivo level. *FEBS Lett* 1991; 285:199-212.
12. Tracey KJ, Lowry SF, Beutler B, et al. Cachectin/tumor necrosis factor mediates changes of skeletal muscle plasma membrane potential. *J Exp Med* 1986; 164:1368-1373.
13. Haussinger D, Lang F, Gerok W. Regulation of cell function by the cellular hydration state. *Am J Physiol* 1994; 30:E343-E355.
14. vom Dahl S, Hallbrucker C, Lang F, Haussinger D. Regulation of liver cell volume by hormones. *Biochem J* 1991; 280:105-09.
15. Parry-Billings M, Bevan SJ, Opara E, Newsholme EA. Effects of changes in cell volume on the rates of glutamine and alanine release from rat skeletal muscle in vitro. *Biochem J* 1991; 276(Pt 2):559-61.
16. Rivas T, Urcelay E, Gonzalez-Manchon C, Parrilla R, Ayuso MS. Role of amino acid-induced changes in ion fluxes in the regulation of hepatic protein synthesis. *J Cell Physiol* 1995; 163(2):277-84.
17. Baquet A, Hue L, Meijer AJ, van Woerkom GM, Plomp PJ. Swelling of rat hepatocytes stimulates glycogen synthesis. *J Biol Chem* 1990; 265(2):955-959.
18. Rennie MJ, Edwards RH, Krywawych S, et al. Effect of exercise on protein turnover in man. *Clin Sci* 1981; 61(5):627-39.
19. Lowell BB, Ruderman NB, Goodman MN. Regulation of myofibrillar protein degradation in rat skeletal muscle during brief and prolonged starvation. *Metabolism* 1986; 35:1121-1127.
20. Li JB, Goldberg AL. Effects of food deprivation on protein synthesis and degradation in rat skeletal muscle. *Am J Physiol* 1984; 246:E32-E37.
21. Dohm GL, Tapscott EB, Barakat HA, et al. Measurement of in vivo protein synthesis in rats during an exercise bout. *Biochem Med* 1982; 27:367-372.
22. Dohm GL, Williams RT, Kasperek GJ. Increased excretion of urea and N tau-methylhistidine by rats and humans after a bout of exercise. *J Appl Physiol: Respir Environ Exerc Physiol* 1982; 52(1):27-33.
23. Millward DJ, Davies CT, Halliday D, Wolman SL, Matthews D, Rennie M. Effect of exercise on protein metabolism in humans as explored with stable isotopes. *Fed Proc* 1982; 41(10):2686-91.
24. Wolfe RR, Wolfe MH, Nadel ER, Shaw JHF. Isotopic determinations of amino acid-urea interactions in exercise. *J Appl Physiol* 1984; 56:221-229.
25. Wolfe RR, Goodenough RD, Wolfe MH, Royle GT, Nadel ER. Isotopic analysis of leucine and urea metabolism in exercising humans. *J Appl Physiol* 1982; 52:458-466.
26. Devlin JT, Brodsky I, Scrimgeour A, Fuller S, Bier DM. Amino acid metabolism after intense exercise. *Am J Physiol* 1990; 258(2 Pt 1):E249-55.
27. *Nutrition in Exercise and Sport,* edited by Ira Wolinsky and James F. Hickson, Jr. 1994 CRC Press, Boca Raton, FL pg. 127.
28. Morgan HE, Earl DCN, Broadus A, Wolpert EB, Giger KE, Jefferson LS: Regulation of protein synthesis in heart muscle. I. Effect of amino acid levels on protein synthesis. *J Biol Chem* 1971; 246:2152-2162.

28a. Zawadzki KM, Yaspelkis BB, Ivy JL. Carbohydrate-protein complex increases the rate of muscle glycogen storage after exercise. *J. Appl. Physiol.* 1992; 72(5):1854-9.

28b. Okamura K, Doi T, Hamada K, et al. Effect of amino acid and glucose administration during post -exercise recovery on protein kinetics in dogs. APS Manuscript Number E386-6. Article publication pending. *Am. J. Physiol.* (Endocrinol. Metab.). Published in APStracts on 5 March 1997.
28c. Biolo G, Tipton K, Klein S, Wolfe RR. An abundant supply of balanced amino acids synergistically enhances protein muscle anabolism after exercise. APS Manuscript Number E426-6. Article publication pending *Am. J. Physiol. (Endocrinol. Metab.).* Published in APStracts on 21 March 1997.
28d. Roy BD, Tarnopolsky MA, Macdougall JD, et al. The effect of glucose supplement timing on protein metabolism following resistance training. APS Manuscript Number A891-6. Article publication pending. *J. Appl. Physiol.* Published in APStracts on 5 March 1997.
29. Borer KT. The effects of exercise on growth. *Sports Med* 1995; 20(6):375-97.
30. Tipton KD, Ferrando AA, Williams BD, Wolfe, RR. Muscle protein metabolism in female swimmers after a combination of resistance and endurance exercise. *J Appl Physiol* 1996; 81(5):2034-2038.
31. Cooper RR. Alterations during immobilization and regeneration of skeletal muscle in cats. *J Bone Joint Surg* 1972; 54A:919-952.
32. Eichner ER, Calabrese LH. Immunology and exercise. Physiology, pathophysiology, and implications for HIV infection. *Med Clin North Am* 1994; 78(2):377-88.
33. Norton JA, Lowry SF, Brennan MF. Effect of work induced hypertrophy on skeletal muscle of tumor and non-tumor bearing rats. *J Appl Physiol* 1979; 46:654-657.
34. Goldberg AL, Etlinger JD, Goldspink DF, Jablecki C. Mechanism of work-induced hypertrophy of skeletal muscle. *Med Sci Sports* 1975; 7(3):185-98.
35. Katzeff HL, Ojamaa KM, Klein I. The effects of long-term aerobic exercise and energy restriction on protein synthesis. *Metab Clin Exp* 1995; 44(2):188-92.
36. Stroud MA, Jackson AA, Waterlow JC. Protein turnover rates of two human subjects during an unassisted crossing of Antarctica. *Br J Nutr* 1996; 76(2):165-74.
37. Donnelly JE, Sharp T, Houmard J, et al. Muscle hypertrophy with large-scale weight loss and resistance training. *Am J Clin Nutr* 1993; 58:561-565.
38. Wood PD, Terry RB, Haskell WL. Metabolism of substrates: diet, lipoprotein metabolism, and exercise. *Fed Proc* 1985; 44:358-363.
39. Gollnick PD. Metabolism of substrates: energy substrate metabolism during exercise and as modified by training. *Fed Proc* 1985; 44:353-357.
40. Dohm GL, Kasperek J, Tapscott EB, Barakat HA. Protein metabolism during endurance exercise. *Fed Proc* 1985; 44:348-352.
41. Castill DL. Carbohydrate nutrition before, during, and after exercise. *Fed Proc* 1985; 44:364-368.
42. Astrand PO, Rodahl K. *Textbook of Work Physiology,* 2nd ed. New York: McGraw-Hill, 1977.
43. Borer KT. Neurohumoral mediation of exercise-induced growth. *Med Sci Sports Exerc* 1994; 26(6):741-54.
44. Goldberg AL. Influence of insulin and contractile activity on muscle size and protein balance. *Diabetes* 1979; 28:18-24.
45. Goldberg AL, Goodman HM. Relationship between cortisone and muscle work in determining muscle size. *J Physiol* 1969; 200(3):667-75.
46. Goldberg AL, Tischler M, Libby P. Regulation of protein degradation in skeletal muscle. *Biochem Soc Trans* 1980; 8(5):497.
47. Goldberg AL. Protein synthesis during work-induced growth of skeletal muscle. *J Cell Biol* 1968; 36(3):653-8.
48. Goldberg AL. Role of insulin in work-induced growth of skeletal muscle. *Endocrinology* 1968; 83(5):1071-3.
49. Goldberg AL, Goodman HM. Relationship between growth hormone and muscular work in determining muscle size. *J Physiol* 1969; 200(3):655-66.
50. Goldberg AL. Protein turnover in skeletal muscle. II. Effects of denervation and cortisone on protein catabolism in skeletal muscle. *J Biol Chem* 1969; 244(12):3223-9.
51. Goldberg AL, Griffin GE. Hormonal control of protein synthesis and degradation in rat skeletal muscle [proceedings]. *J Physiol* 1977; 270(1):51P-52P.
52. Kettelhut IC,Wing SS, Goldberg AL. Endocrine regulation of protein breakdown in skeletal muscle. *Diabetes Metab Rev* 1988; 4:751-772.
53. Goldberg AL, Tischler M, DeMartino G, Griffin G. Hormonal regulation of protein degradation and synthesis in skeletal muscle. *Fed Proc* 1980; 39(1):31-6.
54. McMurray RG, Eubank TK, Hackney AC. Nocturnal hormonal responses to resistance exercise. *Eur J Appl Physiol* 1995; 72:121-126.
55. Goodman HM. Amino acid transport during work-induced growth of skeletal muscle. *Am J Physiol* 1969; 216(5):1111-5.
56. Goldberg AL. Mechanisms of growth and atrophy of skeletal muscle. *Muscle Biol* 1972; 1:89-118.
57. Goldberg AL, Goodman HM. Amino acid transport during work-induced growth of skeletal muscle. *Am J Physiol* 1969; 216(5):1111-5.
58. Goldberg AL. Protein turnover in skeletal muscle. I. Protein catabolism during work-induced hypertrophy and growth induced with growth hormone. *J Biol Chem* 1969; 244(12):3217-22.

59. Dohm GL, Hecker AL, Brown WE, et al. Adaptation of protein metabolism to endurance training. Increased amino acid oxidation in response to training. *Biochem J* 1977; 164: 705-708.
60. Goldberg AL, Etlinger JD, Goldspink DF, Jablecki C. Mechanism of work-induced hypertrophy of skeletal muscle. *Med Sci Sports* Exerc 1971; 7:248-261.
61. Goldberg AL, Etlinger JD, Goldspink DF, Jablecki C. Mechanism of work-induced hypertrophy of skeletal muscle. *Med Sci Sports* 1975; 7(3):185-98.
62. Kuoppasalmi K, Naveri H, Rehunen S, Harkonen M, Adlercreutz H. Effect of strenuous anaerobic running exercise on plasma growth hormone, cortisol, luteinizing hormone, testosterone, androstenedione, estrone and estradiol. *J Steroid Biochem* 1976; 7(10):823-9.
63. Skierska E, Ustupska J, Biczowa B, Lukaszewska J. [Effect of physical exercise on plasma cortisol, testosterone and growth hormone levels in weight lifters]. *Endokrynol Pol* 1976; 27(2):159-65.
64. Morville R, Pesquies PC, Guezennec CY, Serrurier BD, Guignard M. Plasma variations in testicular and adrenal androgens during prolonged physical exercise in man. *Ann Endocrinol* 1979; 40(5):501-10.
65. Gawel MJ, Park DM, Alaghband-Zadeh J, Rose FC. Exercise and hormonal secretion. *Postgrad Med J* 1979; 55(644):373-6.
66. Kuoppasalmi K, Naveri H, Harkonen M, Aldercreuttz H. Plasma cortisol androstenedione, testosterone and luteinizing hormone in running exercise of different intensities. *Scand J Clin Lab Invest* 1980; 40:403-409.
67. Kindermann W, Schnabel A, Schmitt WM, Biro G, Cassens J, Weber F. Catecholamines, growth hormone, cortisol, insulin, and sex hormones in anaerobic and aerobic exercise. *Eur J Appl Physiol Occup Physiol* 1982; 49(3):389-99.
68. Craig BW, Brown R, Everhart J. Effects of progressive resistance training on growth hormone and testosterone levels in young and elderly subjects. *Mech Ageing Dev* 1989; 49:159-169.
69. Kraemer RR, Kilgore JL, Kraemer GR, Castracane VD. Growth hormone, IGF-1, and testosterone responses to resistive exercise. *Med Sci Sports Exerc* 1992; 24(12):1346-52.
70. Kraemer W, Marchitelli L, Gordon S, Fleck S. Hormonal and growth factor responses to heavy resistance exercise protocols. *J Appl Physiol* 1990; 69(4):1442-1450.
71. Kraemer WJ, Gordon SE, Fleck SJ, et al. Endogenous anabolic hormonal and growth factor responses to heavy resistance exercise in males and females. *Int J Sports Med* 1991; 12:228-235.
72. Snegovskaya V, Viru A. Steroid and pituitary hormone responses to rowing: relative significance of exercise intensity and duration and performance level. *Eur J Appl Physiol Occup Physiol* 1993; 67(1):59-65.
73. Lehmann M, Knizia K, Gastmann U, et al. Influence of 6-week, 6 days per week, training on pituitary function in recreational athletes. *Br J Sports Med* 1993; 27(3):186-92.
74. Hickson RC, Hidaka K, Foster C, Falduto MT, Chatterton RT Jr. Successive time courses of strength development and steroid hormone responses to heavy-resistance training. *J Appl Physiol* 1994; 76(2):663-70.
75. Kraemer WJ, Fry AC, Warren BJ, Stone MH, Fleck SJ, Kearney JT, Conroy BP, Maresh CM, Weseman CA, Triplett NT, et al. Acute hormonal responses in elite junior weightlifters. *Int J Sports Med* 1992, 13 (2) p103-9.
76. Lehmann M, Foster C, Keul J. Overtraining in endurance athletes: a brief review. *Med Sci Sports Exerc* 1993; 25(7):854-62.
77. Fry AC, Kraemer WJ, Stone MH, et al. Endocrine responses to overreaching before and after 1 year of weightlifting. *Can J Appl Physiol* 1994; 19(4):400-10.
78. Silverman HG, Mazzeo RS. Hormonal responses to maximal and submaximal exercise in trained and untrained men of various ages. *J Gerontol Ser A Biol Sci Med Sci* 1996; 51(1):B30-7.
79. Mathur RS, Neff MR, Landgrebe SC, et al. Time-related changes in the plasma concentrations of prolactin, gonadotropins, sex hormone-binding globulin, and certain steroid hormones in female runners after a long distance race. *Fertil Steril* 1986; 46:1067.
80. Hale RW, Kosasa T, Kreiger J, Pepper S. A marathon: the immediate effect on female runners' luteinizing hormone, follicle-stimulating hormone, prolactin, testosterone, and cortisol levels. *Am J Obstet Gynecol* 1983; 146:550.
81. Maynar M, Caballero MJ, Mena P, Rodriguez C, Cortes R, Maynar JI. Urine excretion of androgen hormones in professional racing cyclists. *Eur J Appl Physiol Occup Physiol* 1994; 68(3):200-4.
82. Hortobagyi T, Houmard JA, Stevenson JR, Fraser DD, Johns RA, Israel RG. The effects of detraining on power athletes. *Med Sci Sports Exerc* 1993; 25(8):929-35.
83. Zarubina NA, Dobracheva AD, Nekrasova LV. [Pathogenesis of functional retardation of physical and sexual development in adolescents. Status of somatotropic and gonadotropic function]. *Probl Endokrinol* 1989; 35(2):18-22.
84. Kuoppasalmi K, Adlercreutz H. Interaction between catabolic and anabolic steroid hormones in muscular exercise. In K. Fotherby and S. Pal (Eds.): *Exercise Endocrinology.* Walter de Gruyter, New York, 1985. 65-98.
85. Stuart CA, Nagamani M. Insulin infusion acutely augments ovarian androgen production in normal women. *Fertil Steril* 1990; 54(5):788-792.
86. Young GA, Yule AG, Hill GL. Effects of an anabolic steroid on plasma amino acids, proteins, and body composition in patients receiving intravenous hyperalimentation. *J Parenteral Enteral Nutr* 1983; 7:221-225.

87. Michelsen CB, Askanazi J, Kinney JM, et al. Effect of an anabolic steroid on nitrogen balance and amino acid patterns after total hip replacement. *J Trauma* 1982; 22:410-413.
88. Gore DC, Honeycutt D, Jahoor F, et al. Effect of exogenous growth hormone on whole-body and isolated-limb protein kinetics in burned patients. *Arch Surg* 1991; 126:38-43.
89. Ziegler TR, Rombeau JL, Young LS, et al. Recombinant human growth hormone enhances the metabolic efficacy of parenteral nutrition. A double-blind, randomized controlled study. *J Clin Endocrinol Metab* 1992; 74:865-73.
90. Vara-Thorback R, Guerra JA, Ruiz-Requena ME, et al. Effects of growth hormone in patients receiving total parenteral nutrition following major gastrointestinal surgery. *Hepatogastroenterology* 1992; 39:270-5.
91. Woolfson AMJ, Heatley RV, Allison SP. Insulin to inhibit protein catabolism after injury. *N Engl J Med* 1979; 300:14-17.
92. Jeevanandam M. Ornithine alpha-ketoglutarate in trauma situations. *Clin Nutr* 1993; 12:61-65.
93. Wernerman J, Hammarqvist F, von der Decken A, et al. Ornithine alpha ketoglutarate improves skeletal muscle protein synthesis as assessed by ribosome analysis and nitrogen use after surgery. *Ann Surg* 1987; 206:674-678.
94. Cerra FB, Upson D, Angelico R, et al. Branched-chain amino acids support post-operative protein synthesis. *Surgery* 1982; 92:192-199.
95. Bonau RA, Ang SD, Jeevanandam M, et al. High branched-chain amino acid solutions. Relationship of composition to efficacy. JPEN. *J Parenteral Enteral Nutr* 1984; 8:622-628.
96. Furst P, Stehle P. The potential use of parenteral dipeptides in clinical nutrition. *Nutr Clin Pract* 1993; 8:106-114 .
97. Hammarqvist F, Wernerman J, Ali R, et al. Addition of glutamine to total parenteral nutrition after elective abdominal surgery spares free glutamine in muscle, counteracts the fall in muscle protein synthesis, and improves nitrogen balance. *Ann Surg* 1989; 209:455-461.
98. Miki N, Ono M, Miyoshi H, et al. Hypothalamic growth hormone releasing factor (GRF) participates in the negative feedback regulation of growth hormone secretion. *Life Sci* 1988; 44:469-476.
99. Johnston DG. Regulation of GH secretion. *J R Soc Med* 1985; 78:319-24.
100. *Evaluation of Growth Hormone Secretion.* Laron Z, Butenandt O, Eds. S. Karger, New York, 1983.
101. *Growth Hormone and Other Biologically Active Peptides,* Pecile A, Muller E, Eds. Elsevier, New York, 1980.
102. Keller V, Schnell H, Girard J, Stauffacher W. Effect of physiological elevation of plasma growth hormone levels on ketone body kinetics and lipolysis in normal acutely insulin deficient man. *Diabetologia* 1984; 26:103-108.
103. Sonntag WE, Hylka VW, Meites J. Growth hormone restores protein synthesis in skeletal muscle of old male rats. *J Gerontol* 1985; 40:684-694.
104. Cuneo RC, Salomon F, Wiles CM, Hesp R, Sonksen PH. Growth hormone treatment in growth hormone-deficient adults. II. Effects on exercise performance. *J Appl Physiol* 1991; 70:695-700.
105. Crist DM, Peake GT, Loftfield RB, Kraner JC, Egan PA. Supplemental growth hormone alters body composition, muscle protein metabolism and serum lipids in fit adults: characterization of dose-dependent and response-recovery effects. *Mech Ageing Dev* 1991; 58:191-205.
106. Rudman D, Feller AG, Nagraj HS, et al. Effects of human growth hormone in men over 60 years old. *N Engl J Med* 1990; 323:1-5.
107. Revhaug A, Mjaaland M. Growth hormone and surgery. *Horm Res* 1993; 40: 99-101.
108. Jorgensen JO, Moller J, Alberti KG, Schmitz O, Christiansen JS, Orskov H, Moller N. Marked effects of sustained low growth hormone (GH) levels on day-to-day fuel metabolism: studies in GH-deficient patients and healthy untreated subjects. *J Clin Endocrinol Metab* 1993; 77(6):1589-96.
109. Clark RG, Jansson JO, Isaksson O, Robinson IC. Intravenous growth hormone: growth responses to patterned infusions in hypophysectomized rats. *J. Endocrinol* 1985; 104:53-61.
110. Jansson, JO, Albertsson-Wikland, K, Eden, S, Throngren, KG & Isaksson, O. Circumstantial evidence for a role of the secretory pattern of growth hormone in control of body growth. *Acta Endocrinol* 1982; 99:24-30.
111. Crist DM, Peake GT, Loftfield RB, Kraner JC, Egan PA. Supplemental growth hormone alters body composition, muscle protein metabolism and serum lipids in fit adults: characterization of dose-dependent and response-recovery effects. *Mech Ageing Dev* 1991; 58(2-3):191-205.
112. Snyder DK, Underwood LE, Clemmons DR. Anabolic effects of growth hormone in obese diet-restricted subjects are dose dependent. *Am J Clin Nutr* 1990; 52(3):431-7.
113. Seve B, Ballevre O, Ganier P, et al. Recombinant porcine somatotropin and dietary protein enhance protein synthesis in growing pigs. *J Nutr* 1993; 123(3):529-40.
114. Clemmons DR, Snyder DK, Williams R, et al. Growth hormone administration conserves lean body mass during dietary restriction in obese subjects. *J Clin Endocrinol Metab* 1987; 64:878-83.
115. Snyder DK, Clemmons DR, Underwood LE. Treatment of obese, diet-restricted subjects with growth hormone for 11 weeks: effects on anabolism, lipolysis, and body composition. *J Clin Endocrinol Metab* 1988; 67(1):54-61.

116. Ward HC, Halliday D, Sim AJW. Protein and energy metabolism with biosynthetic human growth hormone after gastrointestinal surgery. *Ann Surg* 1983; 206:56-61.
117. Ziegler TR, Young LS, Manson JM, et al. Metabolic effects of recombinant human growth hormone in patients receiving parenteral nutrition *Ann Surg* 1987; 208:6-16.
118. Ponting GA, Halliday D, Teale JD, et al. Postoperative positive nitrogen balance with intravenous hyponutrition and growth hormone. *Lancet* 1988; 1:438,.
119. Jiang ZM, He GZ, Zhang SY, et al. Low-dose growth hormone and hypocaloric nutrition attenuate the protein-catabolic response after major operation. *Ann Surg* 1989; 210:513-24.
120. Douglas RG, Humberstone DA, Haystead A, Shaw JHF. Metabolic effects of recombinant human growth hormone: Isotopic studies in the postabsorptive state and during total parenteral nutrition. *Br J Surg* 1990; 77:785-790.
121. Ziegler TR, Young LS, Ferrari-Baliviera E, Demling RH, Wilmore DW. Use of human growth hormone combined with nutritional support in a critical care unit. JPEN. *J Parenteral Enteral Nutr* 1990; 14:574-81.
122. Gore DC, Honeycutt D, Jahoor F, et al. Effect of exogenous growth hormone on whole-body and isolated-limb protein kinetics in burned patients. *Arch Surg* 1991; 126:38-43.
123. Hammarqvist F, Stromberg C, von der Decken A, et al. Biosynthetic human growth hormone preserves both muscle protein synthesis and the decrease in muscle-free glutamine, and improves whole-body nitrogen economy after operation. *Ann Surg* 1992; 216:184-191.
124. Voerman HJ, Strack van Schijndel RJM, Groeneveld ABJ, et al. Effects of recombinant human growth hormone in patients with severe sepsis. *Ann Surg* 1992; 216:64855.
125. Vara-Thorback R, Guerra JA, Ruiz-Requena ME, et al. Effects of growth hormone in patients receiving total parenteral nutrition following major gastrointestinal surgery. *Hepatogastroenterology* 1992; 39:270-276.
126. Ziegler TR, Rombeau JL, Young LS, et al. Recombinant human growth hormone enhances the metabolic efficacy of parenteral nutrition: A double-blind, randomized controlled study. *J Clin Endocrinol Metab* 1992; 74:865-73.
127. Petersen SR, Holaday, NJ, Jeevanandam M. Enhancement of protein synthesis efficiency in parenterally fed trauma victims by adjuvant recombinant human growth hormone. *J. Trauma* 1994; 36(5):726-733.
128. Koea JB, Breier BH, Douglas RG, Gluckman PD, Shaw JH. Anabolic and cardiovascular effects of recombinant human growth hormone in surgical patients with sepsis. *Br J Surg* 1996; 83(2):196-202.
129. Vara-Thorbeck R, Ruiz-Requena E, Guerrero-Fernandez JA. Effects of human growth hormone on the catabolic state after surgical trauma. *Horm Res* 1996; 45(1-2):55-60.
130. Jeevanandam M, Ramias L, Shamos RF, et al. Decreased growth hormone levels in the catabolic phase of severe injury. *Surgery* 1992; 111:495-502.
131. Petersen SR, Holaday NJ, Jeevanandam M. Enhancement of protein synthesis efficiency in parenterally fed trauma victims by adjuvant recombinant human growth hormone. *J Trauma* 1994; 36(5):726-733.
132. Roth E, Valentini L, Semsroth M, et al. Resistance of nitrogen metabolism to growth hormone treatment in the early phase after injury of patients with multiple injuries. *J Trauma* 1995; 38(1):136-41.
133. Taaffe DR, Jin IH, Vu TH, Hoffman AR, Marcus R. Lack of effect of recombinant human growth hormone (GH) on muscle morphology and GH-insulin-like growth factor expression in resistance-trained elderly men. *J Clin Endocrinol Metab* 1996; 81(1):421-5.
134. Saito H. Inouc T, Fukatsu K, Ming-Tsan L, Inaba T, Fukushima R, Muto T. Growth hormone and the immune response to bacterial infection. *Horm Res* 1996; 45(1-2):50-4.
135. Roth J, Glick SM, Yalow RS, Berson SA. Secretion of human growth hormone: Physiologic and experimental modification. *Metab* 1963; 12:577-579.
136. Nicklas BJ, Ryan AJ, Treuth MM, et al. Testosterone, growth hormone and IGF-1 responses to acute and chronic resistive exercise in men aged 55-70 years. *Int J Sports Med* 1995; 16(7):445-50.
137. Galbo H. *Hormonal and Metabolic Adaptation to Exercise.* New York: Georg Thieme Verlag. 1983
138. VanHelder WP, Goode RC, Radomski MW. Effect of anaerobic and aerobic exercise of equal duration and work expenditure on plasma growth hormone levels. *Eur J Appl Physiol* 1984; 52:255-257.
139. VanHelder WP, Radomski MW, Goode RC. Growth hormone responses during intermittent weight lifting exercise in men. *Eur J Appl Physiol* 1984; 53:31-34.
140. VanHelder WP, Radomski MW, Goode RC, Casey K. Hormonal and metabolic response to three types of exercise of equal duration and external work output. *Eur J Appl Physiol* 1985; 54:337-342.
141. Nguyen NU, Wolf JP, Simon ML, Henriet MT, Dumoulin G, Berthelay S. [Variations in circulating levels of prolactin and growth hormone during physical exercise in man: influence of the intensity of the workout.] *C R Seances Soc Biol Filiales* 1984; 178(4):450-457.
142. Garden G, Hale PJ, Horrocks PM, Crase J, Hammond V, Nattrass M. Metabolic and hormonal responses during squash. *Eur J Appl Physiol Occup Physiol* 1986; 55(4):445-449.
143. Tatar P, Kozlowski S, Vigas M, et al. Endocrine response to physical efforts with equivalent total work loads but different intensities in man. *Endocrinol Exp* 1984; 18(4):233-239.
144. VanHelder WP, Casey K, Radomski MW. Regulation of growth hormone during exercise by oxygen demand and availability. *Eur J Appl Physiol Occup Physiol* 1987; 56(6):628-632.

145. Vanhelder WP, Radomski MW, Goode RC. Growth hormone responses during intermittent weight lifting exercise in men. *Eur J Appl Physiol Occup Physiol* (Berlin, W.G.) 53(1), 1984, 31-34.
146. Kozlowski S, Chwalbinska Moneta J, Vigas M, Kaciuba Vsailko H, Nazar K. Greater serum GH response to arm than to leg exercise performed at equivalent oxygen uptake. *Eur J Appl Physiol Occup Physiol* 52(1), Nov 1983, 131-135.
147. Cappon JP, Ipp E, Brasel JA, Cooper DM. Acute effects of high fat and high glucose meals on the growth hormone response to exercise. *J Clin Endocrinol Metab* 1993; 76(6):1418-22.
148. Nevill ME, Holmyard DJ, Hall GM, et al. Growth hormone responses to treadmill sprinting in sprint- and endurance-training athletes. *Eur J Appl Physiol* 1996; 72:460-467.
149. De Feo P, Perriello G, Torlone E, et al. Demonstration of a role for growth hormone in glucose counter-regulation. *Am J Physiol* 1989; 256:E835-E843.
150. Kostyo JL, Isaksson O. Growth hormone and the regulation of somatic growth. *Int. Rev. Physiol* 1977; 13:255-262.
151. Merimee TJ. Growth hormone: secretion and action. In: De Groot, L.J., *Endocrinology* New York: Grune & Stratton, 1979.
152. Snyder DK, Underwood LE, Clemmons DR. Persistent lipolytic effect of exogenous growth hormone during caloric restriction. Am J Med 1995; 98(2):129-34.
153. Guyton AC. The pituitary hormones and their control by the hypothalamus. In: *Textbook of Medical Physiology,* 8th ed, edited by M.J. Wonsiewicz. Toronto: W.B. Saunders 1991; 819-826.
154. Rabinowitz D, Merimee TJ, Mafezzolo R, Burgess JA. Patterns of hormonal release after glucose, protein and glucose plus protein. *Lancet* 1968; 2: 434-441.
155. Sonntag WE, Forman LJ, Mikki N, Meites J. Growth hormone secretion and neuroendocrine regulation. In: *CRC Handbook of Endocrinology* 1981; 35-59. CRC Press, Boca Raton, FL.
156. Moller N, Moller J, Jorgensen JO, Ovesen P, Schmitz O, Alberti KG. Christiansen JS. Impact of 2 weeks high dose growth hormone treatment on basal and insulin stimulated substrate metabolism in humans. *Clin Endocrinol* 1993; 39(5):577-81.
157. Kelley VC, Ruvalcaba RH. Use of anabolic agents in treatment of short children. *Clin Endocrinol Metab* 1982; 11:25-39.
158. Alen M, Rahkila P, Reinila M, Vihko R. Androgenic -anabolic steroid effects on serum thyroid, pituitary and steroid hormones in athletes. *Am J Sports Med* 1987; 14:357-361.
159. Welbourne TC, Cronin MJ. Growth hormone accelerates tubular acid secretion. *Am J Physiol* 1991; 260:R1036-42.
160. Matzen LE, Andersen BB, Jensen BG, Gjessing HJ, Sindrup SH, Kvetny J. Different short-term effect of protein and carbohydrate intake on TSH, growth hormone (GH), insulin, C-peptide, and glucagon in humans. *Scand J Clin Lab Invest* 1990; 50(7):801-5.
161. Berelowitz M, Szabo M, Frohman LA, et al. Somatostatin-C mediates growth hormone negative feedback by effects on both the hypothalamus and pituitary. *Science* 1981; 212:1279-1281.
162. Berelowitz M, Firestone SL, Frohman LA. Effect of growth hormone excess and deficiency on hypothalamic somatostatin content and release and on tissue somatostatin distribution. *Endocrinology* 1981; 109:714-719.
163. Bercu BB, Diamond F. A determinant of stature: regulation of growth hormone secretion. In: Barness L, ed. *Advances in Pediatrics*. Chicago: Year Book Medical Publishers, 1984: 331-80.
164. Haynes SP. Growth hormone. *Aust J Sci Med Sport* 1986; 18(1):3-10.
165. Bertherat J, Bluet-Pajot MT, Epelbaum J. Neuroendocrine regulation of growth hormone. *Eur. J. Endocrinol* 1995; 132(1):12-24.
166. Bercu BB. Disorders of growth hormone neurosecretory function. Proc Seventh Int Congr Endocrinology. In: Labrie F, Proulx L, eds. *Endocrinology.* New York: Excerpta Medica 1984:753-6.
167. Bercu BB, Diamond F. Growth hormone neurosecretory dysfunction. *Clin Endocrinol Metab* 1986; 15:537-90.
168. Ghigo E, Bellone J, Mazza E, Imperiale E, Procopio M, Valente F, Lala R, De Sanctis C, Camanni F. Arginine potentiates the GHRH- but not the pyridostigmine-induced GH secretion in normal short children. Further evidence for a somatostatin suppressing effect of arginine. *Clin Endocrinol* 1990; 32(6):763-767.
169. Koppeschaar HP, ten Horn CD, Thijssen JH, Page MD, Dieguez C, Scanlon MF. Differential effects of arginine on growth hormone releasing hormone and insulin induced growth hormone secretion. *Clin Endocrinol* 1992; 36(5):487-90.
170. Masuda A, Shibasaki T, Hotta M, Yamauchi N, Ling N, Demura H, Shizume K. Insulin-induced hypoglycemia, L-dopa and arginine stimulate GH secretion through different mechanisms in man. *Regul Pept* 1990; 31(1):53-64.
171. Kelijman M, Frohman LA. The role of the cholinergic pathway in growth hormone feedback. *J Clin Endocrinol Metab* 1991; 72(5):1081-87.
172. Casanueva FF, Villanueva L, Cabranes JA, Cabezas Cerrato J, Fernandez Cruz A. Cholinergic mediation of growth hormone secretion elicited by arginine, clonidine, and physical exercise in man. *J Clin Endocrinol Metab* (Baltimore) 59(3), Sept 1984, 526-530.

173. Mendelson WB, Lantigua RA, Wyatt RJ, Gillin JC, Jacobs LS. Piperidine enhances sleep-related and insulin-induced growth hormone secretion: further evidence for a cholinergic secretory mechanism. *J Clin Endocrinol Metab* 1981; 52(3):409-15.
174. Mazza E, Ghigo E, Bellone J, et al. Effects of alpha and beta adrenergic agonists and antagonists on growth hormone secretion in man. *SO Endocrinol Exp* 1990; 24(1-2):211-9.
175. Muller EE, Cocchi D, Ghigo E, Arvat E, Locatelli V, Camanni F. Growth hormone response to GHRH during lifespan. *J Pediatr Endocrinol* 1993; 6(1):5-13.
176. Vermeulen A. [Neuroendocrinological aspects of aging]. Verhandelingen — Koninklijke Academie voor Geneeskunde van Belgie 1994; 56(4):267-80.
177. Minamitani N, Chihara K, Kaji H, et al. Alpha2-adrenergic control of growth hormone (GH) secretion in conscious male rabbits. Involvement of endogenous GH-releasing factor and somatostatin. *Endocrinology* 1989; 125:2839-2845.
178. Cordido F, Dieguez C, Casanueva FF. Effect of central cholinergic neurotransmission enhancement by pyridostigmine on the growth hormone secretion elicited by clonidine, arginine, or hypoglycemia in normal and obese subjects. *J Clin Endocrinol Metab* 1990; 70(5):1361-1370.
179. Reichardt B, Schrader M, Mojto J, Mehltretter G, Muller OA, Schopohl J. The decrease in growth hormone (GH) response after repeated stimulation with GH-releasing hormone is partly caused by an elevation of somatostatin tonus. *J Clin Endocrinol Metab* 1996; 81(5):1994-8.
180. Malaab SA, Pollak MN, Goodyer CG. Direct effects of tamoxifen on growth hormone secretion by pituitary cells in vitro. *Eur J Cancer* 1992; 28A(4-5):788-93.
181. Tannenbaum GS, Gurd W, Lapointe M, Pollak M. Tamoxifen attenuates pulsatile growth hormone secretion: mediation in part by somatostatin. *Endocrinology* 1992; 130(6):3395-401.
182. O'Sullivan UP, Gluckman D, Breier BH, et al. Insulin-like growth factor-1 (IGF-1) in mice reduces weight loss during starvation. *Endocrinology* 1989; 125:2793-2795.
183. Jacob RE, Barrett G, Plewe KD, et al. Acute effects of insulin-like growth factor-1 on glucose and amino acid metabolism in the awake fasted rat. *J Clin Invest* 1989; 83:1717-1723.
184. Scheiwiller E, Guler HP, Merryweather J, et al. Growth restoration of insulin-deficient diabetic rats by recombinant human insulin-like growth factor-1. *Nature* 1986; 323:169-171.
185. Guler HP, Zapf J, Scheiwiller E, Froesch ER. Recombinant human insulin-like growth factor-1 stimulates growth and has distinct effects on organ size in hypophysectomized rats. *Proc Natl Acad Sci U.S.A.* 1988; 85:4889-4893.
186. Schoenle E, Zapf J, Humbrel RE, Froesch ER. Insulin-like growth factor-1 stimulates growth in hypophysectomized rats. *Nature* 1982; 296:252-253.
187. Zapf JC, Schmid H, Froesch ER. Biological and immunological properties of insulin-like growth factors I and II. *Clin Endocrinol Metab* 1984; 13:3-30.
188. Blundell TL, Bedarkar S, Rinderknecht E, Humbel RE. Insulin-like growth factors: a model for tertiary structure accounting for immunoreactivity and receptor binding. *Proc Natl Acad Sci U.S.A.* 1979; 75:180-184.
189. Underwood LE, D'Ercole AJ, Clemmons DR, Van Wyk JJ. Paracrine functions of somatomedins. *J Clin Endocrinol Metab* 1986; 15:5-77.
190. Fryburg DA. Insulin-like growth factor-1 exerts growth hormone- and insulin-like actions on human muscle protein metabolism. *Am J Physiol* 1994; 267: E331-E336.
191. Zapf J, Schoenle E, Froesch ER. Insulin-like growth factors I and II: some biological actions and receptor binding characteristics of two purified constituents of non-suppressible insulin-like activity of human serum. *Eur J Biochem* 1978; 87:285-296.
192. Poggi C, Le Marchand-Brustel Y, Zapf J, Froesch ER, Freychet P. Effects and binding of insulin-like growth factor-1 in the isolated soleus muscle of lean and obese mice: comparison with insulin. *Endocrinology* 1979; 105:723-730.
193. Bolinder J, Lindblad A, Engfeldt P, Arner P. Studies of acute effects of insulin-like growth factors I and II in human fat cells. *J Clin Endocrinol Metab* 1987; 65:732-737.
194. Zapf J, Hauri C, Waldvogel M, Froesch ER. Acute metabolic effects and half-lives of intravenously administered insulinlike growth factors I and II in normal and hypophysectomized rats. *J Clin Invest* 1986; 77:1768-1775.
195. Guler HP, Zapf J, Froesch FR. Short-term metabolic effects of recombinant human insulin-like growth factor-1 in healthy adults. *N Engl J Med* 1987; 317:137-140.
196. McCarthy TL, Centrella M, Canalis E. Regulatory effects of insulin-like growth factors I and II on bone collagen synthesis in rat calvarial cultures. *Endocrinology* 1989; 124:301-309.
197. Schoenle E, Zapf J, Hauri C, Steiner T, Froesch ER. Comparison of in vivo effects of insulin-like growth factors I and II and of growth hormone in hypophysectomized rats. *Acta Endocrinol* 1985; 108:167-174.
198. Douglas RG, Gluckman PD, Ball K, Breier B, Shaw JH. The effects of infusion of insulinlike growth factor (IGF) I, IGF-2, and insulin on glucose and protein metabolism in fasted lambs. *J Clin Invest* 1991; 88(2):614-22.

199. Haymond MW, Horber FF, Mauras N. Human growth hormone but not insulin-like growth factor-1 positively affects whole-body estimates of protein metabolism. *Horm Res* 1992; 38 Suppl 1:73-5.
200. Huybrechts LM, Decuypere E, Buyse J, Kuhn ER, Tixier Boichard M. Effect of recombinant human insulin-like growth factor-1 on weight gain, fat content, and hormonal parameters in broiler chickens. *Poult Sci* 1992; 71(1):181-7.
201. Yang H, Grahn M, Schalch DS, Ney DM. Anabolic effect of IGF-1 coinfused with total parenteral nutrition in dexamethasone-treated rats. *Am J Physiol* 1994; 266(5 Pt 1):E690-8.
202. Kraemer WJ, Aguilera BA, Terada M, et al. Responses of IGF-1 to endogenous increases in growth hormone after heavy-resistance exercise. *J Appl Physiol* 1995; 79:1310-1315.
203. Tomas FM, Knowles SE, Owens PC, Read LC, Chandler CS, Gargosky SE, Ballard FJ. Increased weight gain, nitrogen retention and muscle protein synthesis following treatment of diabetic rats with insulin-like growth factor (IGF)-1 and des(1-3)IGF-1. *Biochem J* 1991; 276(Pt 2):547-54.
204. Jacob R, et al. IGF-1 stimulation of muscle protein synthesis in the awake rat: permissive role of insulin and amino acids. *Am J Physiol* 1996; 270:E60-E66.
205. Loughna PT, Goldspink DF, Goldspink G. Effects of hypokinesia and hypodynamia upon protein turnover in hindlimb muscles of the rat. *Aviat Space Environ Med* 1987; 58(9 Pt 2):A133-8.
206. Morgan MJ, Loughna PT. Work overload induced changes in fast and slow skeletal muscle myosin heavy chain gene expression. *FEBS Lett* 1989; 255(2):427-30.
207. Loughna PT, Mason P, Bates PC. Regulation of insulin-like growth factor-1 gene expression in skeletal muscle. *Symp Soc Exp Biol* 1992; 46:319-30.
208. Bates PC, Loughna PT, Pell JM, Schulster D, Millward DJ. Interactions between growth hormone and nutrition in hypophysectomized rats: body composition and production of insulin-like growth factor-1. *J Endocrinol* 1993; 139(1):117-26.
209. Loughna PT, Bates PC. Interactions between growth hormone and nutrition in hypophysectomised rats: skeletal muscle myosin heavy chain mRNA levels. *Biochem Biophys Res Commun* 1994; 198(1):97-102.
210. Gulve EA, Dice JF. Regulation of protein synthesis and degradation in L8 myotubes. Effects of serum, insulin and insulin-like growth factors. *Biochem J* 1989; 260(2):377-87.
211. Laager R, Ninnis R, Keller U. Comparison of the effects of recombinant human insulin-like growth factor-1 and insulin on glucose and leucine kinetics in humans, *J Clin Invest* 1993; 92(4):1903-1909.
212. Russell-Jones DL, Umpleby AM, Hennessy TR, et al. Use of a leucine clamp to demonstrate that IGF-1 actively stimulates protein synthesis in normal humans. *Am J Physiol* 1994; 267(4 Pt 1):E591-8.
213. Mauras N, Horber FF, Haymond MW. Low dose recombinant human insulin-like growth factor-1 fails to affect protein anabolism but inhibits islet cell secretion in humans, *J Clin Endocrinol Metab* 1992; 75(5):1192-1197.
214. Haymond MW, Horber FF, De Feo P, Kahn SE, Mauras N. Effect of human growth hormone and insulin-like growth factor-1 on whole-body leucine and estimates of protein metabolism. *Horm Res* 1993; 40(1-3):92-4.
215. Yarasheski KE, Zachweija JJ, Angelopoulos TJ, Bier DM. Short-term growth hormone treatment does not increase muscle protein synthesis in experienced weight lifters. *J Appl Physiol* 1993; 74(6):3073-6.
216. Mauras N, Beaufrere B. Recombinant human insulin-like growth factor-1 enhances whole body protein anabolism and significantly diminishes the protein catabolic effects of prednisone in humans without a diabetogenic effect. *J Clin Endocrinol Metab* 1995; 80(3):869-74.
217. Bondy CA, Underwood LE, Clemmons DR, Guler HP, Bach MA, Skarulis M. Clinical uses of insulin-like growth factor-1. *Ann Intern Med* 1994; 120(7):593-601.
218. Chwals WJ, Bistrian BR. Role of exogenous growth hormone and insulin-like growth factor-1 in malnutrition and acute metabolic stress: A hypothesis. Crit Care Med 1991; 19:1317.
219. Clemmons DR. Use of growth hormone and insulin-like growth factor-1 in catabolism that is induced by negative energy balance. *Horm Res* 1993; 40(1-3):62-67.
220. Lo H, Ney DM. Simultaneous treatment with IGF-1 and GH additively increases anabolism in parenterally fed rats. *Am J Physiol* 1995; 269:E368-E376.
221. Lo H, Ney DM. Gh and IGF-1 differentially increase protein synthesis in skeletal muscle and jejunum of parenterally-fed rats. 1996; 271(5 Pt.1):E872-878.
222. Kupfer SR, Underwood LE, Baxter RC, Clemmons DR. Enhancement of the anabolic effects of growth hormone and insulin-like growth factor-1 by use of both agents simultaneously. *J Clin Invest* 1993; 91(2):391-6.
223. Kupfer SR, Underwood LF, Baxter RC, Clemmons DR. Enhancement of the anabolic effects of growth hormone and insulin-like growth factor-1 by use of both agents simultaneously. *J Clin Invest* 1993; 91:391-396.
224. Mauras N. Combined recombinant human growth hormone and recombinant human insulin-like growth factor-1: lack of synergy on whole body protein anabolism in normally fed subjects. *J Clin Endocrinol Metab* 1995; 80(9):2633-7.
225. Kuhara T, Ikeda S, Ohneda A, Sasaki Y. Effects of intravenous infusion of 17 amino acids on the secretion of GH, glucagon, and insulin in sheep. *Am J Physiol* 1991; 260(1 Pt 1):E21-6.

226. Hundal HS, Rennie MJ, Watt PW. Characteristics of acidic, basic and neutral amino acid transport in the perfused rat hindlimb. *J Physiol* 1989; 408:93-114.
227. Hundal HS, Rennie MJ, Watt PW. Characteristics of L-glutamine transport in perfused rat skeletal muscle. *J Physiol* 1987; 393:283-305.
228. Shotwell MA, Kilberg MS, Oxender DL. The regulation of neutral amino acid transport in mammalian cells. *Biochim Biophys Acta* 1983; 737:267-284.
229. Christensen HN. Role of amino acid transport and countertransport in nutrition and metabolism. *Physiol Rev* 1990; 70:43-77.
230. Natali A, Buzzigoli G, Taddei S, et al. Effects of insulin on hemodynamics and metabolism in human forearm. *Diabetes* 1990; 39:490-500.
231. Pozefsky TP, Felig P, Tobin JD, et al. Amino acid balance across tissues of the forearm in postabsorptive man. Effects of insulin at two dose levels. *J Clin Invest* 1969; 48:2273-2282.
232. Fryburg DA, Jahn LA, Hill SA, Oliveras DM, Barrett EJ. Insulin and insulin-like growth factor-1 enhance human skeletal muscle protein anabolism during hyperaminoacidemia by different mechanisms. *J Clin Invest* 1995; 96(4):1722-9.
233. Biolo G, Declan Fleming RY, Wolfe RR. Physiologic hyperinsulinemia stimulates protein synthesis and enhances transport of selected amino acids in human skeletal muscle. *J Clin Invest* 1995; 95(2):811-9.
234. Gelfand RA, Barrett EJ. Effect of physiologic hyperinsulinemia on skeletal muscle protein synthesis and breakdown in man. *J Clin Invest* 1987; 80:1-7.
235. Florini JR. Hormonal control of muscle growth. *Muscle Nerve* 1987; 10:577-598.
236. Lundholm K, Edstrom L, Ekman L, et al. Protein degradation in human skeletal muscle: the effect of insulin, leucine, amino acids and ions. *Clin Sci* 1981; 60:319-326.
237. Frexes-Steed M, Warner ML, Bulus N, et al. Role of insulin and branched-chain amino acids in regulating protein metabolism during fasting. *Am J Physiol* 1990; 258:E907-E917.
238. Flakoll PJ, Kulaylat M, Frexes-Steed M, et al. Amino acids augment insulin's suppression of whole body proteolysis. *Am J Physiol* 1989; 257:E839-E847.
239. Jefferson LS. Role of insulin in the regulation of protein synthesis. *Diabetes* 1980; 29:487-96.
240. Fukagawa NK, Minaker KL, Rowe JW, Young VR. Plasma tryptophan and total neutral amino acid levels in men: influence of hyperinsulinemia and age. *Metabolism* 1987; 36:683-6.
241. Fukagawa NK, Minaker KL, Young VR, Rowe JW. Insulin dose-dependent reductions in plasma amino acids in man. *Am J Physiol* 1986; 250:E13-17.
242. Fukagawa NK, Minaker KL, Rowe JW, et al. Insulin-mediated reductions of whole body protein breakdown: dose-response effects on leucine metabolism in postabsorptive men. *J Clin Invest* 1985; 76:2306-11.
243. Jefferson LS, Koehler JO, Morgan HE. Effect of insulin on protein synthesis in skeletal muscle of an isolated perfused preparation of rat hemicorpus. *Proc Natl Acad Sci U.S.A.* 1972; 69:816-820.
244. Marshall S, Monzon R. Amino acid regulation of insulin action in isolated adipocytes. Selective ability of amino acids to enhance both insulin sensitivity and maximal insulin responsiveness of the protein synthesis system. *J Biol Chem* 1989; 264:2037-2042.
245. Jefferson LS, Li JB, Rannels SR. Regulation by insulin of amino acid release and protein turnover in the perfused rat hemicorpus. *J Biol Chem* 1977; 252:1476-1483.
246. Airhart J, Arnold JA, Stirewalt WS, Low RB. Insulin stimulation of protein synthesis in cultured skeletal and cardiac muscle cells. *Am J Physiol* 1982; 243:C81-C86.
247. Kimball SR, Jefferson LS. Cellular mechanisms involved in the action of insulin on protein synthesis. *Diabetes Metab Rev* 1988; 4:773-787.
248. Garlick PJ, Fern M, Preedy VR. The effect of insulin infusion and food intake on muscle protein synthesis in postabsorptive rats. *Biochem J* 1983; 210:669-676.
249. Manchester KL, Young FG. The effect of insulin on the incorporation of amino acid into protein of normal rat diaphragm in vitro. *Biochem J* 1958; 70:353-358.
250. Jefferson LS, Li JB, Rannels SR. Regulation by insulin of amino acid release and protein turnover in the perfused rat hemicorpus. *J Biol Chem* 1977; 252(4):1476-83.
251. Bennett WM, Connacher AA, Scringeour CM, Jung RT, Rennie MJ. Euglycemic hyperinsulinemia augments amino acid uptake by human leg tissues during hyperaminoacidemia. *Am J Physiol* 1990; 259:E185-E194.
252. Castellino P, Luzi L, Simonson DC, et al. Effect of insulin and plasma amino acid concentration on leucine metabolism in man: role of substrate availability on estimates of whole body protein synthesis. *J Clin Invest* 1987; 80:1784-1793.
253. Bonadonna RC, Saccomani MP, Cobelli C, et al. Effect of Insulin on System a Amino Acid Transport in Human Skeletal Muscle. *J Clin Invest* 1993; 91(2):514-521.
254. Tessari P, Inchiostro S, Biolo G. Vincenti E, Sabadin L. Effects of acute systemic hyperinsulinemia on forearm muscle proteolysis in healthy man. *J Clin Invest* 1991; 88(1):27-33.
255. Volpi E, Lucidi P, Cruciani G, et al. Contribution of amino acids and insulin to protein anabolism during meal absorption. *Diabetes* 1996; 45(9):1245-52.

256. Tischler ME, Desautels M, Goldberg AL. Does leucine, leucyl-tRNA, or some metabolite of leucine regulate protein synthesis and degradation in skeletal and cardiac muscle? *J Biol Chem* 1982; 257:1613-1621.
257. Jefferson LS. Role of insulin in the regulation of protein synthesis. *Diabetes* 1980; 29:487-496.
258. Nair KS, Ford GC, Ekberg K, et al. Protein dynamics in whole body and in splanchnic and leg tissues in type I diabetic patients. *J Clin Invest* 1995; 95:2926-2937.
259. Biolo G, Declan Fleming RY, Wolfe RR. Physiologic hyperinsulinemia stimulates protein synthesis and enhances transport of selected amino acids in human skeletal muscle. *J Clin Invest* 1995; 95:811-819.
260. Haussinger D, Lang F. Cell volume in the regulation of hepatic function: a mechanism for metabolic control. *Biochem Biophys Acta* 1991; 1071:331-350.
261. Watt PW, Corbett ME, Rennie MJ. Stimulation of protein synthesis in pig skeletal muscle by infusion of amino acids during constant insulin availability. *Am J Physiol* 1992; 263(3 Pt 1):E453-60.
262. Newman E, Heslin MJ, Wolf RF, Pisters PW, Brennan MF. The effect of systemic hyperinsulinemia with concomitant amino acid infusion on skeletal muscle protein turnover in the human forearm. *Metab Clin Exp* 1994; 43(1):70-8.
263. Wolf Rf, Pearlstone DB, Newman E, et al. Growth hormone and insulin reverse net whole body and skeletal muscle protein catabolism in cancer patients. *Ann Surg* 1992; 216:280-290.
264. Scott CD, Baxter RC. Production of insulin-like growth factor-1 and its binding protein in rat hepatocyte cultures from diabetic and insulin-treated diabetic rats. *Endocrinology* 1986; 119: 2346-2352.
265. Johnson TR, Ilan J. Expression of IGF-1 in liver. In: LeRoith D, Raizada MK, eds. *Molecular and Cellular Biology of Insulin-like Growth Factors and Their Receptors,* Plenum Press, New York. 1989:129-139.
266. Pasquali R, Casimirri F, De Iasio R, et al. Insulin regulates testosterone and sex hormone-binding globulin concentrations in adult normal weight and obese men. *J Clin Endocrinol Metab* 1995; 80:654-658.
267. Monder C, Hardy MP, Blanchard RJ, Blanchard DC. Comparative aspects of 11 beta-hydroxysteroid dehydrogenase. Testicular 11 beta-hydroxysteroid dehydrogenase: development of a model for the mediation of Leydig cell function by corticosteroids. *Steroids* 1994; 59(2):69-73.
268. Petrides AS, Luzi L, Reuben A, Riely C, DeFronzo RA. Effect of insulin and plasma amino acid concentration on leucine metabolism in cirrhosis. *Hepatology* 1991; 14(3):432-41.
269. Wolf RF, Heslin MJ, Newman E, Pearlstone DB, Gonenne A, Brennan MF. Growth hormone and insulin combine to improve whole-body and skeletal muscle protein kinetics. *Surgery* 1992; 112(2):284-92.
270. Fryburg DA, Louard RJ, Gerow KE, et al. Growth hormone stimulates skeletal muscle protein synthesis and antagonizes insulin's antiproteolytic action in humans. *Diabetes* 1992; 41:424-429.
271. Louard RJ, Bhushan R, Gelfand RA, et al. Glucocorticoids antagonize insulin's antiproteolytic action on skeletal muscle in humans. *J Clin Endocrinol* 1994; 79:278-284.
272. Tomas FM. Interactive effects of insulin and corticosterone on myofibrillar protein turnover in rats as determined by N-methylhistidine excretion. *Biochem J* 1984; 220:469-479.
273. Ohtsuka A, Hayashi K, Noda T, Tomita Y. Reduction of corticosterone-induced muscle proteolysis and growth retardation by a combined treatment with insulin, testosterone and high-protein-high-fat diet in rats. *J Nutr Sci Vitam* 1992; 38(1):83-92.
274. Rennie MJ, Tadros L, Khogali S, Ahmed A, Taylor PM. Glutamine transport and its metabolic effects. *J Nutr* 1994; 124(8 Suppl):1503S-1508S.
275. Wolf RF, Heslin MJ, Newman E, Pearlstone DB, Gonenne A, Brennan MF. Growth hormone and insulin combine to improve whole-body and skeletal muscle protein kinetics. *Surgery* 1992; 112(2):284-91; discussion 291-2.
276. Wolf RF, Pearlstone DB, Newman E, et al. Growth hormone and insulin reverse net whole body and skeletal muscle protein catabolism in cancer patients. *Ann Surg* 1992; 216(3):280-8; discussion 288-90.
277. Umpleby AM, Shojaee-Moradie F, Thomason MJ, et al. Effects of insulin-like growth factor-1 (IGF-1), insulin, and combined IGF-1-insulin infusions on protein metabolism in dogs, *Eur J Clin Invest* 1994; 24:337-344.
278. Wolf RF, Heslin MJ, Newman E, et al. Growth hormone and insulin combine to improve whole-body and skeletal muscle protein kinetics. *Surgery* 1992; 112:284-292.
279. Russell-Jones DL, Bates AT, Umpleby AM, et al. A comparison of the effects of IGF-1 and Insulin on glucose metabolism, fat metabolism, and the cardiovascular system in normal human volunteers. *Eur J Clin Invest* 1995; 25:403-411.
280. Rosa LF, Safi DA, Curi R. Effect of hypo- and hyperthyroidism on the function and metabolism of macrophages in rats. *Cell Biochem Funct* 1995; 13(2):141-7.
281. Cryer PE. Glucose counterregulation in man. *Diabetes* 1981; 30:261.
282. Gordon GG, Lieber CS. Alcoholic men: Effects of abuse on the endocrine system. *Med Aspects Hum Sex* 1986; 20(2):72-82.
283. Di Paolo T, Rouillard C, Morissette M, et al. Endocrine and neurochemical actions of cocaine. *Can J Physiol Pharmacol* 1989; 67(9):1177-81.

284. Thomas MR, Miell JP, Taylor AM, et al. Endocrine and cardiac paracrine actions of insulin-like growth factor-1 (IGF-1) during thyroid dysfunction in the rat: is IGF-1 implicated in the mechanism of heart weight/body weight change during abnormal thyroid function? *J Mol Endocrinol* 1993; 10(3):313-23.
285. Ruff RL, Weissmann J. Endocrine myopathies. [Review] *Neurol Cli* 1988; 6(3):575-92.
286. Crantz FR, Larsen PR. Rapid thyroxine to 3,5,3′-triiodothyronine conversion and nuclear 3,5,3′-triiodothyronine binding in rat cerebral cortex and cerebellum. *J Clin Invest* 1980; 65:935-941.
287. Eisenstein Z, Hagg S, Vagenakis AG, et al. Effect of starvation on the production and peripheral metabolism of 3,3′,5′-triiodothyronine in euthyroid obese subjects. *J Clin Endocrinol Metab* 1978; 47(4):889-93.
288. Balsam A, Ingbar SH. Observations on the factors that control the generation of triiodothyronine from thyroxine in rat liver and the nature of the defect induced by fasting. *J Clin Invest* 1979; 63(6):1145-56.
289. Chopra IJ. An assessment of daily production and significance of thyroidal secretion of 3,3′,5′-triiodothyronine (reverse T3) in man. *J Clin Invest* 1976; 58(1):32-40.
290. Koppeschaar HP, Meinders AE, Schwarz F. Metabolic responses in grossly obese subjects treated with a very-low-calorie diet with and without triiodothyronine treatment. *Int J Obesity* 1983; 7(2):133-41.
291. Danforth E Jr, Horton ES, O'Connell M, et al. Dietary-induced alterations in thyroid hormone metabolism during overnutrition. *J Clin Invest* 1979; 64(5):1336-47.
292. Becker RA, Wilmore DW, Goodwin CW, et al. Free T4, Free T3 and reverse T3 in critically ill, thermally injured patients. *J Trauma* 1980; 20:713-721.
293. Zumoff B. The low t3, low t4 syndrome of nonthyroidal illness. Adaptive temporary hypothyroidism. *Mt Sinai J Med* 1984; 51:604-609.
294. Vagerakis AG, Buiger A, Portray GI, et al. Diversion of peripheral thyroxin metabolism from activating to inactivating pathway during complete fasting. *J Clin Endocrinol Metab* 1975; 41:191-194.
295. Spaulding SW, Chopra IJ, Sherwin RS, Lyall SS. Effect of caloric restriction and dietary composition on serum T3 and reverse T3 in man. *J Clin Endocrinol Metab* 1976; 42:197-200.
296. Gardner DF, Kaplan MM, Stanley CA, Utiger RD. Effect of tri-iodothyronine replacement on the metabolic and pituitary responses to starvation. *N Engl J Med* 1979; 300(11):579-584.
297. Chopra IJ, Smith SR. Circulating thyroid hormones and thyrotropin in adult patients with protein-calorie malnutrition. *J Clin Endocrinol Metab* 1975; 40:221-227.
298. Nomura S, Pittman CS, Chambers JB Jr. Reduced peripheral conversion of thyroxine to triiodothyronine in patients with hepatic cirrhosis. *J Clin Invest* 1975; 56:6113-6152.
299. Burr WA, Black EG, Griffiths RS, Hoffenberg R, Meinhold H, Wenzel KW. Serum triiodothyronine and reverse triiodothyronine concentrations after surgical operation. *Lancet* 1975; 2:1277-1279.
300. Degrout LJ, Hoye K. Dexamethasone suppression of serum T3 and T4. *J Clin Endocrinol Metab* 1976; 42:976-978.
301. Vaughan GM, Becker RA, Unger RH, et al. Nonthyroidal control of metabolism after burn injury. Possible role of glucagon metabolism. *Metabolism* 1985; 34:637-641.
302. Zaloga GP, Chernow B, Smallridge RC, et al. A longitudinal evaluation of thyroid function in critically ill surgical patients. *Ann Surg* 1985; 201:456-464.
303. Schimmel M, Utiger RD. Thyroidal and peripheral production of thyroid hormones, review of recent findings and their clinical implications. *Ann Intern Med* 1977; 87(6):760-768.
304. Balsam A, Ingbar SH. The influence of fasting, diabetes, and several pharmacological agents on the pathways of thyroxine metabolism in rat liver. *J Clin Invest* 1978; 62(2):415-424.
305. Gardner DF, Kaplan MM, Stanley CA, Utiger RD. Effect of tri-iodothyronine replacement on the metabolic and pituitary responses to starvation. *N Engl J Med* 1979; 300(11):579-584.
306. Schimmel M, Utiger RD. Thyroidal and peripheral production of thyroid hormones, review of recent findings and their clinical implications. *Ann Intern Med* 1977; 87(6):760-768.
307. Balsam A, Ingbar SH. The influence of fasting, diabetes, and several pharmacological agents on the pathways of thyroxine metabolism in rat liver. *J Clin Invest* 1978; 62(2):415-424.
308. Van Gaal LF, De Leeuw IH. Reverse T3 changes during protein supplemented diets. Relation to nutrient combustion rates. *J Endocrinol Invest* 1989; 12(11):799-803.
309. Klingenspor M, Ivemeyer M, Wiesinger H, et al. Biogenesis of thermogenic mitochondria in brown adipose tissue of Djungarian hamsters during cold adaptation. *Biochem J* 1996; 316 (Pt 2):607-13.
310. Danforth E Jr, Horton ES, O'Connell M, et al. Dietary-induced alterations in thyroid hormone metabolism during overnutrition. *J Clin Invest* 1979; 64(5):1336-47.
311. Beckett GJ, Kellett HA, Gow SM, Hussey AJ, Toft AD, et al. Raised plasma glutathione S-transferase values in hyperthyroidism and in hypothyroid patients receiving thyroxine replacement: evidence for hepatic damage. *Br Med J* 1985; 291:427-431.
312. Hasselgren PO, Adlerberth A, Angeras U, Stenstrom G. Protein metabolism in skeletal muscle tissue from hyperthyroid patients after preoperative treatment with antithyroid drug or selective beta-blocking agent. Results from a prospective, randomized study. *J Clin Endocrinol Metab* 1984; 59(5):835-9.

313. Leighton B, Dimitriadis GD, Parry-Billings M, Bond J, Kemp P, Newsholme EA. Thyroid hormone analogue SKF L-94901: effects on amino acid and carbohydrate metabolism in rat skeletal muscle in vitro. *Biochem Pharmacol* 1990; 40(5):1161-4.
314. Muller MJ, Seitz HJ. Thyroid hormone action on intermediary metabolism. Part III. Protein metabolism in hyper- and hypothyroidism. *Klin Wochenschr* 1984; 62(3):97-102.
315. Tauveron I, Charrier S, Champredon C, et al. Response of leucine metabolism to hyperinsulinemia under amino acid replacement in experimental hyperthyroidism. *Am J Physiol* 1995; 269(3 Pt 1):E499-507.
316. Katzeff HL. Ojamaa KM. Klein I. Effects of exercise on protein synthesis and myosin heavy chain gene expression in hypothyroid rats. *Am J Physiol* 1994; 267(1 Pt 1):E63-7.
317. Sonka J, Limanova Z, Neffeova I. Hormonal, metabolic and cardiovascular response to the duration of a combined slimming regimen. *Czech Med* 1991; 14(3):156-63.
318. Pacy PJ, Price GM, Halliday D, et al. Nitrogen homeostasis in man: the diurnal responses of protein synthesis and degradation and amino acid oxidation to diets with increasing protein intakes, *Clin Sci* 1994; 86:103-118.
319. Millward DJ, Bates PC, Brown JG, et al. Role of thyroid, insulin and corticosteroid hormones in the physiological regulation of proteolysis in muscle. *Prog Clin Biol Res* 1985; 180:531-42.
320. Taillandier D, Bigard X, Desplanches D, Attaix D, Guezennec CY, Arnal M. Role of protein intake on protein synthesis and fiber distribution in the unweighted soleus muscle. *J Appl Physiol* 1993; 75(3):1226-32.
321. Pakarinen A, Hakkinen K, Alen M. Serum thyroid hormones, thyrotropin and thyroxine binding globulin in elite athletes during very intense strength training of one week. *J Sports Med Phys Fitness* 1991; 31(2):142-6.
322. Loucks AB, Callister R. Induction and prevention of low-T3 syndrome in exercising women. *Am J Physiol* 1993; 264(5 Pt 2):R924-30.
322a. Kreider RB, Phosphate loading and exercise performance. *J Appl Nutr* 1992; 44(1):29-49.
323. Moav B, McKeown BA. Thyroid hormone increases transcription of growth hormone mRNA in rainbow trout pituitary. *Horm Metabc Res* 1992; 24(1):10-4.
324. Jana NR, Bhattacharya S. Binding of thyroid hormone to the goat testicular Leydig cell induces the generation of a proteinaceous factor which stimulates androgen release. *J Endocrinol* 1994; 143(3):549-56.
325. Bachrach LK, Eggo MC, Hintz RL, Burrow GN. Insulin-like growth factors in sheep thyroid cells: action, receptors and production. *Biochem Biophys Res Commun* 1988; 154(3):861-7.
326. Vigneron P, Dainat J, Bacou F. Properties of skeletal muscle fibers. II. Hormonal influences. *Reprod Nutr Dev* 198929(1):27-53.
327. Schmidely P. [Quantitative bibliographic review on the use of anabolic hormones with steroidogenic action in ruminants for meat production. II. Principal mode of action]. *Reprod Nutr Dev* 1993; 33(4):297-323.
328. Alen M, Rahkila P, Reinilae M, Vihko R. Androgenic anabolic steroid effects on serum thyroid, pituitary and steroid hormones in athletes. *Am J Sports Med* 1987; 15(4):357-361.
329. Deyssig R, Weissel M. Ingestion of androgenic-anabolic steroids induces mild thyroidal impairment in male body builders. *J Clin Endocrinol Metab* 1993; 76(4):1069-1071.
330. Wolthers T, Grofte T, Moller N, Vilstrup H, Jorgensen JO. Effects of long-term growth hormone (GH) and triiodothyronine (T3) administration on functional hepatic nitrogen clearance in normal man. *J Hepatol* 1996; 24(3):313-9.
331. Binnerts A, Swart GR, Wilson JH, et al. The effect of growth hormone administration in growth hormone deficient adults on bone, protein, carbohydrate and lipid homeostasis, as well as on body composition. *Clin Endocrinol* 1992; 37(1):79-87.
332. Prager D, Weber MM, Gebremedhin S, Melmed S. Interaction between insulin and thyroid hormone in rat pituitary tumour cells: insulin attenuates tri-iodothyronine-induced growth hormone mRNA levels. *J Endocrinol* 1993; 137(1):107-14.
333. Sacchi E. A case of infantile gigantism (pedomacrosomia) with a tumor of the testicle. *Riv Sper Freniatr* 1895; 21:149-161.
334. Rowlands RP, Nicholson GW. Growth of left testicle with precocious sexual and bodily development (macrogenitosomia). *Guy's Hosp Rep* 1929; 79:401-408.
335. Kenyon AT. The effect of testosterone propionate on the genitalia, prostrate, secondary sex characters, and body weight in eunuchoidism. *Endocrinology* 1938; 23:121-134.
336. Kenyon AT. The first Josiah Macy Jr. Conference on bone and wound healing, September 1942.
337. Kenyon AT, Knowlton K, Lotwin G, Sandford I. Metabolic response of aged men to testosterone propionate. *J Clin Endocrinol* 1942; 2:690-695.
338. Kenyon AT, Knowlton K, Sandford I. The anabolic effects of the androgens and somatic growth in man. *Ann Intern Med* 1944; 20:632-654.
339. Cartensen H, Terner N, Thoren L, Wide L. Testosterone, luteinizing hormone, and growth hormone in blood following surgical trauma. *Acta Chir Scand* 1972; 138:1-7.
340. Hamanaka Y, Kurachi K, Aono T, Mizutani S, Matsumoto K. Effects of general anesthesia and severity of surgical stress on serum LH and testosterone in males. *Acta Endocrinol* 1975; 78:258-265.
341. Wang C, Chan V, Tse TF, Yeung TT. Effect of acute myocardial infarction on pituitary-testicular function. *Clin Endocrinol* 1978; 9:249-253.

342. Woolfe PD, Hamill RW, McDonald JV, Lee LA, Kelly M. Transient hypogonadotropic hypogonadism caused by critical illness. *J Clin Endocrinol Metab* 1985; 66:444-450.
343. Gebhart SSP, Waltt NB, Clark RV, Umplerrez G, Sgoutas D. Reversible impairment of gonadotropin secretion in critical illness. *Arch Intern Med* 1989; 149:1637-1641.
344. Fahey TD, Rolph R, Moungmee P, et al. Serum testosterone, body composition, and strength of young adults. *Med Sci Sports* 1976; 8:31-34.
345. Weiss LW, Cureton KJ, Thompson FN. Comparison of serum testosterone and androstenedione responses to weight lifting in men and women. *Eur J Appl Physiol* 1983; 50:412-419.
346. Kraemer RR, Kilgore JL, Kraemer GR, Castracane VD. Growth hormone, IGF-1, and testosterone responses to resistive exercise. *Med Sci Sports Exerc* 1992; 24(12):1346-52.
347. Kraemer W, Marchitelli L, Gordon S, and Fleck S. Hormonal and growth factor responses to heavy resistance exercise protocols. *J Appl Physiol* 1990; 69(4):1442-1450.
348. Kraemer WJ, Gordon SE, Fleck SJ, et al. Endogenous anabolic hormonal and growth factor responses to heavy resistance exercise in males and females. *Int J Sports Med* 1991; 12:228-235.
349. Snegovskaya V, Viru A. Steroid and pituitary hormone responses to rowing: relative significance of exercise intensity and duration and performance level. *Eur J Appl Physiol Occup Physiol* 1993; 67(1):59-65.
350. Hakkinen K, Pakarinen A, Alen M, et al. Daily hormonal and neuromuscular response to intensive strength training in 1 week. *Int J Sports Med* 1985; 9:422-428.
351. Hakkinen K, Pakarinen A, Alen M, et al. Neuromuscular and hormonal responses in elite athletes to two successive strength training sessions. *Eur J Appl Physiol* 1988; 57:133-139.
352. Kraemer WJ. Endocrine response to resistance exercise. *Med Sci Sports Exerc* 1988; 20: S152-S157.
353. Hakkinen K, Pakarinen A, Kallinen M. Neuromuscular adaptations and serum hormones in women during short-term intensive strength training. *Eur J Appl Physiol* 1992; 64: 106-111.
354. Griggs RC, Kingston W, Jozefowicz RF, Herr BE, Forbes G, Halliday D. Effect of testosterone on muscle mass and muscle protein synthesis. *J Appl Physiol* 1989; 66(1):498-503.
355. Bhasin S, Storer TW, Berman N, et al. The effect of supraphysiologic doses of testosterone on muscle size and strength in normal men. *N Engl J Med* 1996; 335(1):1-7.
356. Dessypris A. Hormonal responses in long-term physical exercise. *Psychiatr Fennica* 1986; Suppl:45-53.
357. Kindermann W, Schnabel A, Schmitt WM, et al. Catecholamines, growth hormone, cortisol, insulin, and sex hormones in anaerobic and aerobic exercise. *Eur J Appl Physiol Occup Physiol* 1982; 49(3):389-399.
358. Pestell RG, Hurley DM, Vandongen R. Biochemical and hormonal changes during a 1000 km ultramarathon. *Clin Exp Pharmacol Physiol* 1989; 16(5):353-61.
359. Falkel JE, Hagerman FC, Hikida RS. Skeletal muscle adaptations during early phase of heavy-resistance training in men and women. *J Appl Physiol* 1994; 76(3):1247-55.
360. Opstad PK. Circadian rhythm of hormones is extinguished during prolonged physical stress, sleep and energy deficiency in young men. *Eur J Endocrinol* 1994; 131(1):56-66.
361. Bonifazi M, Lupo C. Differential effects of exercise on sex hormone-binding globulin and non-sex hormone-binding globulin-bound testosterone. *Eur J Appl Physiol* 1996; 72:423-429.
362. Erfurth EM, Hagmar LE, Saaf M, Hall K. Serum levels of insulin-like growth factor-1 and insulin-like growth factor-binding protein 1 correlate with serum free testosterone and sex hormone binding globulin levels in healthy young and middle-aged men. *Clin Endocrinol* 1996; 44(6):659-64.
363. Guezennec CY, Ferre P, Serrurier B, Merino D, Aymonod M, Pesquies PC. Metabolic effects of testosterone during prolonged physical exercise and fasting. *Eur J Appl Physiol Occup Physiol* 1984; 52(3):300-4.
364. Donahue LR, Watson G, Beamer WG. Regulation of metabolic water and protein compartments by insulin-like growth factor-1 and testosterone in growth hormone-deficient lit/lit mice, *J Endocrinol* 1993; 139(3):431-439.
365. Alen M, Rahkila P, Reinilae M, Vihko R. Androgenic-anabolic steroid effects on serum thyroid, pituitary and steroid hormones in athletes. *Am J Sports Med* 1987; 15(4):357-361.
366. Weissberger AJ, Ho KK. Activation of the somatotropic axis by testosterone in adult males: evidence for the role of aromatization. *J Clin Endocrinol Metab* 1993; 76(6):1407-12.
367. Lima L, Arce V, Lois N, et al. Growth hormone (GH) responsiveness to GHRH in normal adults is not affected by short-term gonadal blockade. *Acta Endocrinol* 1989; 120(1):31-6.
368. Hobbs CJ, Plymate SR, Rosen CJ, Adler RA. Testosterone administration increases insulin-like growth factor-1 levels in normal men. *J Clin Endocrinol Metab* 1993; 77(3):776-9.
369. Warner BW, Hasselgren PO, Hummel RP, et al. Effect of catabolic hormone infusion on protein turnover and amino acid uptake in skeletal muscle. *Am J Surgery* 1990; 159(3):295-300.
370. Strack AM, Sebastian RJ, Schwartz MW, Dallman MF. Glucocorticoids and insulin: reciprocal signals for energy balance. *Am J Physiol* 1995; 268(1 Pt 2):R142-9.
371. Dallman MF, Strack AM, Akana SF, et al. Feast and famine: critical role of glucocorticoids with insulin in daily energy flow. *Front Neuroendocrinol* 1993; 14(4):303-47.
372. Bessey PQ, Lowe KA. Early hormonal changes affect the catabolic response to trauma. *Ann Surg* 1993; 218(4):476-89; discussion 489-91.

373. Gelfand RA, Matthews DE, Bier DM, Sherwin KS. Role of counterregulatory hormones in the catabolic response to stress. *J Clin Invest* 1984; 74:2238-2248.
374. Bessey PQ, Watters JM, Aoki TT, Wilmore DW. Combined hormonal infusion stimulates the metabolic response to injury. *Ann Surg* 1984; 200:264-280.
375. Shamoon H, Hendler R, Sherwin RS. Synergistic interactions among anti-insulin hormones in the pathogenesis of stress hyperglycemia in humans. *J Clin Endocrinol Metab* 1981; 52:1235-1241.
376. Darmaun D, Matthews DE, Bier DM. Physiological hypercortisolemia increases proteolysis, glutamine, and alanine production. *Am J Physiol* 1988; 255(3 Pt 1):E366-73.
377. Warner BW, Hasselgren PO, Hummel RP, et al. Effect of catabolic hormone infusion on protein turnover and amino acid uptake in skeletal muscle. *Am J Surg* 1990; 159(3):295-300.
378. Gore DC, Jahoor F, Wolfe RR, Herndon DN. Acute response of human muscle protein to catabolic hormones. *Ann Surg* 1993; 218(5):679-84.
379. Gelfand RA, Matthews DE, Bier DM, Sherwin KS. Role of counterregulatory hormones in the catabolic response to stress. *J Clin Invest* 1984; 74:2238-2248.
380. Pomposelli JJ, Flores EA, Bistrian RR. Role of biochemical mediators in clinical nutrition and surgical metabolism. *JPEN* 1988; 12:212-218.
381. Xi T, Shi X, Guo D, Dong X, Xu X, Zhu D. Biological activities of human tumor necrosis factor-alpha and its novel mutants. *Biochem Mol Biol Int* 1996; 38(4):855-62.
382. Woolf PD, Hamill RW, Lee LA, McDonald JV. Free and total catecholamines in critical illness. *Am J Physiol* 1988; 254:E287-E291.
383. Davies CL, Malyneuf SG, Newman RJ. HPLC determination of plasma catecholamines in road accident casualties. *Br J Clin Pharmacol* 1981; 13:P283.
384. Frayn KN, Little RA, Maycock PF, Stoner HB. The relationship of plasma catecholamines to acute metabolic and hormonal responses to injury in man. *Circ Shock* 1985; 16:229-240.
385. Benedict CR, Grahame-Smith DG. Plasma noradrenaline and adrenaline concentrations and dopamine beta hydroxylase activity in patients with shock due to septicemia, trauma, and hemorrhage. *J Med* 1978; 185:1-20.
386. Jaattela A, Alho A, Avikainen V, Karaharju E, Kataja V, Lahdensuu M, Lepisto P, Rokkanen P, Terio T. Plasma catecholamines in severely injured patients. A prospective study on 45 patients with multiple injuries. *Br J Surg* 1975; 62:177-181.
387. Davies CL, Newman RJ, Molyneux SG, Grahame-Smith DG. The relationship between plasma catecholamines and severity of injury in man. *J Trauma* 1984; 24:99-105.
388. Nistrup-Madsen S, Fog-Moller F, Christiansen C, Verster-Anderson T, Engquist A. Cyclic AMP, adrenaline, and non-adrenaline in plasma during surgery. *Br J Surg* 1978; 65:191-193.
389. Esler M. Assessment of sympathetic nervous function in humans from norepinephrine plasma kinetics. *Clin Sci* 1982; 62:247-254.
390. Waldhaus WK, Gasic S, Bratusch-Marrain P, Komjati M, Korn A. Effect of stress hormones on splanchnic substrate and insulin disposal after glucose ingestion in healthy humans. *Diabetes* 1987; 36:127-135.
391. Deibert DC, DeFronzo RA. Epinephrine-induced insulin resistance in man. *J Clin Invest* 1980; 65:717-721.
392. Hendler RG, Sherwin RS. Epinephrine-stimulated glucose production is not diminished by starvation. Evidence for an effect on gluconeogenesis. *J Clin Endocrinol Metab* 1984; 58:1014-1021.
393. Sigal RJ, Fisher S, Halter JB, Vranic M, Marliss EB. The roles of catecholamines in glucoregulation in intense exercise as defined by the islet cell clamp technique. *Diabetes* 1996; 45(2):148-56.
394. Galbo H, Holst JJ, Christensen NJ. Glucagon and plasma catecholamine responses to graded and prolonged exercise in man. *J Appl Physiol* 1975; 38:70-76.
395. Frayn KN, Little RA, Maycock PF, HB Stoner. The relationship of plasma catecholamines to acute metabolic and hormonal responses to injury in man. *Circ Shock* 1985; 16:229-240.
396. Rizza RA, Cryer PE, Haymond MW, Gerich JE. Adrenergic mechanism for the effects of epinephrine on glucose production and clearance in man. *J Clin Invest* 1980; 65:682-689.
397. Clutter W, Bier D, Shah S, Cryer P. Epinephrine plasma metabolic clearance rates and physiologic threshold for metabolic and hemodynamic actions in man. *J Clin Invest* 1980; 66:94-101.
398. Schade DS, Eaton RP. The regulation of plasma ketone body concentration by counterregulatory hormones in man. III. Effects of norepinephrine in normal man. *Diabetes* 1979; 28:5-10.
399. Keller U, Oberhaensli RD, Stauffacher W. Adrenergic regulation of ketone body kinetics and lipolysis. In *Substrate and Energy Metabolism* 1985. Garrow JS, Halliday D; editors. John Libbey & Co. Ltd., London. 37-45.
400. Shaw JHF, Hodaway CM, Humberstone DA. Metabolic intervention in surgical patients: The effects of alpha- and beta-blockade on glucose and protein metabolism in surgical patients receiving total parenteral nutrition. *Surgery* 1988; 03:52-55.
401. Miles JM, Nissen SL, Gerich JE, Haymond MW. Effects of epinephrine infusion on leucine and alanine kinetics in humans. *Am J Physiol* 1984; 247:E166-E172.
402. Shamoon HR, Jacob R, Sherwin RS. Epinephrine-induced hypoaminoacidemia in normal and diabetic subjects: Effect of beta blockade. *Diabetes* 1980; 29:875-881.

403. Shamoon HR, Jacob R, Sherwin RS. Epinephrine-induced hypoaminoacidemia in normal and diabetic human subjects. *Diabetes* 1980; 29:875-881.
404. Miles JM, Nissen SL, Gerich JE, Haymond MW. Effects of epinephrine infusion on leucine and alanine kinetics in humans. *Am J Physiol* 1984; 247:E166-E172.
405. Garber AJ, Karl IE, Kipnis KM. Alanine and glutamine synthesis and release from skeletal muscle. IV. Beta-adrenergic inhibition of amino-acid release. *J Biol Chem* 1976; 251:851-857.
406. Li JB, Jefferson LS. Effect of isoproterenol on amino-acid levels and protein turnover in skeletal muscle. *Am J Physiol* 1977; 234:E243-E249.
407. Tischler ME. Minireview: hormonal regulation of protein degradation in skeletal and cardiac muscle. *Life Sci* 1981; 28:2569-2576.
408. Kraenzlin M, Keller E, Keller U, et al. Elevation of plasma epinephrine concentrations inhibits proteolysis and leucine oxidation in man via beta-adrenergic mechanisms. *J Clin Invest* 1989; 84(2):388-393.
409. Baltzan MA, Andres R, Cader G, Zierler KL. Effects of epinephrine on forearm blood flow and metabolism in man. *J Clin Invest* 1965; 44:80-92.
410. Hjemdahl P, Linde B. Influence of circulating norepinephrine and epinephrine on adipose tissue vascular resistance and lipolysis in humans. *Am J Physiol* 1983; 245:H447-H452.
411. Tessari P, Nissen SL, Miles JM, Haymond MW. Inverse relationship of leucine flux and oxidation to free fatty acid availability in vivo. *J Clin Invest* 1986; 77:575-581.
412. Weiss M, Keller U, Stauffacher W. Effect of epinephrine and somatostatin-induced insulin deficiency on ketone body kinetics and lipolysis in man. *Diabetes* 1984; 33:738-744.
413. Tessari P, Inchiostro S, Biolo G, et al. Differential effects on hyperinsulinemia and hyperaminoacidemia in leucine-carbon metabolism in vivo. Evidence for distinct mechanisms in regulation of net amino acid deposition. *J Clin Invest* 1987; 79:1062-1069.
414. Buse MG, Biggers JF, Drier C, Buse JF. The effect of epinephrine, glucagon, and the nutritional state on the oxidation of branched chain amino acids and pyruvate by isolated hearts and diaphragms of the rat. *J Biol Chem* 1973; 248:697-706.
415. Kadowaki M, Kamata T, Noguchi T. Acute effect of epinephrine on muscle proteolysis in perfused rat hindquarters. *J Appl Physiol* 1996; 270(6Pt.1):E961-E967.
416. Foster DF. From glycogen to ketones and back. *Diabetes* 1984; 33:1188-1199.
417. Pacy PJ, Cheng KN, Ford GC, Halliday D. Influence of glucagon on protein and leucine metabolism: a study in fasting man with induced insulin resistance [see comments]. *Br J Surg* 1990; 77(7):791-4.
418. Tessari P, Inchiostro S, Barazzoni R, et al. Hyperglucagonemia stimulates phenylalanine oxidation in humans. *Diabetes* 1996; 45(4):463-70.
419. Charlton MR, Adey DB, Nair KS. Evidence for a catabolic role of glucagon during an amino acid load. *J Clin Invest* 1996; 98(1):90-9.
420. Lyengar R, Schwartz TL, Brinbaumer L. Coupling of glucagon receptors to adenylcyclase. *J Biol Chem* 1979; 254:1119-1123.
421. Farah AE. Glucagon and the circulation. *Pharmacol Rev* 1983; 35:181-217.
422. Wise JK, Hendler R, Felig P. Influence of glucocorticoids on glucagon secretion and plasma amino acid concentrations in man. *J Clin Invest* 1973; 52:2774-2782.
423. Unger RH, Orce L. Glucagon and the A cell. *N Engl J Med* 1981; 304:4518-4575.
424. Russell RCG, Walker CJ, Bloom SR. Hyperglucagonemia in the surgical patient. *Br Med J* 1975; 1:10-12.
425. Shamoon H, Hendler R, Sherwin RS. Synergistic interactions among anti-insulin hormones in the pathogenesis of stress hyperglycemia in humans. *J Clin Endocrinol Metab* 1981; 52:1235-1241.
426. Peret J, Foustock S, Chanez M, Bois-Joyeux B, Assan R. Plasma glucagon and insulin concentrations and hepatic phosphoenolpyruvate carboxykinase and pyruvate kinase activities during and upon adaptation of rats to a high-protein diet. *J Nutr* 1981; 111(7):1173-84.
427. Russell RCG, Walker CJ, Bloom SR. Hyperglucagonemia in the surgical patient. *Br Med J* 1975; 1:10-12.
428. Engquist A, Fog-Moller F, Christiansen C, Thode J, Anderson T, Nistrup-Madsen S. Influence of epidural analgesia on the catecholamine and cyclic AMP response to surgery. *Acta Anaesthesiol Scand* 1980; 24:17-21.
429. Sanchez A, Hubbard RW. Plasma amino acids and the insulin/glucagon ratio as an explanation for the dietary protein modulation of atherosclerosis. *Med Hypotheses* 1991; 35(4):324-9.
430. Sanchez A, Hubbard RW, Smit E, Hilton GF. Testing a mechanism of control in human cholesterol metabolism: relation of arginine and glycine to insulin and glucagon. *Atherosclerosis* 1988; 71(1):87-92.
431. Kuhara T, Ikeda S, Ohneda A, Sasaki Y. Effects of intravenous infusion of 17 amino acids on the secretion of GH, glucagon, and insulin in sheep. *Am J Physiol* 1991; 260(1 Pt 1):E21-6.
432. Albisser AM, Cheng DC, Yamasaki Y, Marliss EB, Zinman B. Changes in blood amino acids account for the insulin and glucagon responses to mixed meals in dogs. *Diabetes Res Clin Exp* 1985; 2(1):49-55.
433. Ganong WF. The stress response: A dynamic overview. *Hosp Pract* 1988; 23:155-171.
434. Simmons PS, Miles JM, Gerich JE, Haymond MW: Increased proteolysis. An effect of increases in plasma cortisol within the physiologic range. *J Clin Invest* 1984; 73:412-420.

435. Brown AD, Wallace P, Breachtel G. In vivo regulation of non-insulin mediated and insulin mediated glucose uptake by cortisol. *Diabetes* 1987; 36:1230-1237.
436. Rizza RA, Mandarino LJ, Gerich JE. Cortisol-induced insulin resistance in man. Impaired suppression of glucose production and stimulation of glucose utilization due to a post receptor defect of insulin action. *J Clin Endocrinol Metab* 1982; 54:131-138.
437. Raff H, Flemma RJ, Findling JW, Nelson DK. Fast cortisol-induced inhibition of the adrenocorticotropin response to surgery in humans. *J Clin Endocrinol Metab* 1988; 67:1146-1148.
438. Axelrod J, Reisine TD. Stress hormones. Their interaction and regulation. *Science* 1984; 224:452-459.
439. Lendingham IM, Watt I. Influence of sedation on mortality in critically ill multiple trauma patient. *Lancet* 1983; 1:1270.
440. Moore RA, Allen MC, Wood PJ, Rees LH, Sear JW. Perioperative endocrine effects of etomidate. *Anaesthesia* 1985; 40:124-130.
441. Wagner RL, White PF, Kan PB, Rosenthal MH, Feldman D. Inhibition of adrenal steroidogenesis by the anesthetic etomidate. *N Engl J Med* 1984; 310:1415-1421.
442. Brillon DJ, Zheng B, Campbell RG, Matthews DE. Effect of cortisol on energy expenditure and amino acid metabolism in humans. *Am J Physiol* 1995; 268(3 Pt 1):E501-13.
443. Ottosson M, Vikman-Adolfsson K, Enerback S, Olivecrona G, Bjorntorp P. The effects of cortisol on the regulation of lipoprotein lipase activity in human adipose tissue. *J Clin Endocrinol Metab* 1994; 79:820-825.
444. Hickson RC, Kurowski TT, Andrews GH, et al. Glucocorticoid cytosol binding in exercise-induced sparing of muscle atrophy. *J Appl Physiol* 1986; 60:1413-1419.
445. Hickson RC, Czerwinski SM. Falduto MT. Young AP. Glucocorticoid antagonism by exercise and androgenic-anabolic steroids. *Med Sci Sports Exerc* 1990; 22:331-340.
446. Horber FF, Haymond MW. Human growth hormone prevents the protein catabolic side effects of prednisone in humans. *J Clin Invest* 1990; 86:265-272.
447. Dinan TG, Thakore J. O'Keane V. Lowering cortisol enhances growth hormone response to growth hormone releasing hormone in healthy subjects. *Acta Physiol Scand* 1994; 151: 413-416.
448. Mauras N, Beaufrere B. Recombinant human insulin-like growth factor-1 enhances whole body protein anabolism and significantly diminishes the protein catabolic effects of prednisone in humans without a diabetogenic effect. *J Clin Endocrinol Metab* 1995; 80(3):869-874.
449. Swolin D, Brantsing C, Matejka G, Ohlsson C. Cortisol decreases IGF-1 mRNA levels in human osteoblast-like cells. *J Endocrinol* 1996; 149(3):397-403.
450. Hickson RC, Czerwinski SM, Wegrzyn LE. Glutamine prevents downregulation of myosin heavy chain synthesis and muscle atrophy from glucocorticoids. *Am J Physiol* 1995; 268(4 Pt 1):E730-E734.
451. Ohtsuka A, Hayashi K, Noda T, Tomita Y. Reduction of corticosterone-induced muscle proteolysis and growth retardation by a combined treatment with insulin, testosterone, and high protein, high fat diets in rats. *J Nutr Sci Vitaminol* 1992; 38:83-92.
452. Dinneen S, Alzaid A, Miles J, Rizza R. Metabolic effects of the nocturnal rise in cortisol on carbohydrate metabolism in normal humans. *J Clin Invest* 1993; 92(5):2283-90.
453. Simmons PS, Miles JM, Gerich JE et al. Increased proteolysis: an effect of increases in plasma cortisol within the physiological range. *J Clin Invest* 1984; 73:412-420.
454. Shamoon H, Soman V, Sherwin RS. The influence of acute physiological increments of cortisol on fuel metabolism and insulin binding in monocytes in normal humans. *J Clin Endocrinol Metab* 1980; 50:495-501.
455. Morrison D, Capewell S, Reynolds SP, et al. Testosterone levels during systemic and inhaled corticosteroid therapy. *Respir Med* 1994; 88(9):659-63.
456. MacAdams MR, White RH, Chipps BE. Reduction of serum testosterone levels during chronic glucocorticoid therapy. *Ann Intern Med* 1986; 104:648-651 .
457. Monder C, Hardy MP, Blanchard RJ, Blanchard DC. Comparative aspects of 11 beta-hydroxysteroid dehydrogenase. Testicular 11 beta-hydroxysteroid dehydrogenase: development of a model for the mediation of Leydig cell function by corticosteroids. *Steroids* 1994; 59(2):69-73.
458. Schaison G, Durand F, Mowszowicz I. Effect of glucocorticoids on plasma testosterone in men. *Acta Endocrinol (Copenh)* 1978; 89:126-31.
459. Deschenes MR, Kraemer WJ, Maresh CM, Crivello JF. Exercise-induced hormonal changes and their effects upon skeletal muscle tissue. *Sports Med* 1991; 12:80-93.
459a. Hoogeveen AR, Zonderland ML. Relationships between testosterone, cortisol and performance in professional cyclists. *Int J Sports Med* 1996; 17(6):423-428.
460. Forest MG. Age-related response of plasma testosterone, delta 4-androstenedione, and cortisol to adrenocorticotropin in infants, children, and adults. *J Clin Endocrinol Metab* 1978; 47(5):931-7.
461. Kemppainen RJ, Thompson FN, Lorenz MD, Munnell JF, Chakraborty PK. Effects of prednisone on thyroid and gonadal endocrine function in dogs. *J Endocrinol* 1983; 96(2):293-302.
462. Juniewicz PE, Keeney DS, Ewing LL. Effect of adrenocorticotropin and other proopiomelanocortin-derived peptides on testosterone secretion by the in vitro perfused testis. *Endocrinology* 1988; 122(3):891-8.

463. Juniewicz PE, Johnson BH, Bolt DJ. Effect of adrenal steroids on testosterone and luteinizing hormone secretion in the ram. *J Androl* 1987; 8(3):190-6.
464. Mann DR, Free C, Nelson C, Scott C, Collins DC. Mutually independent effects of adrenocorticotropin on luteinizing hormone and testosterone secretion. *Endocrinology* 1987; 120(4):1542-50.
465. Kuhn JM, Gay D, Lemercier JP, Pugeat M, Legrand A, Wolf LM. [Testicular function during prolonged corticotherapy] Fonction testiculaire au cours de la corticotherapie prolongee. *Presse Med* 1986; 15(12):559-62.
466. MacAdams MR, White RH, Chipps BE. Reduction of serum testosterone levels during chronic glucocorticoid therapy. *Ann Intern Med* 1986; 104:648-651 .
467. Danhaive PA, Rousseau GG. Evidence for sex-dependent anabolic response to androgenic steroids mediated by muscle glucocorticoid receptors in the rat. *J Steroid Biochem* 1988; 29(6):575-581.
468. Wilson JD. Androgen abuse by athletes. *Endocrinol Rev* 1988; 9:950-954.
469. Marinelli M, Roi GS, Giacometti M, Bonini P, Banfi G. Cortisol, testosterone, and free testosterone in athletes performing a marathon at 4,000 m altitude. *Horm Res* 1994; 41(5-6):225-9.
470. Banfi G, Marinelli M, Roi GS, Agape V. Usefulness of free testosterone/cortisol ratio during a season of elite speed skating athletes. *Int J Sports Med* 1993; 14(7):373-9.
471. Urhausen A, Gabriel H, Kindermann W. Blood hormones as markers of training stress and overtraining. *Sports Med* 1995; 20(4):251-76.
472. Wing SS, Goldberg AL. Glucocorticoids activate the ATP-ubiquitin-dependent proteolytic system in skeletal muscle during fasting. *Am J Physiol* 1993; 264:E668-E676.
473. Soares MJ, Piers LS, Shetty PS, et al. Whole body protein turnover in chronically undernourished individuals, *Clin Sci* 1994; 86:441-446.
474. Yahya ZA, Tirapegui JO, Bates PC, Millward DJ. Influence of dietary protein, energy and corticosteroids on protein turnover, proteoglycan sulfation and growth of long bone and skeletal muscle in the rat. *Clin Sci* 1994; 87(5):607-18.
475. Kern W, Perras B, Wodick R, Fehm HL, Born J. Hormonal secretion during nighttime sleep indicating stress of daytime exercise. *J Appl Physiol* 1995; 79(5):1461-8.
476. Hakkinen K, Pakarinen A, Alen M, et al. Relationships between training volume, physical performance capacity, and serum hormone concentrations during prolonged training in elite weight lifters. *Int J Sports Med* 1987; 8:61-65.
477. Kraemer WJ, Marchitelli L, Gordon SE, et al. Hormonal and growth factor responses to heavy resistance exercise protocols. *J Appl Physiol* 1990; 69(4):1442-50.
478. Kraemer WJ, Gordon SE, Fleck SJ, et al. Endogenous anabolic hormonal and growth factor responses to heavy resistance exercise in males and females. *Int J Sports Med* 1991; 12(2):228-35.
478a. Ohtsuka A, Hayashi K, Noda T, Tomita Y. Reduction of corticosterone-induced muscle proteolysis and growth retardation by a combined treatment with insulin, testosterone, and high protein, high fat diets in rats. *J Nutr Sci Vitaminol* 1992; 38:83-92.
478b. Dorgan JF, Judd JT, Longcope C, et al. Effects of dietary fat and fiber on plasma and urine androgens and estrogens in men: a controlled feeding study. *Am. J. Clin. Nutr.* 1996; 64(6):850-5.
478c. Hamalainen E, Adlercreutz H, Puska P, Pietinen P. Diet and serum sex hormones in healthy men. *J Steroid Biochem* 1984; 20(1):459-464.
478d. Raben A, Kiens B, Ritchter EA, et al. Serum sex hormones and endurance performance after a lacto-ovo vegetarian and a mixed diet. *Med Sci Sports Exercise* 1992; 24:1290-1297.
478e. Anderson KE, Rosner W, Khan MS, et al. Diet-hormone interactions: protein/carbohydrate ratio alters reciprocally the plasma levels of testosterone and cortisol and their respective binding globulins in man. *Life Sci* 1987; 40:1761-1768
478f. Hamalainen E, Aldercreutz H, Puska P, Pietinen P. Diet and serum sex hormones in healthy men. *J Steroid Biochem* 1984; 20:459-464.
478g. Volek JS, Kraemer WJ, Bush JA, Incledon T, Boetes M. Testosterone and cortisol in relationship to dietary nutrients and resistance exercise. *J Appl Physiol* 1997; 82(1):49-54.
479. Shaw JF, Wildbore M, Wolfe RR. Whole body protein kinetics in severely septic patients. *Ann Surg* 1987; 205:288-294.
480. Jahoor F, Wolfe RR. Regulation of protein catabolism. *Kidney Int* 1987; 82(suppl 22):581-593.
481. Jahoor F, Desai M, Herndon DN, Wolfe RR. Dynamics of the protein metabolic response to burn injury. *Metabolism* 1988; 37:330-337.
482. Downey RS, Monafo WW, Karl IE, Matthews DE, Bier DM. Protein dynamics in skeletal muscle after trauma: Local and systemic effects. *Surgery* 1986; 90:265-274.
483. Stahl WM. Acute phase protein response to tissue injury. *Crit Care Med* 1987; 15:545-550.
484. Andus T, Geiger T, Hirano T. Action of recombinant human Interleukin 6, Interleukin 1B, and tumor necrosis factor alpha on the m-RNA reduction of acute phase proteins. *Eur J Immunol* 1988; 18:739-746.
485. Perlmutter DH, Dinarello CD, Pupsai PI. Cachectin/tumor necrosis factor regulates hepatic acute phase gene expression. *J Clin Invest* 1986; 78:1349-1354.

486. Ramadori G, Mitsch A, Rieder H, Meyer zum Buschenfelde KH. Alpha and gamma-interferon but not Interleukin 1 modulates synthesis and secretion of beta 2-microglobulin by hepatocytes. *Eur J Clin Invest* 1988; 18:343-351.
487. Castell JV, Gomez-Lechon MJ, David M, et al. Interleukin-6 is the major regulator of acute phase protein synthesis in adult human hepatocytes. *FEBS Lett* 1989; 24:237-239.
488. Espat NJ, Auffenberg T, Rosenberg JJ, et al. Ciliary neurotrophic factor is catabolic and shares with IL-6 the capacity to induce an acute phase response. *Am J Physiol* 1996; 271(1 Pt 2):R185-90.
489. Carraro F, Hartl WH, Stuart CA, Layman DK, Jahoor F, Wolfe RR. Whole body and plasma protein synthesis in exercise and recovery in human subjects. *Am J Physiol* 1990; 258(5 Pt 1):E821-31.
490. Tayek JA. Effects of tumor necrosis factor alpha on skeletal muscle amino acid metabolism studied in vivo. *J Am Coll Nutr* 1996; 15(2):164-8.
491. Tracey KJ, Wei H, Manogue KR, et al. Cachectin/tumor necrosis factor induces cachexia, anemia and inflammation. *J Exp Med* 1988; 167:1211-1227.
492. Warren RS, Starnes HF, Gabrilove JL, et al. The acute metabolic effects of tumor necrosis factor administration. *Arch Surg* 1987; 122:1396-1400.
493. Klasing KC, Johnstone BJ. Monokines in growth and development. *Poult Sci* 1991; 70(8):1781-9.
494. Gray JB, Martinovic AM. Eicosanoids and essential fatty acid modulation in chronic disease and the chronic fatigue syndrome. *Med Hypotheses* 1994; 43(1):31-42.
495. Suchner U, Senftleben U. Immune modulation by polyunsaturated fatty acids during nutritional therapy: interactions with synthesis and effects of eicosanoids. *Infusionsther Transfusionsmed* 1994; 21(3):167-82.
496. Kinsella JE, Lokesh B, Broughton S, Whelan J. Dietary polyunsaturated fatty acids and eicosanoids: potential effects on the modulation of inflammatory and immune cells: an overview. *Nutrition* 1990; 6:24-44.
497. Young MR. Eicosanoids and the immunology of cancer. *Cancer Metastasis Rev* 1994; 13(3-4):337-48.
498. Foley P, Kazazi F, Biti R, Sorrell TC, Cunningham AL. HIV infection of monocytes inhibits the T-lymphocyte proliferative response to recall antigens, via production of eicosanoids. *Immunology* 1992; 75(3):391-7.
499. Juzan M, Hostein I, Gualde N. Role of thymus-eicosanoids in the immune response. *Prostaglandins Leukotrienes Essential Fatty Acids* 1992; 46(4):247-55.
500. Zurier RB. Fatty acids, inflammation and immune responses. *Prostaglandins Leukotrienes Essential Fatty Acids* 1993; 48(1):57-62.
501. Makheja AN. Atherosclerosis: the eicosanoid connection. *Mol Cell Biochem* 1992; 111(1-2):137-42.
502. Buchanan MR, Brister SJ, Bertomeu MC. Eicosanoids, other fatty acid metabolites and the cardiovascular system: are the present antithrombotic approaches rational?. *Agents Actions* — Supplements 1992; 37:273-81.
503. Schror K, Hohlfeld T. Inotropic actions of eicosanoids [editorial]. *Basic Res Cardiol* 1992; 87(1):2-11.
504. Muller B. Pharmacology of thromboxane A2, prostacyclin and other eicosanoids in the cardiovascular system. *Therapie* 1991; 46(3):217-21.
505. Sessa WC, Halushka PV, Okwu A, Nasjletti A. Characterization of the vascular thromboxane A sub 2/prostaglandin endoperoxide receptor in rabbit aorta: Regulation by dexamethasone. *Circ Res* 1990; 67:1562-1569.
506. Fitzgerald DJ, FitzGerald GA: Eicosanoids in myocardial ischemia and injury, in Halushka PV, Mais DE (eds): *Eicosanoids in the Cardiovascular and Renal System.* Norwell, Mass, MTP Press 1988; 128-158.
507. Saadi-M, Gerozissis-K, Dray-F. Release of luteinizing hormone-releasing hormone: Interrelations between eicosanoids and catecholamines. *Brain Res* 1989; 488(1-2):97-104.
508. Bernardini R, Chiarenza A, Calogero AE, Gold PW, Chrousos GP. Arachidonic acid metabolites modulate rat hypothalamic corticotropin-releasing hormone secretion in vitro. *Neuroendocrinology* 1989. 50(6):708-715.
509. Ojeda SR, Dissen GA, Junier MP. Neurotrophic factors and female sexual development. *Front Neuroendocrinol* 1992; 13(2):120-62.
510. Bandyopadhyay GK, Lee LY, Guzman RC, Nandi S. Effect of reproductive states on lipid mobilization and linoleic acid metabolism in mammary glands. *Lipids* 1995; 30(2):155-62.
511. Lopez Bernal A, Newman GE, Phizackerley PJ, Bryant-Greenwood G, Keeling JW. Human placental phospholipase A2 activity in term and preterm labour. *Eur J Obstet Gynecol Reprod Biol* 1992; 43(3):185-92.
512. Toth P, Li X, Rao CV, Lincoln SR, Sanfilippo JS, Spinnato JA 2nd, Yussman MA. Expression of functional human chorionic gonadotropin/human luteinizing hormone receptor gene in human uterine arteries. *J Clin Endocrinol Metab* 1994; 79(1):307-15.
513. Dray F. [Prostaglandins and reproduction. I. Physiological aspects]. [French] *J Gynecol Obstet Biol Reprod* 1991; 20(1):7-17.
514. Griffin DE, Wesselingh SL, McArthur JC. Elevated central nervous system prostaglandins in human immunodeficiency virus-associated dementia. *Ann Neurol* 1994; 35(5):592-7.
515. Lindsberg PJ, Hallenbeck JM, Feuerstein G. Platelet-activating factor in stroke and brain injury. *Ann Neurol* 1991; 30(2):117-29.
516. Piomelli D. Eicosanoids in synaptic transmission. *Crit Rev Neurobiol* 1994; 8(1-2):65-83.
517. Serhan CN. Lipoxins: eicosanoids carrying intra- and intercellular messages. *J Bioenerget Biomembr* 1991; 23(1):105-22.

518. Rosenthal MD, Rzigalinski BA, Blackmore PF, Franson RC. Cellular regulation of arachidonate mobilization and metabolism. *Prostaglandins Leukotrienes Essential Fatty Acids* 1995; 52(2-3):93-8.
519. Shimizu N, Nakamura T. Prostaglandins as hormones. *Dig Dis Sci* 1985; 30(Suppl):109-13S.
520. Schror K. Converting enzyme inhibitors and the interaction between kinins and eicosanoids. *J Cardiovasc Pharmacol* 1990; 15 Suppl 6:S60-8.
521. Das UN. Interaction(s) between essential fatty acids, eicosanoids, cytokines, growth factors and free radicals: relevance to new therapeutic strategies in rheumatoid arthritis and other collagen vascular diseases. *Prostaglandins Leukotrienes Essential Fatty Acids* 1991; 44(4):201-10.
522. Schaison G. [LHRH in man. Current data]. *Ann Endocrinol* 1982; 43(4):247-58.
523. Konturek SJ. Role of growth factors in gastroduodenal protection and healing of peptic ulcers. *Gastroenterol Clin North Am* 1990; 19(1):41-65.
524. Dray F, Kouznetzova B, Harris D, Brazeau P. Role of prostaglandins on growth hormone secretion: PGE2 a physiological stimulator. *Adv Prostaglandin Thromboxane Res* 1980; 8:1321-8.
525. Zacharieva S, Borissova AM, Popova J, Andonova K. Role of prostaglandin E2 (PGE2) in the growth hormone releasing hormone action on growth hormone, insulin and C-peptide in normal men. *Diabete Metab* 1992; 18(3):202-8.
526. Raisz LG, Fall PM, Gabbitas BY, McCarthy TL, Kream BE, Canalis E. Effects of prostaglandin E2 on bone formation in cultured fetal rat calvariae: role of insulin-like growth factor-1. *Endocrinology* 1993; 133(4):1504-10.
527. Wade MG, Van der Kraak G. Arachidonic acid and prostaglandin E2 stimulate testosterone production by goldfish testis in vitro. *Gen Comp Endocrinol* 1993; 90(1):109-18.
528. Zakar T, Hirst JJ, Mijovic JE, Olson DM. Glucocorticoids stimulate the expression of prostaglandin endoperoxide H synthase-2 in amnion cells. *Endocrinology* 1995; 136(4):1610-9.
529. Delany AM, Pash JM, Canalis E. Cellular and clinical perspectives on skeletal insulin-like growth factor-1. *J Cell Biochem* 1994; 55(3):328-33.
530. Conte D, Falaschi P, Proietti A, et al. Role of arachidonate metabolism on the in vitro release of luteinizing hormone and prolactin from the anterior pituitary gland: possible involvement of lipoxygenase pathway. *Neuroendocrinology* 1986; 43(3):428-34.
531. Sarvas K, Angervo M, Koistinen R, Tiitinen A, Seppala M. Prostaglandin F2 alpha stimulates release of insulin-like growth factor binding protein-3 from cultured human granulosa-luteal cells. *Hum Reprod* 1994; 9(9):1643-6.
532. Phair RD, Pek SB, Lands WE. Arachidonic acid induced release of insulin and glucagon: role of endogenous prostaglandins in pancreatic hormone secretion. *Diabete Metabolisme* 1984; 10(2):71-7.
533. Zalin RJ. The role of hormones and prostanoids in the in vitro proliferation and differentiation of human myoblasts. *Exp Cell Res* 1987; 172(2):265-81.
534. Fletcher JR, Eicosanoids. Critical agents in the physiological process and cellular injury. *Arch Surg* 1993; 128(11):1192-6.
535. Pomposelli JJ, Flores EA, Bistrian RR. Role of biochemical mediators in clinical nutrition and surgical metabolism. *JPEN* 1988; 12:212-218.
536. Baracos V, Rodeman P, Dinarell CA, Goldberg AL. Stimulation of muscle degradation and prostaglandin E2 release by leukocytes pyrogen (Interleukin 1). *N Engl J Med* 1983; 308:553-558.
537. Asoh T, Shirosaka C, Uchida I, Tsudi H. Effects of indomethacin on endocrine responses and nitrogen loss after surgery. *Ann Surg* 1987; 206:770-776.
538. Hasselgren RO, Warner BW, Hummel R, James JH, Ogle CK, Fischer JE. Further evidence that accelerated muscle protein breakdown during sepsis is not mediated by prostaglandin E2. *Ann Surg* 1988; 207:399-406.
539. Hasselgren PO, Talamini M, Lafrance R, James JH, Peters JC, Fischer JE. Effect of indomethacin on proteolysis in septic muscle 1982; *Ann Surg* 202:557-562.
540. Marcus AJ, Hajjar DP. Vascular transcellular signaling. *J Lipid Res* 1993; 34(12):2017-31.
541. Goddard DH, Grossman SL, Newton R, Clark MA, Bomalaski JS. Regulation of synovial cell growth: basic fibroblast growth factor synergizes with interleukin 1 beta stimulating phospholipase A2 enzyme activity, phospholipase A2 activating protein production and release of prostaglandin E2 by rheumatoid arthritis synovial cells in culture. *Cytokine* 1992; 4(5):377-84.
542. Molnar M, Romero R, Hertelendy F. Interleukin-1 and tumor necrosis factor stimulate arachidonic acid release and phospholipid metabolism in human myometrial cells. *Am J Obstet Gynecol* 1993; 169(4):825-9.
543. Bergstrom S, Carlson LA, Weeks JR. The prostaglandins: a family of biologically active lipids. *Pharmacol Rev* 1968; 20:1-48.
544. Samuelson B, Goldyne M, Granstrom E, et al., Prostaglandins and thromboxanes, *Annu Rev Biochem* 1978; 47:995-1029.
545. Rodemann HP, Waxman L, Goldberg AL. The stimulation of protein degradation in muscle by Ca^{2+} is mediated by prostaglandin E2 and does not require the calcium-activated protease. *J Biol Chem* 1982; 257(15):8716-23.

546. Baracos V, Rodemann HP, Dinarello CA, Goldberg AL. Stimulation of muscle protein degradation and prostaglandin E2 release by leukocytic pyrogen (interleukin-1). A mechanism for the increased degradation of muscle proteins during fever. *N Engl J Med* 1983; 308(10):553-8.
547. Rodemann HP, Goldberg AL. Arachidonic acid, prostaglandin E2 and F2 influence rates of protein turnover in skeletal and cardiac muscle. *J Biol Chem* 1982; 257:1632-1638.
548. Baracos V, Greenberg RE, Goldberg AL. Influence of calcium and other divalent cations on protein turnover in rat skeletal muscle. *Am J Physiol* 1986; 250:E702-E710.
549. Turinsky J. Phospholipids, prostaglandin E2, and proteolysis in derived muscle. *Am J Physiol* 1986; 251:R165-R173.
550. Goldberg AL, Baracos V, Rodemann P, et al. Control of protein degradation in muscle by prostaglandins, Ca^{2+} and leukocytic pyrogen (interleukin 1). *Fed Proc* 1984; 43(5):1301-1306.
551. Smith RH, Palmer RM, Reeds PJ. Protein synthesis in isolated rabbit forelimb muscles. *Biochem J* 1983; 214:153-161.
552. Palmer RM. Prostaglandins and the control of muscle protein synthesis and degradation. *Prostaglandins Leukotrienes Essential Fatty Acids* 1990; 39:95-104.
553. Palmer RM, Reeds PJ, Atkinson T, et al. The influence of changes in tension on protein synthesis and prostaglandin release in isolated rabbit muscles. *Biochem J* 1983; 214:1011-1014.
554. Vandenburgh HH, Hatfaludy S, Sohar L, et al. Stretch-induced prostaglandins and protein turnover in cultured skeletal muscle. *Am J Physiol* 1990; 259:C232-C240.
555. Templeton GH, Padalino M, Moss R. Influences of inactivity and indomethacin on soleus phosphatidylethanolamine and size. *Prostaglandins* 1986; 31:545-559.
556. Irvine, How is the level of free arachidonic acid controlled in mammalian cells? *Biochem J* 204 (1982): 3-16.
557. Wennmalm A, Fitzgerald G. Excretion of prostacyclin and thromboxane A2 metabolites during leg exercise in humans. *Am J Physiol* 1988; 255:H15-H18.
558. JD Symons, SJ Theodossy, JC Longhurst et al., "Intramuscular accumulation of prostaglandins during static contraction of the cat triceps surae," *J Appl Physiol* 71 (1991): 1837-1842.
559. Sawada T, Asada M, Mori J. Effects of single and repeated administration of prostaglandin F2 alpha on secretion of testosterone by male rats. *Prostaglandins* 1994; 47(5):345-52.
560. Reddy GP, Prasad M, Sailesh S, Kumar YV, Reddanna P. Arachidonic acid metabolites as intratesticular factors controlling androgen production. *Int J Androl* 1993; 16(3):227-33.
561. Romanelli F, Valenca M, Conte D, Isidori A, Negro-Vilar A. Arachidonic acid and its metabolites effects on testosterone production by rat Leydig cells. *J Endocrinol Invest* 1995; 18(3):186-93.
562. Conte D, Nordio M, Fillo S,De Giorgio G, Isidori A, Romanelli F. Aspirin inhibition of naloxone-induced luteinizing hormone secretion in man. *J Clin Endocrinol Metab* 1996; 81(5):1772-5.
563. Rieger GM, Hein R, Adelmann-Grill BC, Ruzicka T, Krieg T. Influence of eicosanoids on fibroblast chemotaxis and protein synthesis in vitro. *J Dermatol Sci* 1990; 1(5):347-54.
564. Bruggeman LA, Horigan EA, Horikoshi S, Ray PE, Klotman PE. Thromboxane stimulates synthesis of extracellular matrix proteins in vitro. *Am J Physiol* 1991; 261(3 Pt 2):F488-94.
565. Mene P, Taranta A, Pugliese F, Cinotti GA, D'Agostino A. Thromboxane A2 regulates protein synthesis of cultured human mesangial cells [see comments]. *J Lab Clin Med* 1992; 120(1):48-56.
566. Liu S, Baracos VE, Quinney HA, Clandinin MT. Dietary omega-3 and polyunsaturated fatty acids modify fatty acyl composition and insulin binding in skeletal-muscle sarcolemma. *Biochem J* 1994; 299(Pt 3):831-837.
567. Kruger MC. Eicosapentaenoic acid and docosahexaenoic acid supplementation increases calcium balance. *Nutr Res* 1995; 15; 211-219.
568. Graham J, Franks S, Bonney RC. In vivo and in vitro effects of gamma-linolenic acid and eicosapentaenoic acid on prostaglandin production and arachidonic acid uptake by human endometrium. *Prostaglandins Leukotrienes Essential Fatty Acids* 1994; 50(6):321-9.
569. MacDonald ID, Graff G, Anderson LA, Dunford HB. Optical spectra and kinetics of reactions of prostaglandin H synthase: effects of the substrates 13-hydroperoxyoctadeca-9,11-dienoic acid, arachidonic acid, N,N,N',N'-tetramethyl-p-phenylenediamine, and phenol and of the nonsteroidal anti-inflammatory drugs aspirin, indomethacin, phenylbutazone, and bromfenac. *Arch Biochem Biophys* 1989; 272(1):194-202.
570. Simon LS, Mills JA. Nonsteroidal anti-inflammatory drugs. *N Engl J Med.* 1980; 302:1179-85.
571. Kobayashi K, Arakawa T, Satoh H et al. Effect of indomethacin, tiaprofenic acid and dicrofenac (sic) on rat gastric mucosal damage and content of prostacyclin and prostaglandin E2. *Prostaglandins* 1985; 30:609-18.
572. Oliw E, Lunden I, Anggard E. In vivo inhibition of prostaglandin synthesis in rabbit kidney by non-steroidal anti-inflammatory drugs. *Acta Pharmacol Toxicol* 1978; 42:179-84.
573. Furst DE. Are There Differences Among Nonsteroidal Antiinflammatory Drugs? Comparing Acetylated Salicylates, Nonacetylated Salicylates, and Nonacetylated Nonsteroidal Antiinflammatory Drugs. *Arthritis Rheum* 1994; 37: 1-9.
574. Sukkar MJ, Hunter WM, Passmore R. Changes in plasma levels of insulin and growth hormone levels after a protein meal. *Lancet* 1967; 2:1020-1022.

575. Carli G, Bonifazi M, Lodi L, et al. Changes in the exercise-induced hormone response to branched chain amino acid administration. *Eur J Appl Physiol* 1992; 64:272-277.
576. Pitkow HS, Brekke M, Harte G, Labbad ZG, Bitar MS. 1994 William J. Stickel Bronze Award. Amino acids, dipeptides, and leg skeletal muscle wound healing in diabetes. *J Am Podiatr Med Assoc* 1994; 84(11):564-73.
577. Jepson MM, Bates PC, Millward DJ. The role of insulin and thyroid hormones in the regulation of muscle growth and protein turnover in response to dietary protein in the rat. *Br J Nutr* 1988; 59(3):397-415.
578. Lardeux BR, Mortimore GE. Amino acid and hormonal control of macromolecular turnover in perfused rat liver. Evidence for selective autophagy. *J Biol Chem* 1987; 262(30):14514-9.
579. Mortimore GE, Lardeux BR, Heydrick SJ. Mechanism and control of protein and RNA degradation in the rat hepatocyte: two modes of autophagic sequestration. *Rev Sobre Biol Cel* 1989; 20:79-96.
580. Balavoine S, Feldmann G, Lardeux B. Rates of RNA degradation in isolated rat hepatocytes. Effects of amino acids and inhibitors of lysosomal function. *Eur J Biochem* 1990; 189:617-623.
581. Balavoine S, Feldmann G, Lardeux B. Regulation of RNA degradation in cultured rat hepatocytes: effects of specific amino acids and insulin. *J Cell Physiol* 1993; 156(1):56-62.
582. Stoll B, Gerok W, Lang F, Haussinger D. Liver cell volume and protein synthesis. *Biochem J* 1992; 287(Pt 1):217-22
583. Freed DLJ, Banks AJ, Longson D, Burley DM. Anabolic steroids in athelics: crossover double-blind trial on weightlifters. *Br Med J* 1975; 2(5969):471-473.
584. Chandler RM, Byrne HK, Patterson JG, Ivy JL. Dietary supplements affect the anabolic hormones after weight-training exercise. *J Appl Physiol* 1994; 76(2):839-45.
585. Biolo G, Maggi SP, Williams BD, Tipton KD, Wolfe RR. Increased rates of muscle protein turnover and amino acid transport after resistance exercise in humans. *Am J Physiol* 1995; 268(3 Pt 1):E514-20.
586. Finley RJ, Inculet RI, Pace R, et al. Major operative trauma increases peripheral amino acid release during the steady-state infusion of total parenteral nutrition in man. *Surgery* 1986; 99(4):491-500.
587. Hammarqvist F, von der Decken A, Vinnars E, Wernerman J. Stress hormone and amino acid infusion in healthy volunteers: short-term effects on protein synthesis and amino acid metabolism in skeletal muscle. *Metab Clin Exp* 1994; 43(9):1158-63.
588. Wernerman J, Botta D, Hammarqvist F, et al. Stress hormones given to healthy volunteers alter the concentration and configuration of ribosomes in skeletal muscle, reflecting changes in protein synthesis. *Clin Sci* 1989; 77(6):611-6.
589. Souba WW, Smith RJ, Wilmore DW. Glutamine metabolism by the intestinal tract. *JPEN* 1985; 9:608-617.
590. Souba WW, Wilmore DW. Gut-liver interaction during accelerated gluconeogenesis. *Arch Surg* 1985; 120:66-70.
591. Mourier A, Bigard AX, de Kerviler E, Roger B, Legrand H, Guezennec CY. Combined effects of caloric restriction and branched-chain amino acid supplementation on body composition and exercise performance in elite wrestlers. *Int J Sports Med* 1997; 18(1):47-55.
591. Ferreira M, Kreider R, Wilson M, et al. Effects of Ingesting a supplement designed to enhance creatine uptake on strength and sprint capacity. Presented May 30, 1997 at the American College of Sports Medicine Annual Meeting.
592. Piatti PM, Monti LD, Pacchioni M, Pontiroli AE, Pozza G. Forearm insulin- and non-insulin-mediated glucose uptake and muscle metabolism in man: role of free fatty acids and blood glucose levels. *Metab Clin Exp* 1991; 40(9):926-33.
593. Felig P, Wahren J, Sherwin R, Palaiologos G. Amino acid and protein metabolism in diabetes mellitus. *Arch Intern Med* 1977; 137(4):507-13.
594. Favier RJ, Koubi HE, Mayet MH, Sempore B, Simi B, Flandrois R. Effects of gluconeogenic precursor flux alterations on glycogen resynthesis. after prolonged exercise. *J Appl Physiol* 1987; 63(5)p1733-8.
595. Azzout B, Bois-Joyeux B, Chanez M, Peret J. Development of gluconeogenesis from various precursors in isolated rat hepatocytes during starvation or after feeding a high protein, carbohydrate-free diet. *J Nutr* 1987; 117(1):164-9.
596. Jahoor F, Peters EJ, Wolfe RR. The relationship between gluconeogenic substrate supply and glucose production in humans. *Am J Physiol* 1990; 258(2 Pt 1):E288-96.
597. Amiel SA, Archibald HR, Chusney G, Williams AJ, Gale EA. Ketone infusion lowers hormonal responses to hypoglycaemia: evidence for acute cerebral utilization of a non-glucose fuel. *Clin Sci* 1991; 81(2):189-94.
598. Cori CF. Mammalian carbohydrate metabolism. *Physiol Rev* 1931; 11: 143-275.
599. Reichard GA Jr, Moury FN Jr, Hochella NJ, Patterson AL, Weinhouse S. Quantitative estimation of the Cori cycle in the human. *J Biol Chem* 1963; 238:495-501.
600. Gerich JE. Control of glycaemia. 7(3):551-86, 1993 Jul. *Baillieres Clin Endocrinol Metab* 1993; 7(3):551-86.
601. Nurjhan N, Bucci A, Perriello G, et al. Glutamine: a major gluconeogenic precursor and vehicle for interorgan carbon transport in man. *J Clin Invest* 1995; 95(1):272-7.
602. Kaloyianni M, Freedland RA. Contribution of several amino acids and lactate to gluconeogenesis in hepatocytes isolated from rats fed various diets. *J Nutr* 1990; 120(1):116-22.

603. Widhalm K, Zwiauer K, Hayde M, Roth E. Plasma concentrations of free amino acids during 3 weeks treatment of massively obese children with a very low calorie diet. *Eur J Pediatr* 1989; 149(1):43-7.
604. Pozefsky T, Tancredi RG, Moxley RT, Dupre J, Tobin JD. Effects of brief starvation on muscle amino acid metabolism in nonobese man. *J Clin Invest* 1976; 57(2):444-9.
605. Fery F, Bourdoux P, Christophe J, Balasse EO. Hormonal and metabolic changes induced by an isocaloric isoproteinic ketogenic diet in healthy subjects. *Diabete Metab* 1982; 8(4):299-305.
606. Cynober L. Amino acid metabolism in thermal burns. Jpen: J Parenteral Enteral Nutr 1989; 13(2):196-205.
607. Lemon PW, Nagle FJ. Effects of exercise on protein and amino acid metabolism. *Med Sci Sports Exerc* 1981; 13(3):141-9.
608. Rothman DL, Magnusson I, Katz LD, Shulman RG, Shulman GI. Quantitation of hepatic glycogenolysis and gluconeogenesis in fasting humans with (sup 13) C NMR. *Science* 1991; 254:573-6.
609. Jungas RL, Halperin ML, Brosnan JT. Quantitative analysis of amino acid oxidation and related gluconeogenesis in humans. *Physiol Rev* 1992; 72(2):419-48.
610. Hochachka PW, Dressendorfer RH. Succinate accumulation in man during exercise. *Eur J Appl Physiol* 1976; 35(4):235-242.
611. Pisarenko OI, Solomatina ES, Studneva IM. Formation of the intermediate products of the tricarboxylic acid cycle and ammonia from free amino acids in anoxic heart muscle. *Biokhimiia* 1986; 51(8):1276-85.
612. Wiesner RJ, Ruegg JC, Grieshaber MK. The anaerobic heart: succinate formation and mechanical performance of cat papillary muscle. *Exp Biol* 1986; 45(1):55-64.
613. Camici P, Marraccini P, Lorenzoni R, et al. Metabolic markers of stress-induced myocardial ischemia. *Circulation* 1991; 83(5 Suppl):III8-13.
614. Hutson SM, Wallin R, Hall TR. Identification of mitochondrial branched chain aminotransferase and its isoforms in rat tissues. *J Biol Chem* 1992; 267(22):15681-6.
615. Fisher AG, Jensen CR. *Scientific Basis of Athletic Conditioning,* Lea & Febiger, Philadelphia. 1991.
616. Wagenmakers AJ. Amino acid metabolism, muscular fatigue and muscle wasting. Speculations on adaptations at high altitude. [Review] *Int J Sports Med* 1992; 13 Suppl 1:S110-3.
617. Kuhn E. [The effect of work load on amino acid metabolism]. [Czech] *Vnitr Lek* 1994; 40(7):411-5.
618. Brown JA, Gore DC, Jahoor F. Catabolic hormones alone fail to reproduce the stress-induced efflux of amino acids. *Arch Surg* 1994; 129(8):819-24.
619. Brown J, Gore DC, Lee R. Dichloroacetate inhibits peripheral efflux of pyruvate and alanine during hormonally simulated catabolic stress. *J Surg Res* 1993; 54(6):592-6.
620. Carlin JI, Olson EB Jr, Peters HA, Reddan WG. The effects of post-exercise glucose and alanine ingestion on plasma carnitine and ketosis in humans. *J Physiol* 1987; 390:295-303.
621. Newsholme EA, Crabtree B, Ardawi MS. The role of high rates of glycolysis and glutamine utilization in rapidly dividing cells. Bioscience Reports 1985; 5(5):393-400.
622. Felig P. The glucose-alanine cycle. *Metabolism* 1973; 22:179-207.
623. Ahlborg G, Hagenfeldt L, Wahren J. Substrate turnover during prolonged exercise in man. *J Clin Invest* 1974; 53:1080 -1090.
624. Lemon PWR, Mullin JP. Effect of initial muscle glycogen levels on protein catabolism during exercise. *J Appl Physiol* 1980; 48: 624-629.
625. Lemon PW, Nagle FJ. Effects of exercise on protein and amino acid metabolism. *Med Sci Sports Exerc* 1981; 13(3):141-9.
626. Brooks GA. Amino acid and protein metabolism during exercise and recovery. *Med Sci Sports Exerc* 1987; 19(5 Suppl):S150-6.
627. Wolfe RR, Jahoor F, Herndon DN, Miyoshi H. Isotopic evaluation of the metabolism of pyruvate and related substrates in normal adult volunteers and severely burned children: effect of dichloroacetate and glucose infusion. *Surgery* 1991; 110(1):54-67.
628. Sewell DA, Harris RC. Adenine nucleotide degradation in the thoroughbred horse with increasing exercise duration. *Eur J Appl Physiol Occup Physiol* 1992; 65(3):271-7.
629. Sewell DA, Gleeson M, Blannin AK. Hyperammonaemia in relation to high-intensity exercise duration in man. *Eur J Appl Physiol Occup Physiol* 1994; 69(4):350-4.
630. Sahlin, Broberg S. Adenine nucleotide depletion in human muscle during exercise: causality and significance of AMP deamination. *Int J Sports Med* 1990; 11 Suppl 2:S62-7.
631. van Hall G, van der Vusse GJ, Soderlund K, Wagenmakers AJ. Deamination of amino acids as a source for ammonia production in human skeletal muscle during prolonged exercise. *J Physiol* 1995; 489(Pt 1):251-61.
632. Graham TE, MacLean DA. Ammonia and amino acid metabolism in human skeletal muscle during exercise. *Can J Physiol Pharmacol* 1992; 70(1):132-41.
633. Wagenmakers AJ, Beckers EJ, Brouns F, Kuipers H, Soeters PB, van der Vusse GJ, Saris WH. Carbohydrate supplementation, glycogen depletion, and amino acid metabolism during exercise. *Am J Physiol* 1991; 260(6 Pt 1):E883-90.
634. MacLean DA, Graham TE, Saltin B. Branched-chain amino acids augment ammonia metabolism while attenuating protein breakdown during exercise. *Am J Physiol* 1994; 267:E1010-E1022.

635. Peters JC, Harper AE. Protein and energy consumption, plasma amino acid ratios, and brain neurotransmitter concentrations. *Physiol Behav* 1981; 27(2):287-98.
636. Peters JC, Harper AE. Influence of dietary protein level on protein self-selection and plasma and brain amino acid concentrations. *Physiol Behav* 1984; 33(5):783-90.
637. Peters JC, Harper AE. Adaptation of rats to diets containing different levels of protein: effects on food intake, plasma and brain amino acid concentrations and brain neurotransmitter metabolism. *J Nutr* 1985; 115(3):382-98.
638. Fernstrom JD. Dietary effects on brain serotonin synthesis: relationship to appetite regulation. *Am J Clin Nutr* 1985; 42(5 Suppl):1072-82.
639. Peters JC, Harper AE. Acute effects of dietary protein on food intake, tissue amino acids, and brain serotonin. *Am J Physiol* 1987; 252(5 Pt 2):R902-14.
640. Wurtman RJ, Wurtman JJ. Brain serotonin, carbohydrate-craving, obesity and depression. *Obesity Res* 1995; 3 Suppl 4:477S-480S.
641. Wurtman RJ, Wurtman JJ. Do carbohydrates affect food intake via neurotransmitter activity?. *Appetite* 1988; 11 Suppl 1:42-7.
642. Harper AE, Peters JC. Protein intake, brain amino acid and serotonin concentrations and protein self-selection. *J Nutr* 1989; 119(5):677-89.
643. Vandewater K, Vickers Z. Higher-protein foods produce greater sensory-specific satiety. *Physiol Behav* 1996; 59(3):579-83.
644. Hazum E. Neuroendocrine peptides in milk. *Trends Endocrinol Metab* 1991; Jan/Feb:25-8.
645. Roberts PR, Zaloga GP. Dietary bioactive peptides. *New Horizons* 1994; 2(2):237-43.
646. Matthews DM, Crampton RF, Lis MT. Sites of maximal intestinal absorptive capacity for amino acids and peptides: evidence for an independent peptide uptake system or systems. *J Clin Pathol* 1971; 24(9):882-3.
647. Crampton RF, Gangolli SD, Simson P, Matthews DM. Rates of absorption by rat intestine of pancreatic hydrolysates of proteins and their corresponding amino acid mixtures. *Clin Sci* 1971; 41(5):409-17.
648. Mitchell HH. Some species and age differences in amino acid requirements. In: Albanese AA, ed., *Protein and Amino Acid Requirements of Mammals.* Academic Press, New York 1950; 1-32.
649. Mitchell HH. *Comparative Nutrition of Man and Domestic Animals.* Vol 1. Academic Press, New York. 1962. Page 166.
650. Frexes-Steed M, Lacy DB, Collins J, Abumrad NN. Role of leucine and other amino acids in regulating protein metabolism in vivo. *Am J Physiol* 1992; 262(6 Pt 1):E925-35.
651. Marchini JS, Cortiella J, Hiramatsu T, Chapman TE, Young VR. Requirements for indispensable amino acids in adult humans: longer-term amino acid kinetic study with support for the adequacy of the Massachusetts Institute of Technology amino acid requirement pattern. *Am J Clin Nutr* 1993; 58(5):670-83.
652. Marchini JS, Cortiella J, Hiramatsu T, Castillo L. Chapman TE. Young VR. Phenylalanine and tyrosine kinetics for different patterns and indispensable amino acid intakes in adult humans. *Am J Clin Nutr* 1994; 60(1):79-86.
653. Young VR. Adult amino acid requirements: the case for a major revision in current recommendations. *J Nutr* 1994; 124(8 Suppl):1517S-1523S.
654. Iapichino G. Ronzoni G. Bonetti G. Corti M. Grugni L. Guarnerio C. Palandi A. Pasetti G. Rotelli S. Savioli M. [Determination of the best amino acid input after orthotopic liver transplantation]. *Minerva Anestesiol* 1992; 58(9):503-8.
655. Furst P, Stehle P. Are intravenous amino acid solutions unbalanced?. *New Horizons* 1994; 2(2):215-23.
656. Swendseid ME, Kopple JD. Amino acid requirements and non-specific nitrogen. *Infusionsther Klin Ernahrung* 1975; 2(3):203-7.
657. Sturman JA. Chesney RW. Taurine in pediatric nutrition. *Pediatr Clin North Am* 1995; 42(4):879-97.
658. Motil KJ, Thotathuchery M, Montandon CM, et al. Insulin, cortisol and thyroid hormones modulate maternal protein status and milk production and composition in humans. *J Nutr* 1994; 124(8):1248-57.
659. Rudman D, Kutner M, Ansley J, Jansen R, Chipponi J, Bain RP. Hypotyrosinemia, hypocystinemia and failure to retain nitrogen during total parenteral nutrition of cirrhotic patients. *Gastroenterology* 1981; 81: 1025-35.
660. Kies C. Nonspecific nitrogen in the nutrition of human beings. *Fed Proc* 1972; 31:1172-77.
661. Kies C. Comparative value of various sources of nonspecific nitrogen for the human. *J Agric Food Chem* 1974; 22:190-193.
662. Young VR, El-Khoury AE. The notion of the nutritional essentiality fo amino acids, revisited, with a note on the indespensible amino acid requirements in adults. In *Amino Acid Metabolism and Therapy in Health and Nutritional Disease* edited by Cynober LA. CRC Press. Boca Raton, Florida. 1995.
663. Davidsson L, Almgren A, Sandstrom B, Juillerat M, Hurrell RF. Zinc absorption in adult humans: the effect of protein sources added to liquid test meals. *Br J Nutr* 1996; 75(4):607-13.
664. Draper A, Lewis J, Malhotra N, Wheeler E. The energy and nutrient intakes of different types of vegetarian: a case for supplements? [published erratum appears in *Br J Nutr* 1993; 70(3):812]. *Br J Nutr* 1993; 69(1):3-19.

665. Young VR. Pellett PL. Plant proteins in relation to human protein and amino acid nutrition. *Am J Clin Nutr.* 59(5 Suppl):1203S-1212S, 1994 May.
666. Graham GG, Lembcke J, Lancho E, Morales E. Quality protein maize: digestibility and utilization by recovering malnourished infants. *Pediatrics* 1989 Mar; 83(3); P 416-21.
667. Bressani. R, Elias LG, Gomez Brenes RA. Improvement of protein quality by amino acid and protein supplementation. In: Bigwood EJ, ed. *Protein and Amino Acid Functions*. Vol. 11. Oxford, UK: Pergamon Press, 1972; 475-540.
668. Food and Agriculture Organization/World Health Organization/United Nations University. Energy and protein requirements. Report of joint FAO/WHO/UNU expert consultation. Geneva: World Health Organization. 1985. (WHO Tech rep ser no. 724)
669. Geiger E. The role of the time factor in feeding supplementary proteins. *J Nutr* 1948; 36:813-9.
670. Geiger E. Experiments with delayed supplementation of incomplete amino acid mixtures. *J Nutr* 1947; 34:97-111.
671. Batterham ES, O'Neill GH. The effect of frequency of feeding on the response by growing pigs to supplements of free lysine. *Br J Nutr* 1978; 39:265-70.
672. Taylor YSM, Young VR, Murray E, Pencharz PB, Scrimshaw. Daily protein and meal patterns affecting young men fed adequate and restricted energy intakes. *Am J Clin Nutr* 1973; 26:1216-22.
673. Scrimshaw NS, Behar M, Wilson D, Viteri F, Arroyave G, Bressani R. Volume 9, 1961: All-vegetable protein mixtures for human feeding. *Nutr Rev* 1989; 47(11):346-9.
674. Nissen S, Haymond MW. Changes in leucine kinetics during meal absorption: effects of dietary leucine availability. *Am J Physiol* 1986; 250(6 Pt 1):E695-701.
675. Erbersdobler HF. Protein reactions during food processing and storage — their relevance to human nutrition. *Bibl Nutr Dieta*; 1989; 36(43); P 140-55.
676. Furst P. Regulation of intracellular metabolism of amino acids. In: F Bozzetti and R Dionigi, eds. *Nutrition in Cancer and Trauma Sepsis* Karger, New York 1985; 21-53.
677. Hernandez M, Montalvo I, Sousa V, Sotelo A. The protein efficiency ratios of 30:70 mixtures of animal:vegetable protein are similar or higher than those of the animal foods alone. *J Nutr* 1996; 126(2):574-81.
678. Whitney EN, Hamilton EMN, Rolfes SR. *Understanding Nutrition.* Fifth Edition, West Publishing Company, St. Paul, Minnesota 1990; J3-J4.
679. Krajcovicova-Kudlackova M, Ozdin L. [The effect of a vegetarian diet on protein and fat metabolism values in rats of various ages]. *Vet Med* 1993; 38(7):413-25.
680. Sarwar G, McDonough FE. Evaluation of protein digestibility-corrected amino acid score method for assessing protein quality of foods. [Review] *J Assoc Off Anal Chem* 1990; 73(3):347-56.
681. Holt S. Soya for Health. *The Definitive Medical Guide.* Mary Ann Liebert, Inc., Larchmont NY, 1996, 83-85.
682. Yu YM, Yang RD, Matthews DE, et al. Quantitative aspects of glycine and alanine nitrogen metabolism in postabsorptive young men: effects of level of nitrogen and dispensable amino acid intake. *J Nutr* 1985; 115(3):399-410.
683. National Research Council. *Recommended Dietary Allowances,* 10th ed. Washington, D.C., National Academy of Sciences, 1989.
684. von Liebig J. *Animal Chemistry or Organic Chemistry and Its Application to Physiology and Pathology* (translated by W Gregory). London, Taylor, and Walton 1842; p 144.
685. Fick A, Wislicenus J. On the origin of muscular power. *Philos Mag J Sci* 1866; 41:485-503.
686. Cathcart EP. Influence of muscle work on protein metabolism. *Physiol Rev* 1925; 5: 225-243.
687. Astrand PO, Rodahl K. *Textbook of Work Physiology,* 3rd ed. McGraw-Hill, New York, 1986.
688. Lemon PWR. Do athletes need more dietary protein and amino acids? *Int J Sport Nutr* 1995; 5:S39-S61.
689. Kleiner SM, Bazzarre TL, Ainsworth BE. Nutritional status of nationally ranked elite bodybuilders. *Int J Sport Nutr* 1994; 4(1):54-69.
690. Darden E. Protein. *Nautilus Mag* 1981; 3(1):12-17.
691. Dohm GL. Protein nutrition for the athlete. *Clin Sports Med* 1984; 3(3):595-604.
692. Lemon PW. Maximizing performance with nutrition: protein and exercise: update 1987. *Med Sci Sports Exerc* 1987; 19(5):S179-S190.
693. Burke LM, Read RS. Sports nutrition. Approaching the nineties. *Sports Med* 1989; 8(2):80-100.
694. Lemon PW, Proctor DN. Protein intake and athletic performance. *Sports Med* 1991; 12(5):313-325.
695. Lemon PW. Protein requirements of soccer. *J Sports Sci* 1994; 12:S17-22.
696. Lemon PW. Do athletes need more dietary protein and amino acids? *Int J Sport Med* 1995; 5:S39-S61.
697. Phillips SM, Atkinson SA, Tarnopolsky MA, et al. Gender differences in leucine kinetics and nitrogen balance in endurance athletes. *J Appl Physiol* 1993; 75:2134-2141.
698. Butterfield GE. Whole body protein utilization in humans, *Med Sci Sports Exerc* 1987; 19:S157-S165.
699. Piatti PM, Monti LD, Magni F, et al. Hypocaloric high-protein diet improves glucose oxidation and spares lean body mass: comparison to hypocaloric high-carbohydrate diet. *Metabolism* 1994; 43:1481-1487.
700. Fern EB, Bielinski RN, Schutz Y. Effects of exaggerated amino acid and protein supply in man. *Experientia* 1991; 47(2):168-72.

701. Bigard AX, Satabin P, Lavier P, et al. Effects of protein supplementation during prolonged exercise at moderate altitude on performance and plasma amino acid pattern. *Eur J Appl Physiol Occup Physiol* 1993; 66(1):5-10.
702. Dohm GL, Tapscott EB, Kasperek GJ. Protein degradation during endurance exercise and recovery. *Med Sci Sports Exerc* 1987; 19(5):S166-S171.
703. Henriksson J. Effect of exercise on amino acid concentrations in skeletal muscle and plasma. *J Exp Biol* 1991; 160:149-65.
704. Millward DJ, Bates PC, Brown JG, et al. Role of thyroid, insulin and corticosteroid hormones in the physiological regulation of proteolysis in muscle. *Prog Clin Biol Res* 1985; 180:531-42.
705. Lemon PW. Protein requirements of soccer. *J Sports Sci* 1994; 12:S17-22.
706. Manz F, Remer T, Decher-Splicthoff E, et al. Effects of a high protein intake on renal acid excretion in bodybuilders. *Z Ernahrungswiss* 1995; 34(1):10-5.
707. Sterck JG, Ritskes-Hoitinga J, Beynen AC. Inhibitory effect of high protein intake on nephrocalcinogenesis in female rats. *Br J Nutr* 1992; 67(2):223-33.
708. Wolfe BM, Giovannetti PM. Short-term effects of substituting protein for carbohydrate in the diets of moderately hypercholesterolemic human subjects. *Metab Clin Exp* 1991; 40(4):338-43.
709. Campbell TC, Hayes JR. The effect of quantity and quality of dietary protein on drug metabolism. *Fed Proc* 1976; 35(13):2470-2474.
710. Maiter D, Maes M, Underwood LE, Fliesen T. Gerard G. Ketelslegers JM. Early changes in serum concentrations of somatomedin-C induced by dietary protein deprivation in rats: contributions of growth hormone receptor and post-receptor defects. *J Endocrinol* 1988; 118(1):113-20.
711. Lopes J, Russell DMcR, Whitwell J, Jeejeeboy K. Skeletal muscle function and malnutrition. *Am J Clin Nutr* 1982; 36: 602-10.
712. Hymsfield SB, Stevens V, Noel R, McManus C, Smith J, Nixon D. Biochemical composition of muscle in normal and semi starved human subjects: relevance to anthropometric measurements. *Am J Clin Nutr* 1982; 36:131-42.
713. Russell DMcR, Leiter LA, Whitwell J. Marliss EB, Jeejeeboy KN. Skeletal muscle function during hypocaloric diets and fasting: a comparison with standard nutritional assessment parameters. *Am J Clin Nutr* 1983; 37:133-8.
714. Millward DJ, Jepson MM. Omer A. Muscle glutamine concentration and protein turnover in vivo in malnutrition and in endotoxemia. *Metab Clin Exp* 1989; 38(8 Suppl 1):6-13.
715. Young VR, Munro HN, Fukagawa NK. Protein and functional consequences of deficiency. In: Horwitz A, Macfadyen DM, Munro H, Scrimshaw NS, Steen B, Williams TF, eds. *Nutrition in the Elderly.* New York: Oxford University Press, 1989.
716. Hoffer LJ, Forse RA. Protein metabolic effects of a prolonged fast and hypocaloric refeeding. *Am J Physiol* 1990; 258(5 Pt 1):E832-40.
717. Sullivan DA, Vaerman JP, Soo C. Influence of severe protein malnutrition on rat lacrimal, salivary and gastrointestinal immune expression during development, adulthood and ageing. *Immunology* 1993; 78(2):308-317.
718. Yahya ZA, Tirapegui JO, Bates PC, Millward DJ. Influence of dietary protein, energy and corticosteroids on protein turnover, proteoglycan sulfation and growth of long bone and skeletal muscle in the rat. *Clin Sci* 1994; 87(5):607-618.
719. Bouziane M, Prost J, Belleville J. Dietary protein deficiency affects n-3 and n-6 polyunsaturated fatty acids hepatic storage and very low density lipoprotein transport in rats on different diets. *Lipids* 1994; 29(4):265-72.
720. Munro HN. Regulation of protein metabolism in relation to adequacy of intake. *Infusionsther Klin Ernahrung* 1975; 2(2):112-7.
721. Young VR, Marchini JS. Mechanisms and nutritional significance of metabolic responses to altered intakes of protein and amino acids, with reference to nutritional adaptation in humans. *Am J Clin Nutr* 1990; 51:270-89.
722. Tawa NE Jr, Goldberg AL. Suppression of muscle protein turnover and amino acid degradation by dietary protein deficiency. *Am J Physiol* 1992; 263(2 Pt 1):E317-25.
723. Tawa NE Jr, Kettelhut IC, Goldberg AL. Dietary protein deficiency reduces lysosomal and nonlysosomal ATP-dependent proteolysis in muscle. *Am J Physiol* 1992; 263(2 Pt 1):E326-34.
724. Attaix D, Taillandier D, Temparis S, Larbaud D. Aurousseau E. Combaret L. Voisin L. Regulation of ATP-ubiquitin-dependent proteolysis in muscle wasting. *Reprod Nutr Dev* 1994; 34(6):583-97.
725. Peret J, Chanez M, Cota J, Macaire I. Effects of quantity and quality of dietary protein and variation in certain enzyme activities on glucose metabolism in the rat. *J Nutr* 1975; 105(12):1525-34.
726. Szepesi B, Freedland RA. Alterations in the activities of several rat liver enzymes at various times after initiation of a high protein regimen. *J Nutr* 1967; 93(3):301-6.
727. Szepesi B, Freedland RA. Time-course of changes in rat liver enzyme activities after initiation of a high protein regimen. *J Nutr* 1968; 94(4):463-8.

728. Fafournoux P, Remesy C, Demigne C. Fluxes and membrane transport of amino acids in rat liver under different protein diets. *Am J Physiol* 1990; 259(5 Pt 1):E614-25.
729. Munro HN. Regulation of protein metabolism in relation to adequacy of intake. *Infusionsther Klin Ernahrung* 1975; 2(2):112-7.
730. Ljungqvist BG, Svanberg US, Young VR. Plasma amino acid response to single test meals in humans. II. Healthy young adults given synthetic amino acid mixtures. *Res Exp Med* 1978; 174(1):13-28.
731. Fujita Y, Yamamoto T, Rikimaru T, Ebisawa H, Inoue G. Effect of quality and quantity of dietary protein on free amino acids in plasma and tissues of adult rats. *J Nutr Sci Vitam* 1981; 27(2):129-47.
732. Tews JK, Rogers QR, Morris JG, Harper AE. Effect of dietary protein and GABA on food intake, growth and tissue amino acids in cats. *Physiol Behav* 1984; 32(2):301-8.
733. Yokogoshi H, Hayase K, Yoshida A. The quality and quantity of dietary protein affect brain protein synthesis in rats. *J Nutr* 1992; 122(11):2210-7.
734. Soemitro S, Block KP, Crowell PL, Harper AE. Activities of branched-chain amino acid — degrading enzymes in liver from rats fed different dietary levels of protein. *J Nutr* 1989; 119(8):1203-12.
735. Anderson SA, Tews JK, Harper AE. Dietary branched-chain amino acids and protein selection by rats. *J Nutr* 1990; 120(1):52-63.
736. Maher TJ, Glaeser BS, Wurtman RJ. Diurnal variations in plasma concentrations of basic and neutral amino acids and in red cell concentrations of aspartate and glutamate: effects of dietary protein intake. *Am J Clin Nutr* 1984; 39(5):722-9.
737. Frexes-Steed M, Lacy DB, Collins J, Abumrad NN. Role of leucine and other amino acids in regulating protein metabolism in vivo. *Am J Physiol* 1992; 262(6 Pt 1):E925-35.
738. Block KP, Harper AE. High levels of dietary amino and branched-chain alpha-keto acids alter plasma and brain amino acid concentrations in rats. *J Nutr* 1991; 121(5):663-71.
739. Powanda MC, Dinterman RE, Wannemacher RW Jr, Beisel WR. Tryptophan metabolism in relation to amino acid alterations during typhoid fever. *Acta Vitam Enzymol* 1975; 29(1-6):164-8.
740. Hoerr RA, Matthews DE, Bier DM, Young VR. Effects of protein restriction and acute refeeding on leucine and lysine kinetics in young men. *Am J Physiol* 1993; 264(4 Pt 1):E567-75.
741. Eisenstein RS, Harper AE. Relationship between protein intake and hepatic protein synthesis in rats. *J Nutr* 1991; 121(10):1581-90.
742. Tawa NE Jr, Goldberg AL. Suppression of muscle protein turnover and amino acid degradation by dietary protein deficiency. *Am J Physiol* 1992; 263(2 Pt 1):E317-25.
743. Yokogoshi H, Yoshida A. Some factors affecting the nitrogen sparing action of methionine and threonine in rats fed a protein free diet. *J Nutr* 1976; 106(1):48-57.
744. Frexes-Steed M, Lacy DB, Collins J, Abumrad NN. Role of leucine and other amino acids in regulating protein metabolism in vivo. *Am J Physiol* 1992; 262(6 Pt 1):E925-35.
745. Young VR, Marchini JS. Mechanisms and nutritional significance of metabolic responses to altered intakes of protein and amino acids, with reference to nutritional adaptation in humans. *Am J Clin Nutr* 1990; 51(2):270-89.
746. Kadowaki M, Nagasawa T, Hirata T, Noguchi T, Naito H. Effects of insulin, amino acids and fasting on myofibrillar protein degradation in perfused hindquarters of rats. *J Nutr Sci Vitam* 1985; 31(4):431-40.
747. Taveroff A, Lapin H, Hoffer LJ. Mechanism governing short-term fed-state adaptation to dietary protein restriction. *Metab Clin Exp* 1994; 43(3):320-7.
748. Millward DJ, Price GM, Pacy PJH, et al. Maintenance protein requirements: the need for conceptual re-evaluation. *Proc Nutr Soc* 1990; 49:473-487.
749. Yokogoshi H, Hayase K, Yoshida A. The quality and quantity of dietary protein affect brain protein synthesis in rats. *J Nutr* 1992; 122(11):2210-7.
750. Viru A. Mobilisation of structural proteins during exercise. *Sports Med* 1987; 4(2):95-128.
751. Millward DJ, Price GM, Pacy PJH, et al. Maintenance protein requirements: the need for conceptual re-evaluation. *Proc Nutr Soc* 1990; 49:473-487.
752. Bennet WM, Connacher AA, Scrimgeour CM, et al. Increase in anterior tibialis muscle protein synthesis in healthy man during mixed amino acid infusion: studies of incorporation of [1-13C]leucine. *Clin Sci* 1989 76:447-454.
753. Bennet WM, Connacher AA, Scrimgeour CM, et al. The effect of amino acid infusion on leg protein turnover assessed by L-[1-15N]phenylalanine and L-[13C]leucine exchange. *Eur J Clin Invest* 1990; 20:41-50.
754. Millward DJ, Rivers JP. The need for indispensable amino acids: the concept of the anabolic drive. *Diabetes Metab Rev* 1989; 5(2):191-211.
755. Castellino P, Luzi L, Simonson DC, Haymond M, DeFronzo RA. Effect of insulin and plasma amino acid concentrations on leucine metabolism in man. Role of substrate availability on estimates of whole body protein synthesis. *J Clin Invest* 1987; 80(6):1784-93.
756. Tessari P, Inchiostro S, Biolo G, et al. Differential effects of hyperinsulinemia and hyperaminoacidemia on leucine-carbon metabolism in vivo. Evidence for distinct mechanisms in regulation of net amino acid deposition. *J Clin Invest* 1987; 79(4):1062-9.

757. Pacy PJ, Price GM, Halliday D, et al. Nitrogen homeostasis in man: the diurnal responses of protein synthesis and degradation and amino acid oxidation to diets with increasing protein intakes, *Clin Sci* 1994; 86:103-118.
758. Price GM, Halliday D, Pacy PJ, et al. Nitrogen homeostasis in man: influence of protein intake on the amplitude of diurnal cycling of body nitrogen. *Clin Sci* 1994; 86:91-102.
759. Tovar AR, Tews JK, Torres N, Harper AE. Neutral amino acid transport into rat skeletal muscle: competition, adaptive regulation, and effects of insulin. *Metab Clin Exp* 1991; 40(4):410-9.
760. Edozien JC, Switzer BR. Influence of diet on growth in the rat. *J Nutr* 1978; 108(2):282-90.
761. Moundras C, Remesy C, Demigne C. Dietary protein paradox: decrease of amino acid availability induced by high-protein diets. *Am J Physiol* 1993; 264:G1057-G1065.
762. Tews JK, Kim YW, Harper AE. Induction of threonine imbalance by dispensable amino acids: relation to competition for amino acid transport into brain. *J Nutr* 1979; 109(2):304-15.
763. Kim SW, Morris JG, Rogers QR. Dietary soybean protein decreases plasma taurine in cats. *J Nutr* 1995; 125(11):2831-7.
764. Moundras C, Remesy C, Demigne C. Dietary protein paradox: decrease of amino acid availability induced by high-protein diets. *Am J Physiol* 1993; 264:G1057-G1065.
765. Bistrian BR, Hoffer J, Young VR, et al. Metabolic effects of very-low-calorie weight reduction diets. *J Clin Invest* 1984; 73:750-758.
766. Czarnowski D, Langfort J, Pilis W, Gorski J. Effect of a low-carbohydrate diet on plasma and sweat ammonia concentrations during prolonged nonexhausting exercise. *Eur J Appl Physiol Occup Physiol* 1995; 70(1):70-4.
767. Hickson JF Jr, Johnson TE, Lee W, Sidor RJ Nutrition and the precontest preparations of a male bodybuilder. *J Am Diet Assoc* 1990; 90(2):264-7.
768. Shimazu M, Aoki H. [Amino acid metabolism in surgical stress]. Nippon Rinsho — *Jpn J Clin Med* 1992; 50(7):1626-30.
769. Kaimachnikov NP, Maevskii EI. [Model of regulating blood glucose level during physical load]. *Biofizika* 1982; 27(4):698-702.
770. Kuhn E. [The effect of work load on amino acid metabolism]. *Vnitr Lek* 1994; 40(7):411-5.
771. Felig P, Pozefsky T, Marliss E, Cahill Jr GF. Alanine: key role in gluconeogenesis. *Science* 1970; 167:1003-1004.
772. Felig P. The glucose-alanine cycle. *Metabolism* 1973; 22:179-207.
773. Labadie P. [Glucose-alanine cycle]. *Rev Prat* 1976; 26(43):3023-30.
774. Brodan V, Kuhn E, Pechar J, Tomkova D. Changes of free amino acids in plasma of healthy subjects induced by physical exercise. *Eur J Appl Physiol Occup Physiol* 1976; 35(1):69-77.
775. Chochinov RH, Perlman K, Moorhouse JA. Circulating alanine production and disposal in healthy subjects. *Diabetes* 1978; 27(3):287-95.
776. Sharmanov TSh, Mukhamedzhanov EK. [Synthesis, transport and utilization of alanine (alanine-glucose cycle)]. *Vopr Med Khim* 1981; 27(3):300-10.
777. Miller-Graber P, Lawrence L, Fisher M, Bump K, Foreman J, Kurcz E. Metabolic responses to ammonium acetate infusion in exercising horses. *Cornell Vet* 1991; 81(4):397-410.
778. Viru A, Litvinova L. Viru M. Smirnova T. Glucocorticoids in metabolic control during exercise: alanine metabolism. *J Appl Physiol* 1994 76(2):801-5, .
779. Consoli A, Nurjhan N, Reilly JJ Jr, Bier DM, Gerich JE. Contribution of liver and skeletal muscle to alanine and lactate metabolism in humans. *Am J Physiol* 1990; 259:E677-E684.
780. Hoffer LJ. Cori cycle contribution to plasma glucose appearance in man. *J Parenteral Enteral Nutr* 1990; 14(6):646-8.
781. Lee WN, Sorou S, Bergner EA. Glucose isotope, carbon recycling, and gluconeogenesis using [U-13C]glucose and mass isotopomer analysis. *Biochem Med Metab Biol* 1991; 45(3):298-309.
782. Brodan V, Kuhn E, Pechar J, Tomkova D. Changes of free amino acids in plasma of healthy subjects induced by physical exercise. *Eur J Appl Physiol Occup Physiol* 1976; 35(1):69-77.
783. Perriello G, Jorde R, Nurjhan N, Stumvoll M, Dailey G. Jenssen T. Bier DM. Gerich JE. Estimation of glucose-alanine-lactate-glutamine cycles in postabsorptive humans: role of skeletal muscle. *Am J Physiol* 1995; 269(3 Pt 1):E443-50.
784. Cuezva JM, Valcarce C, Chamorro M, Franco A, Mayor F. Alanine and lactate as gluconeogenic substrates during late gestation. *FEBS Lett* 1986; 194(2):219-23.
785. Abernethy PJ, Thayer R, Taylor AW. Acute and chronic responses of skeletal muscle to endurance and sprint exercise. A review. *Sports Med* 1990; 10(6):365-389.
786. Felig P. Amino acid metabolism in exercise. *Ann N Y Acad Sci* 1977; 301:56-63.
787. Lemon PW, Nagle FJ. Effects of exercise on protein and amino acid metabolism. *Med Sci Sports Exerc* 1981; 13(3):141-9.
788. Yang RD, Matthews DE, Bier DM, Wen ZM, Young VR. Response of alanine metabolism in humans to manipulation of dietary protein and energy intakes. *Am J Physiol* 1986; 250(1 Pt 1):E39-46.
789. Goldstein L, Newsholme EA. The formation of alanine from amino acids in diaphragm muscle of the rat. *Biochem J* 1976; 154:555-8.

790. Palmer TN, Caldecourt MA, Snell K, Sugden MC. Alanine and inter-organ relationships in branched-chain amino and 2-oxo acid metabolism. Review. *Biosci Rep* 1985; 5(12):1015-33.
791. Carraro F, Naldini A, Weber JM, Wolfe RR. Alanine kinetics in humans during low-intensity exercise. *Med Sci Sports Exerc* 1994; 26(3):348-53.
792. Einspahr KJ, Tharp G. Influence of endurance training on plasma amino acid concentrations in humans at rest and after intense exercise. *Int J Sports Med* 1989; 10(4):233-236.
793. Felig P, Pozefsky T, Marliss E, Cahill Jr GF. Alanine: key role in gluconeogenesis. *Science* 1970; 167:1003-1004.
794. Dohm GL, Tapscott EB, Kasperek GJ. Protein degradation during endurance exercise and recovery. *Med Sci Sports Exerc* 1987; 19(5 Suppl):pS166-71.
795. Dohm GL, Williams RT, Kasperek GJ, et al. Increased excretion of urea and N tau-methylhistidine by rats and humans after a bout of exercise. *J Appl Physiol: Respir Environ Exerc Physiol* 1982; 52(1):27-33.
796. Wiethop BV, Cryer PE. Glycemic actions of alanine and terbutaline in IDDM. *Diabetes* Care 1993; 16(8):1124-30.
797. Wiethop BV, Cryer PE. Alanine and terbutaline in treatment of hypoglycemia in IDDM. *Diabetes Care* 1993; 16(8):1131-6.
798. Venerando R, Miotto G, Kadowaki M, Siliprandi N, Mortimore GE. Multiphasic control of proteolysis by leucine and alanine in the isolated rat hepatocyte. *Am J Physiol* 1994; 266(2 Pt 1):C455-61.
799. Seglen PO, Solheim AE. Effects of aminooxyacetate, alanine and other amino acids on protein synthesis in isolated rat hepatocytes. *Biochim Biophys Acta* 1978; 520(3):630-41.
800. Rivas T, Urcelay E, Gonzalez-Manchon C, Parrilla R, Ayuso MS. Role of amino acid-induced changes in ion fluxes in the regulation of hepatic protein synthesis. *J Cell Physiol.* 1995; 163(2):277-84.
801. Dragan GI, Wagner W, Ploesteanu E. Studies concerning the ergogenic value of protein supply and L-carnitine in elite junior cyclists. *Physiologie* 1988; 25(3):129-132.
802. Dragan GI, Vasiliu A, Georgescu E. Research concerning the effects of Refit on elite weightlifters. *J Sports Med Phys Fitness* 1985; 25(4):246-250.
803. Dragan GI, Vasiliu A, Georgescu E. Effects of Refit on Olympic (sic) athletes. *Sportorvosi Szemle/Hung Rev Sports Med* 1985; 26(2):107-113.
804. Dragan I, Stroescu V, Stoian I, Georgescu E, Baloescu R. Studies regarding the efficiency of Supro isolated soy protein in Olympic athletes. *Rev Roum Physiol* 1992; 29(3-4):63-70.
805. Dragan GI, Ploesteanu E, Selejan V. Studies concerning the ergogenic value of Cantamega-2000 supply in top junior cyclists. *Rev Roum Physiol* 1991; 28(1-2):13-6.
806. Kreider RB, Klesges KH, Grindstaff P, et al. Effects of ingesting supplements designed to promote lean tissue accretion on body composition during resistance training. *Int J Sports Nutr* 1996; 6:234-246.
807. Lowenthal DT, Karni Y. The nutritional needs of athletes, In: V Herbert and GJ Subak-Sharpe, eds. *Total Nutrition: The Only Guide You'll Ever Need.* St. Martin's Press, New York 1995; 406.
808. Belford DA, Rogers ML, Regester GO, et al. Milk-derived growth factors as serum supplements for the growth of fibroblast and epithelial cells. *In Vitro Cell Dev Biol Anim* 1995; 31(10):752-60.
809. Horton BS. Commercial utilization of minor milk components in the health and food industries. *J Dairy Sci* 1995; 78(11):2584-9.
810. Bounous G, Gervais F, Amer V, Batist G, Gold P. The influence of dietary whey protein on tissue glutathione and the diseases of aging. *Clin Invest Med* 1989; 12(6):343-9.
811. Bounous G, Gold P. The biological activity of undenatured dietary whey proteins: role of glutathione. *Clin Invest Med* 1991; 14(4):296-309.
812. Bounous G, Batist G, Gold P. Immunoenhancing property of dietary whey protein in mice: role of glutathione. *Clin Invest Med* 1989 Jun; 12(3); 154-61.
813. Costantino-AM, Balzola-F, Bounous-G. [Changes in biliary secretory immunoglobulins A in mice fed whey proteins] *Minerva Dietol Gastroenterol* 1989 Oct-Dec; 35(4): 241-5.
814. Zhang X, Beynen AC, Lowering effect of dietary milk-whey protein v. casein on plasma and liver cholesterol concentrations in rats. *Br J Nutr* 1993; 70(1):139-46.
815. Bosselaers IE, Caessens PW, Van Boekel MA, Alink GM. Differential effects of milk proteins, BSA and soy protein on 4NQO- or MNNG-induced SCEs in V79 cells. *Food Chem Toxicol* 1994; 32(10):905-9.
816. Boza JJ, Martinez-Augustin O, Baro L, Suarez MD, Gil A. Protein v. enzymic protein hydrolysates. Nitrogen utilization in starved rats. *Br J Nutr* 1995; 73(1):65-71.
817. Baro L, Guadix EM, Martinez-Augustin O, Boza JJ, Gil A. Serum amino acid concentrations in growing rats fed intact protein vs. enzymatic protein hydrolysate-based diets. *Biol Neonate* 1995; 68(1):55-61.
818. Battermann W. Whey protein for athletes. *Dtsch Milchwirtsch* 1986; 37(33):1010-1012.
819. Boza JJ, Jimenez J, Martinez O, Suarez MD, Gil A. Nutritional value and antigenicity of two milk protein hydrolysates in rats and guinea pigs. *J Nutr* 1994; 124(10):1978-86.
820. Poullain MG, Cezard JP, Roger L, Mendy F. Effect of whey proteins, their oligopeptide hydrolysates and free amino acid mixtures on growth and nitrogen retention in fed and starved rats [published erratum appears in JPEN 1989; 13(6):595]. Jpen: *J Parenteral Enteral Nutr* 1989; 13(4):382-6.

821. Blackburn GL. Nutrition and inflammatory events: highly unsaturated fatty acids (omega-3 vs. omega-6) in surgical injury. *Proc Soc Exp Biol Med* 1992; 200(2): 183-188.
822. Oxidative muscular injury and its relevance to hyperthyroidism. Asayama-K, Kato-K *Free Radic Biol Med* 1990; 8(3): 293-303
823. Clarkson PM. Antioxidants and physical performance. *Crit Rev Food Sci Nutr* 1995; 35(1-2):131-41.
824. Sastre J, Asensi M, Gasco E, Pallardo FV, Ferrero JA. Furukawa T. Vina J. Exhaustive physical exercise causes oxidation of glutathione status in blood: prevention by antioxidant administration. *Am J Physiol* 1992; 263(5 Pt 2):R992-5.
825. Rowe B, Kudsk K, Borum P, et al. Effects of whey- and casein-based diets on glutathione and cysteine metabolism in ICU patients. *J Am Coll Nutr* 1994; 254: 535.
826. Odze RD, Wershil BK. Allergic colitis in infants. *J Pediatr* 1995; 126:163-170.
827. Gmoshinskii IV, Kruglik VI, Samenkova NF, Krzhechkovskaia VV. Zorin SN. Mazo VK. [Characteristics of peptide preparations obtained during enzymatic hydrolysis and ultrafiltration of milk proteins for use in specialized nutrition products]. *Vopr Pitan* 1991; (3):21-7.
828. Lee YH. Food-processing approaches to altering allergenic potential of milk-based formula. *J Pediatr* 1992; 121(5 Pt 2):S47-50.
829. Schmidt DG, Meijer RJ, Slangen CJ, van Beresteijn EC. Raising the pH of the pepsin-catalysed hydrolysis of bovine whey proteins increases the antigenicity of the hydrolysates. *Clin Exp Allergy* 1995; 25(10):1007-17.
830. Vandenplas Y, Hauser B, Van den Borre C, et al. Clybouw C. The long-term effect of a partial whey hydrolysate formula on the prophylaxis of atopic disease. *Eur J Pediatr* 1995; 154(6):488-94.
831. Boza JJ, Jimenez J, Martinez O, Suarez MD, Gil A. Nutritional value and antigenicity of two milk protein hydrolysates in rats and guinea pigs. *J Nutr* 1994; 124(10):1978-86.
832. McLeish CM, MacDonald A, Booth IW. Comparison of an elemental with a hydrolysed whey formula in intolerance to cows' milk. *Arch Dis Child* 1995; 73(3):211-5.
833. Grimble GK, Silk DB. The optimum form of dietary nitrogen in gastrointestinal disease: proteins, peptides or amino acids?. *Verh Dtsch Ges Inn Med* 1986; 92:674-85.
834. Grimble GK, Rees RG, Keohane PP, Cartwright T. Desreumaux M. Silk DB. Effect of peptide chain length on absorption of egg protein hydrolysates in the normal human jejunum. *Gastroenterology* 1987; 92(1):136-42.
835. Steinhardt HJ, Adibi SA. Kinetics and characteristics of absorption from an equimolar mixture of 12 glycyl-dipeptides in human jejunum. *Gastroenterology* 1986; 90(3):577-82.
836. Rerat A, Nunes CS, Mendy F, Roger L. Amino acid absorption and production of pancreatic hormones in non-anaesthetized pigs after duodenal infusions of a milk enzymic hydrolysate or of free amino acids. *Br J Nutr* 1988; 60(1):121-36.
837. Monchi M, Rerat AA. Comparison of net protein utilization of milk protein mild enzymatic hydrolysates and free amino acid mixtures with a close pattern in the rat. Jpen: *J Parenteral Enteral Nutr* 1993; 17(4):355-63.
838. Rerat A, Simoes-Nunes C, Mendy F, Vaissade P, Vaugelade P. Splanchnic fluxes of amino acids after duodenal infusion of carbohydrate solutions containing free amino acids or oligopeptides in the non-anaesthetized pig. *Br J Nutr* 1992; 68(1):111-38.
839. Ziegler F, Ollivier JM, Cynober L, Masini JP. Coudray-Lucas C. Levy E. Giboudeau J. Efficiency of enteral nitrogen support in surgical patients: small peptides v non-degraded proteins. *Gut* 1990; 31(11):1277-83.
840. Moriarty KJ, Hegarty JE, Fairclough PD, Kelly MJ, Clark ML. Dawson AM. Relative nutritional value of whole protein, hydrolysed protein and free amino acids in man. *Gut* 1985; 26(7):694-9.
841. Charlton MR, Adey DB, Nair KS. Evidence for a catabolic role of glucagon during an amino acid load. *J Clin Invest* 1996; 98(1):90-9.
842. May ME, Buse MG. Effects of branched-chain amino acids on protein turnover. *Diabetes Metab Rev*; 1989; 5(3):227-245.
843. Herrling PL. Synaptic physiology of excitatory amino acids. *Arzneim Forsch* 1992; 42(2A):202-8.
844. Watkins JC. Some chemical highlights in the development of excitatory amino acid pharmacology. *Can J Physiol Pharmacol* 1991; 69(7):1064-75.
845. Tsumoto T. Excitatory amino acid transmitters and their receptors in neural circuits of the cerebral neocortex. *Neurosci Res* 1990; 9(2):79-102.
846. Nieoullon A. [Excitatory amino acids, central nervous system neurotransmitters]. *Therapie* 1990; 45(3):281-5.
847. McEntee WJ, Crook TH. Glutamate: its role in learning, memory, and the aging brain. *Psychopharmacology* 1993; 111(4):391-401.
848. Danbolt NC. The high affinity uptake system for excitatory amino acids in the brain. *Prog Neurobiol* 44(4):377-96, 1994 Nov.
849. Headley PM, Grillner S. Excitatory amino acids and synaptic transmission: the evidence for a physiological function. *Trends Pharmacol Sci* 11(5):205-11, 1990 May.
850. Shinozaki H, Ishida M. Excitatory amino acids: physiological and pharmacological probes for neuroscience research. *Acta Neurobiol Exp* 53(1):43-51, 1993.

851. Krebs MO. [Excitatory amino-acids, a new class of neurotransmitters. Pharmacology and functional properties]. *Encephale* 18(3):271-9, 1992 May-Jun.
852. D'Angelo E, Rossi P. Excitatory amino acid regulation of neuronal functions. *Funct Neurol* 7(2):145-61, 1992 Mar-Apr.
853. Farooqui AA, Horrocks LA. Excitatory amino acid receptors, neural membrane phospholipid metabolism and neurological disorders. *Brain Res Brain Res Rev* 16(2):171-91, 1991 May-Aug.
854. Rothstein JD, Kuncl R, Chaudhry V, et al. Excitatory amino acids in amyotrophic lateral sclerosis: an update. *Ann Neurol* 1991; 30:224-5.
855. Fonnum F. Glutamate: a neurotransmitter in mammalian brain. *J Neurochem* 1984; 42:1-11.
856. Nicholls D, Attwell D. The release and uptake of excitatory amino acids. *Trends Pharmacol Sci* 1990; 11:462-8.
857. Haber SN. Neurotransmitters in the human and nonhuman primate basal ganglia. *Hum Neurobiol* 5(3):159-68, 1986.
858. D'Souza SW, Slater P. Excitatory amino acids in neonatal brain: contributions to pathology and therapeutic strategies. *Arch Dis Child* Fetal & Neonatal Edition. 72(3):F147-50, 1995 May.
859. Singewald N, Zhou GY, Schneider C. Release of excitatory and inhibitory amino acids from the locus coeruleus of conscious rats by cardiovascular stimuli and various forms of acute stress. *Brain Res* 704(1):42-50, 1995 Dec 15.
860. Gietzen DW, Dixon KD, Truong BG, Jones AC, Barrett JA, Washburn DS. Indispensable amino acid deficiency and increased seizure susceptibility in rats. *Am J Physiol* 271(1 Pt 2):R18-24, 1996 Jul.
861. Ostroverkhov GE, Khokhlov AP, Maliugin EF, Terent'eva VB, Rykov VI. [Hepatoprotective effect of glutamine]. *Ter Arkh* 1974; 46 (1):89-96.
862. Kendler BS. Taurine: an overview of its role in preventive medicine. *Prev Med* 1989; 18 (1):79-100.
863. Johnson P, Hammer JL. Histidine dipeptide levels in ageing and hypertensive rat skeletal and cardiac muscles. *Comp Biochem Physiol B Comp Biochem* 1992; 103/4:981-984.
864. Brooks GA. Amino acid and protein metabolism during exercise and recovery. *Med Sci Sports Exerc* 1987; 19(5):S150-S156.
865. Algert SJ; Stubblefield NE; Grasse BJ; Shragg GP; Connor JD. Assessment of dietary intake of lysine and arginine in patients with herpes simplex. *J Am Diet Assoc* 1987; 87(11):1560-1561.
866. Mgbodile MUK, Holscher M, Neal RA. Possible protective role for reduced glutathione in aflatoxin B1 toxicity: effect of pretreatment of rats with phenobarbital and 3-methylcholanthrene on aflatoxin toxicity. *Toxicol Appl Pharmacol* 1975; 34:128-142.
867. Ryle PR, Chakraborty J, Thomson AD. Effects of cysteine and antioxidants on the hepatic redox-state, acetaldehyde and triglyceride levels after acute ethanol dosing. *Alcohol* 1987, Suppl 1:289-293.
868. Buse MG, Reid SS. Leucine: a possible regulator of protein turnover in muscle. *J Clin Invest* 1975; 56:1250.
869. Rogers PJ, Blundell JE. Reanalysis of the effects of phenylalanine, alanine, and aspartame on food intake in human subjects [comment]. *Physiol Behav* 1994; 56(2):247-50.
870. Cooke JP, Singer AH, Tsao P, Zera P, Rowan RA, Billingham ME. Antiatherogenic effects of L-arginine in the hypercholesterolemic rabbit. *J Clin Invest* 1992; 90:1168-72.
871. Pitkow HS, Rainieri JJ, Dwyer P. Hormone potentiating capability of amino acids on lactational performance in rats injected with 7,12-dimethylbenzanthracene (DMBA) during gestation. *Drug Chem Toxicol* 1986; 9:15-23.
872. Cynober L. [Role of new nitrogen substrates during peri-operative artificial nutrition in adults]. [French] *Ann Fr Anesthes Reanimation* 1995; 14(Suppl 2):102-6.
873. Castellino P, Levin R; Shohat J, DeFronzo RA. Effect of specific amino acid groups on renal hemodynamics in humans. *Am J Physiol Renal Fluid Electrolyte Physiol* 1990; 258(4):F992-F997.
874. Svanberg E, Moller-Loswick AC, Matthews DE, et al. Effects of amino acids on synthesis and degradation of skeletal muscle proteins in humans. *Am J Physiol* 1996; 271(4 Pt 1):E718-E724.
875. Parry-Billings M, Blomstrand E, McAndrew N, Newsholme EA. A communicational link between skeletal muscle, brain, and cells of the immune system. *Int J Sports Med* 1990; 11(Suppl 2):S122-8.
876. Fernstrom JD. Dietary amino acids and brain function. *J Am Diet Assoc* 1994; 94(1):71-7.
877. Richard JW, Martin CL. Exercise, Plasma Composition, and Neurotransmission. Brouns F (ed): Advances in Nutrition and Top Sports. *Med Sport Sci* 1991; 32:94-109.
878. Lehnert H, Wurtman RJ. Amino acid control of neurotransmitter synthesis and release: physiological and clinical implications. *Psychother Psychosom* 1993; 60(1):18-32.
879. Harper AE, Peters JC. Protein intake, brain amino acid and serotonin concentrations and protein self-selection. *J Nutr* 1989; 119(5):677-89.
880. Pogson CI, Knowles RG, Salter M AF. The control of aromatic amino acid catabolism and its relationship to neurotransmitter amine synthesis. *Crit Rev Neurobiol* 1989; 5(1):29-64.
881. Currie PJ, Chang N, Luo S, Anderson GH. Microdialysis as a tool to measure dietary and regional effects on the complete profile of extracellular amino acids in the hypothalamus of rats. *Life Sci* 1995; 57(21):1911-23.

882. Rasmussen D. Effects of tyrosine and tryptophan ingestion on plasma catechloamine concentrations. *J Clin Endoerinol Metab* 1983; 57(4):760-763.
883. Lehnert H, Beyer J, Cloer E, Gutberlet I, Hellhammer DH. Effects of L-tryptophan and various diets on behavioral functions in essential hypertensives. *Neuropsychobiology* 1989; 21(2):84-9.
884. Feinberg SS, Halbreich U. Treatment-resistant depression. Part 3. Emerging options. *Drug Ther* 1985; 15:106-107; 110-111; 115-118 .
885. Crawford PM, Lloyd KG, Chadwick DW. CSF gradients for amino acid neurotransmitters. *J Neurol Neurosurg Psychiatry* 1988; 51(9):1193-1200.
886. Huxtable RJ. Taurine in the central nervous system and the mammalian actions of taurine. Prog Neurobiol 1989; 32(6):471-533.
887. Cavagnini F, Benetti G, Invitti C, Ramella G, Pinto M, Lazza M, Dubini A, Marelli A, Muller EE. Effect of gamma-aminobutyric acid on growth hormone and prolactin secretion in man: influence of pimozide and domperidone. *J Clin Endocrinol Metab* 1980; 51(4):789-792.
888. Merimee TJ, Rabinowitz D, Fineberg SE. Arginine-initiated release of human growth hormone. *N Engl J Med* 1969; 280(26):1434-1438.
889. Martin J. Neuroendocrine regulation of growth hormone secretion. *Pediatr Adolesc Endocrinol* 1983; 12:1-26.
890. Jacobson B. Effect of amino acids on growth hormone release. *Phys Sportsmed* 1990; 18(1):63-70.
891. Merimee TJ, Lillicrap DA, Rabinowitz D. Effect of arginine on serum-levels of growth-hormone. *Lancet* 1965; 2:668.
892. Merimee TJ, Rabinowitz D, Riggs L, et al. Plasma growth hormone after arginine infusion: clinical experiences. *N Engl J Med* 1967; 276:434.
893. Knopf RF, Conn JW, Fajans SS, et al. Plasma growth hormone response to intravenous administration of amino acids. *J Clin Endocrinol Metab* 1965; 25:1140.
894. Bucci LR, Hickson JF Jr, Pivarnik JM, et al. Ornithine ingestion and growth hormone release in bodybuilders. *Nutr Res* 1990; 10(3):239-245.
895. Iwasaki K, Mano K, Ishihara M, Yugari Y, Matsuzawa T. Effects of ornithine or arginine administration on serum amino acid levels. *Biochem Int* 1987; 14(5):971-976.
896. Bucci LR, Hickson JF Jr, Wolinsky I, Pivarnik JM. Ornithine supplementation and insulin release in bodybuilders. *Int J Sport Nutr* 1992; 2(3):287-91.
897. Fogelholm GM, Naveri HK, Kiilavuori KT, Harkonen MH. Low-dose amino acid supplementation: no effects on serum human growth hormone and insulin in male weightlifters. *Int J Sport Nutr* 1993; 3(3):290-7.
898. Lambert MI, Hefer JA, Millar RP, Macfarlane PW. Failure of commercial oral amino acid supplements to increase serum growth hormone concentrations in male body-builders. *Int J Sport Nutr* 1993; 3(3):298-305.
899. Rodriguez DOL, Valeron MC, Carrillo DA, et al. [Evaluation of growth hormone stimulation tests using clonidine, glucagon, propanolol, hypoglycemia, arginine and L-dopa in 267 children of short stature]. *Rev Clin Esp* 1984; 173(2):113-116.
900. Ghigo E, Bellone J, Mazza E, et al. Arginine potentiates the GHRH- but not the pyridostigmine-induced GH secretion in normal short children. Further evidence for a somatostatin suppressing effect of arginine. *Clin Endocrinol* 1990; 32(6):763-767.
901. Masuda A, Shibasaki T, Hotta M, et al. Insulin-induced hypoglycemia, L-dopa and arginine stimulate GH secretion through different mechanisms in man. *Regul Pept* 1990; 31(1):53-64.
902. Vance MA, Gray PD, Tolman KG. Effect of glycine on valproate toxicity in rat hepatocytes. *Epilepsia* 1994; 35(5):101-22.
903. Nichols JC, Bronk SF, Mellgren RL, Gores GJ. Inhibition of nonlysosomal calcium-dependent proteolysis by glycine during anoxic injury of rat hepatocytes. *Gastroenterology* 1994; 106(1):168-76.
904. den Butter G, Lindell SL, et al. Effect of glycine in dog and rat liver transplantation. *Transplantation* 1993; 56(4):817-22.
905. Endre ZH, Cowin GJ, Stewart-Richardson P, Cross M. Willgoss DA. Duggleby RG. 23Na NMR detects protection by glycine and alanine against hypoxic injury in the isolated perfused rat kidney. *Biochem Biophys Res Commun* 1994; 202(3):1639-44.
906. Rouse K, Nwokedi E, Woodliff JE, Epstein J, Klimberg VS. Glutamine enhances selectivity of chemotherapy through changes in glutathione metabolism. *Ann Surg* 1995; 221(4):420-6.
907. Dragan I, Georgescu E, Bendiu P. Comparative studies concerning the efficiency of some hepatotropic drugs in top athletes, suffering from chronic hepatitis. *Med Sport* 1988; 62(4):199-201.
908. May ME, Buse MG. Effects of branched-chain amino acids on protein turnover. *Diabetes Metab Rev* 1989; 5(3):227-245.
909. Nair KS, Schwartz RG, Welle S. Leucine as a regulator of whole body and skeletal muscle protein metabolism in humans. *Am J Physiol* 1992; 263(5 Pt 1):E928-34.
910. Shinnick FL, Harper AE. Effects of branched-chain amino acid antagonism in the rat on tissue amino acid and keto acid concentrations. *J Nutr* 1977; 107(5):887-95.
911. Boirie Y, Gachon P, Corny S, et al. Acute postprandial changes in leucine metabolism as assessed with an intrinsically labeled milk protein. Am. J. Physiol. 1996; 271(6 Pt 1):E1083-91.

912. Louard RJ, Barrett EJ, Gelfand RA. Effect of infused branched-chain amino acids on muscle and whole-body amino acid metabolism in man. *Clin Sci* 1990; 79:457-466.
913. Candeloro N, Bertini I, Melchiorri G, De Lorenzo A. [Effects of prolonged administration of branched-chain amino acids on body composition and physical fitness]. [Italian] *Minerva Endocrinol* 1995; 20(4):217-23.
914. Palmer TN, Gossain S, Sugden MC. Partial oxidation of leucine in skeletal muscle. *Biochem Mol Biol Int* 1993; 29(2):255-62.
915. Sherwin RS, Hendler RG, Felig P. Effect of ketone infusions on amino acids and nitrogen metabolism in man. *J Clin Invest* 1975; 55:1382-1390.
916. Pawan GL, Semple SJ. Effect of 3-Hydroxybutyrate in obese subjects on very-low-energy diets. *Lancet* 1983; 1(8):15-18.
917. Thompson JR, Wu G. The effect of ketone bodies on nitrogen metabolism in skeletal muscle. *Comp Biochem Physiol* 1991; 100(2):209-16.
918. Alvestrand A, Hagenfeldt L, Merli M, Oureshi A, Eriksson LS. Influence of leucine infusion on intracellular amino acids in humans. *Eur J Clin Invest* 1990; 20(3):293-8.
919. Blomstrand E, Newsholme EA. Effect of branched-chain amino acid supplementation on the exercise-induced change in aromatic amino acid concentration in human muscle. *Acta Physiol Scand* 1992; 146:293-298.
920. Montoya A, Gomez-Lechon MJ, Castell JV. Influence of branched-chain amino acid composition of culture media on the synthesis of plasma proteins by serum-free cultured rat hepatocytes. *In Vitro Cell Dev Biol* 1989; 25(4):358-364.
921. Hunter DC, Weintraub M, Blackburn GL, Bistrian BR. Branched chain amino acids as the protein component of parenteral nutrition in cancer cachexia. *Br J Surg* 1989; 76(2):149-153.
922. Schott KJ, Gehrmann J, Potter U, Neuhoff V. On the role of branched-chain amino acids in protein turnover of skeletal muscle. Studies in vivo with L-norleucine. *Z Naturforsch [C]* 1985; 40(5-6):427-437.
923. Dohm GL, Beecher GR, Warren RQ, Williams RT. Influence of exercise on free amino acid concentrations in rat tissues. *J Appl Physiol: Respir Environ Exerc Physiol* 1981; 50(1):41-4.
924. Askanazi JYA, Carpentier CB, et al. Muscle and Plasma Amino Acids Following Injury: Influence of Intercurrent Infection. *Ann Surg* 1980: 192:78-85.
925. Henriksson J. Effect of exercise on amino acid concentrations in skeletal muscle and plasma. *J Exp Biol* 1991; 160:149-165.
926. Adibi SA. *Metabolism* of branched-chain amino acids in altered nutrition. *Metab Clin Exp* 1976; 25(11):1287-302.
927. Carli G, Bonifazi M, Lodi L, et al. Changes in the exercise-induced hormone response to branched chain amino acid administration. *Eur J Appl Physiol* 1992; 64:272-277.
928. Carli G, Bonifazi M, Lodi L, et al. Changes in the exercise-induced hormone response to branched chain amino acid administration. *Eur J Appl Physiol* 1992; 64:272-277.
929. Buse MG. In vivo effects of branched chain amino acids on muscle protein synthesis in fasted rats. *Horm Metab Res* 1981; 13:502-505.
930. Kraemer WJ. Endocrine response to resistance exercise. *Med Sci Sports Exerc* 1988; 20:S152-S157.
931. Essen P, Heys SD, Garlick P, Wernerman J. The separate and combined effect of leucine and insulin on muscle free amino acids. *Clin Physiol* 1994; 14(5):513-25.
932. Torres N, Tovar AR, Harper AE. Leucine affects the metabolism of valine by isolated perfused rat hearts: relation to branched-chain amino acid antagonism. *J Nutr* 1995; 125(7):1884-93.
933. Blomstrand E, Newsholme EA. Effect of branched-chain amino acid supplementation on the exercise-induced change in aromatic amino acid concentration in human muscle. *Acta Physiol Scand* 1992; 146:293-298.
934. Blomstrand E, Celsing F, Newsholme EA. Changes in plasma concentrations of aromatic and branched-chain amino acids during sustained exercise in man and their possible role in fatigue. *Acta Physiol Scand* 1988; 133:115-122.
935. Ji LL, Miller RH, Nagle FJ, Lardy HA, Stratman FW. Amino acid metabolism during exercise in trained rats: the potential role of carnitine in the metabolic fate of branched-chain amino acids. *Metabolism* 1987; 36(8):748-52.
936. Fukagawa NK, Minaker KL, Young VR, Rowe JW. Insulin dose-dependent reductions in plasma amino acids in man. *Am J Physiol* 1986; 250(1 Pt 1):E13-7.
937. Buckspan, R. Alpha-Ketoiso-Caproate is superior to leucine in sparing glucose utilization in humans. *Am J Physiol* 1986; 251:E648-653.
938. Laouari G. Efficacy of substituation of 2-ketoisocaproic acid and 2-ketoisovaleric acid in the diet of normal and uremic growing rats. *Am J Clin Nutr* 1986; 44:832-846.
939. Alvestrand A, Hagenfeldt L, Merli M, Oureshi A, Eriksson LS. Influence of leucine infusion on intracellular amino acids in humans. *Eur J Clin Invest* 1990; 20(3):293-8.
940. Flakoll PJ, VandeHaar MJ, Kuhlman G, Nissen S. Influence of alpha-ketoisocaproate on lamb growth, feed conversion, and carcass composition. *J Anim Sci* 1991; 69(4):1461-7.
941. Riedel E, Hampl H, Nundel M, Farshidfar G. Essential branched-chain amino acids and alpha-ketoanalogues in haemodialysis patients. *Nephrol Dialysis Transplant* 1992; 7(2):117-20.

942. Mitch WE, Clark AS. Specificity of the effects of leucine and its metabolites on protein degradation in skeletal muscle. *Biochem J* 1984; 222:579-586.
943. Stewart PM, Walser M, Drachman DB. *Muscle Nerve* 1982; 5:197-201.
944. Young VR, Munro HN. N-Methylhistidine (3-methylhistidine) and muscle protein turnover: an overview, *Fed Proc* 1978; 37:2291-2300.
945. Tischler ME, Desautels M, Goldberg AL. Does leucine, leucyl-tRNA, or some metabolite of leucine regulate protein synthesis and degradation in skeletal and cardiac muscle? *J Biol Chem* 1982; 257:1613-1621.
946. Brouwer AE, Carroll PB, Atwater IJ. Effects of leucine on insulin secretion and beta cell membrane potential in mouse islets of Langerhans. *Pancreas* 1991; 6(2):221-8.
947. Van Koevering M, Nissen S. Oxidation of leucine and alpha-ketoisocaproate to beta-hydroxy-beta-methylbutyrate in vivo. *Am J Physiol* 1992; 262(1 Pt 1):E27-31.
948. Nissen S, Fuller JC Jr, Sell J, Ferket PR, Rives DV. The effect of beta-hydroxy-beta-methylbutyrate on growth, mortality, and carcass qualities of broiler chickens. *Poult Sci* 1994; 73(1):137-55.
949. Gatnau R, Zimmerman DR, Nissen SL, Wannemuehler M, Ewan RC. Effects of excess dietary leucine and leucine catabolites on growth and immune responses in weanling pigs. *J Anim Sci* 1995; 73(1):159-65.
950. Nissen S, Faidley TD, Zimmerman DR, Izard R, Fisher CT. Colostral milk fat percentage and pig performance are enhanced by feeding the leucine metabolite beta-hydroxy-beta-methyl butyrate to sows. *J Anim Sci* 1994; 72(9):2331-7.
951. Van Koevering MT, Dolezal HG, Gill DR, Owens FN, Strasia CA, Buchanan DS, Lake R, Nissen S. Effects of beta-hydroxy-beta-methyl butyrate on performance and carcass quality of feedlot steers. *J Anim Sci* 1994; 72(8):1927-35.
952. Nonnecke BJ, Franklin ST, Nissen SL. Leucine and its catabolites alter mitogen-stimulated DNA synthesis by bovine lymphocytes. *J Nutr* 1991; 121(10):1665-72.
953. Nissen S, Sharp R, Ray M, et al. Effect of leucine metabolite beta-hydroxy-beta-methylbutyrate on muscle metabolism during resistance-exercise training. *J Appl Physiol* 1996; 81(5):2095-2104.
953a. Abstract numbers 875, 2167, 2168, 2172, 2175, 2204. *FASEB J.* 11.3, 1997: A150, A374-A376, A381.
954. Kayser BEJ, Hoppeler J, Claassen H, et al. Muscle ultrastructure and performance capacity of Himalayan Simpas. *J Appl Physiol* 1991; 74:1938-192.
955. Schena F, Guerrini F, Tregnaghi P, et al., Branched-chain amino acid supplementation during trekking at high altitude. *Eur J Appl Physiol* 1992; 65:394-398.
956. Bennet WM, Connacher AA, Scrimgeour CM, et al. Euglycemic hyperinsulinemia augments amino acid uptake by human leg tissues during hyperaminoacidemia. *Am J Physiol* 1990; 259:E185-E194.
957. Bennet WM, Connacher AA, Scrimgeour CM, et al. The effect of amino acid infusion on leg protein turnover assessed by L-[15N]phenylalanine and L-[l-13C]leucine exchange. *Eur J Clin Invest* 1990; 20:41-50.
958. Bennet WM, Conacher AA, Scrimgeour CM, et al. Increase in anterior tibialis protein synthesis in healthy man during mixed amino acid infusion: studies of incorporation of [l-13C]leucine. *Clin Sci* 1989; 76:447-454.
959. Kettlehut IC, Wing SS, Goldberg AL. Endocrine regulation of protein breakdown in skeletal muscle. *Diabetes Metab Rev* 1988; 8:441-448.
960. Mercer LP, Dodds SJ, Schweisthal MR, Dunn JD. Brain histidine and food intake in rats fed diets deficient in single amino acids. *J Nutr* 1989; 119(1):66-74.
961. Reeve VE, Bosnic M, Rozinova E. Carnosine (beta alanylhistidine) protects from the suppression of contact hypersensitivity by ultraviolet B (280-320 nm) radiation or by cis urocanic acid. *Immunology* 1993; 78(1):99-104.
962. Boldyrev AA, Koldobski A, Kurella E, Maltseva V, Stvolinski S. Natural histidine-containing dipeptide carnosine as a potent hydrophilic antioxidant with membrane stabilizing function. A biomedical aspect. *Mol Chem Neuropathol* 1993; 19(1-2):185-92.
963. Hipkiss AR, Michaelis J, Syrris P, Kumar S, Lam Y. Carnosine protects proteins against in vitro glycation and cross-linking. *Biochem Soc Trans* 1994; 22(4):399S.
964. Stvolinskii SL, Kotlobai AA, Boldyrev AA. [The pharmacological activity of carnosine]. *Eksp Klin Farmakol* 1995; 58(2):66-74.
965. Babizhayev MA, Seguin MC, Gueyne J, Evstigneeva RP, Ageyeva EA, Zheltukhina GA. L-carnosine (beta-alanyl-L-histidine) and carcinine (beta-alanylhistamine) act as natural antioxidants with hydroxyl-radical-scavenging and lipid-peroxidase activities. *Biochem J* 1994; 304(Pt 2):509-16.
966. Johnson P, Hammer JL. Histidine dipeptide levels in ageing and hypertensive rat skeletal and cardiac muscles. *Comp Biochem Physiol B Comp Biochem* 1992; 103(4):981-984.
967. Chan WK, Decker EA, Chow CK, Boissonneault GA. Effect of dietary carnosine on plasma and tissue antioxidant concentrations and on lipid oxidation in rat skeletal muscle. *Lipids* 1994; 29(7):461-6.
968. Boldyrev A, Abe H, Stvolinsky S, Tyulina O. Effects of carnosine and related compounds on generation of free oxygen species: a comparative study. *Comp Biochem Physiol B Biochem Mol Biol* 1995; 112(3):481-5.
969. Boldyrev AA. [Carnosine metabolism in excitable tissues: biological significance]. *Vestn Ross Akad Med Nauk* 1995; (6):3-7.

970. Dupin AM. Bemanandzara M. Stvolinskii SL. Boldyrev AA. Severin SE. [Muscle dipeptides — natural inhibitors of lipid peroxidation]. [Russian] *Biokhimiia* 1987; 52(5):782-7.
971. Boldyrev AA, Severin SE. The histidine-containing dipeptides, carnosine and anserine: distribution, properties and biological significance. *Adv Enzyme Regul* 1990; 30:175-94.
972. Tesch PA, Colliander EB, Kaiser P. Muscle metabolism during intense, heavy-resistance exercise. *Eur J Appl Physiol* 1986; 55(4):362-366.
973. Norman B, Sollevi A, Kaijser L, Jansson E. ATP breakdown products in human skeletal muscle during prolonged exercise to exhaustion. *Clin Physiol* 1987; 7(6):503-10.
974. Ballmer PE, McNurlan MA, Hulter HN, Anderson SE, Garlick PJ, Krapf R. Chronic metabolic acidosis decreases albumin synthesis and induces negative nitrogen balance in humans. *J Clin Invest* 1995; 95(1):39-45.
975. Layzer RB. Muscle metabolism during fatigue and work. Baillieres *Clin Endocrinol Metab* 1990; 4(3):441-59.
976. Degroot M, Massie BM, Boska M, Gober J, Miller RG, Weiner MW. Dissociation of [H^+] from fatigue in human muscle detected by high time resolution 31P-NMR. *Muscle Nerve* 1993; 16(1):91-8.
977. Mainwood GW, Renaud JM. The effect of acid-base balance on fatigue of skeletal muscle. *Can J Physiol Pharmacol* 1985; 63(5):403-16.
978. Le Rumeur E, Le Moyec L, Toulouse P, Le Bars R, de Certaines JD. Muscle fatigue unrelated to phosphocreatine and pH: an "in vivo" 31-P NMR spectroscopy study. *Muscle Nerve* 1990; 13(5):438-44.
979. Fujimoto T, Nishizono H. Involvement of membrane excitation failure in fatigue induced by intermittent submaximal voluntary contraction of the first dorsal interosseous muscle. *J Sports Med Phys Fitness* 1993; 33(2):107-17.
980. Sjogaard G. Role of exercise-induced potassium fluxes underlying muscle fatigue: a brief review. *Can J Physiol Pharmacol* 1991; 69(2):238-45.
981. Kossler F, Caffier G, Lange F. [Problems of muscular fatigue — relationship to stimulation conduction velocity and K(+) concentration]. *Z Gesamte Hyg Ihre Grenzgeb* 1990; 36(7):354-6.
982. Juel C, Bangsbo J, Graham T, Saltin B. Lactate and potassium fluxes from human skeletal muscle during and after intense, dynamic, knee extensor exercise. *Acta Physiol Scand* 1990; 140(2):147-59.
983. Reaich D, Channon SM, Scrimgeour CM, Goodship TH. Ammonium chloride-induced acidosis increases protein breakdown and amino acid oxidation in humans. *Am J Physiol* 1992; 263(4 Pt 1):E735-9.
984. Parkhouse WS, McKenzie DC. Possible contribution of skeletal muscle buffers to enhanced anaerobic performance: a brief review. *Med Sci Sports Exerc* 1984; 16(4):328-338.
985. Duffy DJ, Conlee RK. Effects of phosphate loading on leg power and high intensity treadmill exercise. *Med Sci Sports Exerc* 1986; 18(6):674-677.
986. Chan KM, Decker EA. Endogenous skeletal muscle antioxidants. *Crit Rev Food Sci Nutr* 1994; 34(4):403-26.
987. Jackson MC, Lenney JF. The distribution of carnosine and related dipeptides in rat and human tissues. *Inflammation Research* 1996; 45(3):132-5.
988. Hong H, Johnson P. Histidine dipeptide levels in exercised and hypertensive rat muscles. *Biochem Soc Trans* 1995; 23(4):542S.
989. Bakardjiev A, Bauer K. Transport of beta-alanine and biosynthesis of carnosine by skeletal muscle cells in primary culture. *Eur J Biochem* 1994; 225(2):617-23.
990. Bauer K, Schulz M. Biosynthesis of carnosine and related peptides by skeletal muscle cells in primary culture. *Eur J Biochem* 1994; 219(1-2):43-7.
991. Cade R, Conte M, Zauner C, et al. Effects of phosphate loading on 2,3-diphosphoglycerate and maximal oxygen uptake. *Med Sci Sports Exerc* 1984; 16:263.
992. Kraemer WJ, Gordon SE, Lynch JM, Pop ME, Clark KL. Effects of multibuffer supplementation on acid-base balance and 2,3-diphosphoglycerate following repetitive anaerobic exercise. *Int J Sport Nutr* 1995; 5(4):300-14.
993. Goldfinch J, McNaughton L, Davies P. Induced metabolic alkalosis and its effects on 400-m racing time. *Eur J Appl Physiol Occup Physiol* 1988; 57(1):45-48.
994. Rupp JC, Bartels RL, Zuelzer W, Fox EL, Clark RN. Effect of sodium bicarbonate ingestion on blood and muscle pH and exercise performance. *Med Sci Sports Exerc* 1983; 15:115-122.
995. Gordon SE, Kraemer WJ, Pedro JG. Increased acid-base buffering capacity via dietary supplementation: Anaerobic exercise implications. *J Appl Nutr* 1991; 43(1):40-48.
996. Ayala E, Krikorian DJ. Effect of L-lysine monohydrochloride on cutaneous herpes simplex virus in the guinea pig. *J Med Virol* May 1989, 28 (1) p16-20.
997. Bach A. [Carnitine biosynthesis in mammals]. [French] *Reprod Nutr Dev* 1982; 22(4):583-96.
998. Gilbert EF. Carnitine deficiency. *Pathology* 1985; 17(2):161-71.
999. Fernandez Ortega MF. Effect of dietary lysine level and protein restriction on the lipids and carnitine levels in the liver of pregnant rats. *Ann Nutr Metab* 1989; 33(3):162-9.
1000. Rebouche CJ, Bosch EP, Chenard CA, Schabold KJ, Nelson SE. Utilization of dietary precursors for carnitine synthesis in human adults. *J Nutr* 1989; 119(12):1907-13.

1001. Berner YN, Larchian WA, Lowry SF, Nicroa RR, Brennan MF, Shike M. Low plasma carnitine in patients on prolonged total parenteral nutrition: association with low plasma lysine. *J Parenteral Enteral Nutr* 1990 May-Jun; 14(3):255-8.
1002. Borum PR, Broquist HP. Lysine deficiency and carnitine in male and female rats. *J Nutr* 1977; 107(7):1209-15.
1003. Khan L, Bamji MS. Tissue carnitine deficiency due to dietary lysine deficiency: triglyceride accumulation and concomitant impairment in fatty acid oxidation. *J Nutr* 1979; 109(1):24-31.
1004. Dunn WA, Rettura G, Seifter E, Englard S. Carnitine biosynthesis from gamma-butyrobetaine and from exogenous protein-bound 6-N-trimethyl-L-lysine by the perfused guinea pig liver. Effect of ascorbate deficiency on the in situ activity of gamma-butyrobetaine hydroxylase. *J Biol Chem* 1984; 259(17):10764-70.
1005. Nelson PJ, Pruitt RE, Henderson LL, Jenness R, Henderson LM. Effect of ascorbic acid deficiency on the in vivo synthesis of carnitine. *Biochim Biophys Acta* 1981; 672(1):123-7.
1006. Rebouche CJ, Bosch EP, Chenard CA, Schabold KJ, Nelson SE. Utilization of dietary precursors for carnitine synthesis in human adults. *J Nutr* 1989; 119(12):1907-13.
1007. Choi YR, Fogle PJ, Bieber LL. The effect of long-term fasting on the branched chain acylcarnitines and branched chain carnitine acyltransferases. *J Nutr* 1979; 109(1):155-61.
1008. Rubaltelli FF, Orzali A, Rinaldo P, Donzelli F, Carnielli V. Carnitine and the premature. *Biol Neonate* 1987; 52 Suppl 1:65-77.
1009. Di Pasquale MG. L-Carnitine and Ketones. *Drugs Sports* 1992; 1(4):6-8.
1010. Paul HS, Adibi SA. Effect of carnitine on branched-chain amino acid oxidation by liver and skeletal muscle. *Am J Physiol* 1978; 234(5):E494-9.
1011. Paulson DJ, Hoganson GE, Traxler J, Sufit R, Peters H, Shug AL. Ketogenic effects of carnitine in patients with muscular dystrophy and cytochrome oxidase deficiency. *Biochem Med Metab Biol* 1988; 39(1):40-47.
1012. Sherwin RS, Hendler RG, Felig P. Effect of ketone infusions on amino acids and nitrogen metabolism in man. *J Clin Invest* 1975; 55:1382-1390.
1013. Pawan GL, Semple SJ. Effect of 3-Hydroxybutyrate in obese subjects on very-low-energy diets. *Lancet*, 1983; l(8):15-18.
1014. Fain, J, N. Biochemical aspects of drug and hormone action on adipose tissue *Pharmacol Rev* 25 67-118 Mar 1973.
1015. Tanphaichitr V, Zaklama MS, Brogquist HP. Dietary lysine and carnitine: relation to growth and fatty livers in rats. *J Nutr* 1976; 106:111-117.
1016. Khan L, Bamji M. Tissue carnitine deficiency due to dietary lysine deficiency: Triglyceride accumulation and concomitant impairment in fatty acid oxidation. *J Nutr* 1979; 109:24-31.
1017. Bernardini I, Rizzo WB, Dalakas M, et al. Plasma and muscle free carnitine deficiency due to renal Fanconi syndrome. *J Clin Invest* 1985; 75:1124-1130.
1018. Jacob C, Belleville F. [L-carnitine: metabolism, functions and value in pathology]. *Pathol Biol* 1992; 40(9):910-9.
1019. Jacob C, Belleville F. [L-carnitine: metabolism, functions and value in pathology]. *Pathol Biol* 1992; 40(9):910-9.
1020. Slonim AE, Borum PR, Tanaka K, et al. Dietary dependent carnitine deficiency as a cause of nonketotic hypoglycemia in an infant. *J Pediatr* 1981; 99:551-556.
1021. Helms RA, Whitington PF, Mauer EC, et al. Enhanced lipid utilization in infants receiving oral L-carnitine during long-term parenteral nutrition. *J Pediatr* 1986; 109:984-988.
1022. Vijayasarathy C, Khan-Siddiqui L, Murthy SN, Bamji MS. Rise in plasma trimethyllysine levels in humans after oral lysine load. *Am J Clin Nutr* 1987; 46(5):772-7.
1023. Bohmer-T, Weddington-S-C, Hansson-V. Effect of testosterone propionate on levels of carnitine and testicular androgen binding protein (ABP) in rat epididymis. *Endocrinology* 1977; 100(3):835-8.
1024. Carter AL, Stratman FW. Sex steroid regulation of urinary excretion of carnitine in rats. *J Steroid Biochem* 1982; 17(2):211-6.
1025. Krahenbuhl S. [Carnitine: vitamin or doping?]. *Ther Umsch* 1995; 52(10):687-92.
1026. Cerretelli P, Marconi C. L-carnitine supplementation in humans. The effects on physical performance. *Int J Sports Med* 1990; 11(1):1-14.
1027. Goa KL, Brogden RN. L-Carnitine. A preliminary review of its pharmacokinetics, and its therapeutic use in ischaemic cardiac disease and primary and secondary carnitine deficiencies in relationship to its role in fatty acid metabolism. *Drugs* 1987; 34(1):1-24.
1028. Hirata K, Yoshioka F, Eto Y, Suzuki K, Yokochi K, Kato H; Ohta K; Terasawa M. [Carnitine deficiency: a treatable cardiomyopathy]. *J Cardiogr* 1986; 16(1):217-225.
1029. Miyajima H, Sakamoto M, Takahashi Y, Mizoguchi K, Nishimura Y. [Muscle carnitine deficiency associated with myalgia and rhabdomyolysis following exercise] *Rinsho Shinkeigaku* 1989; 29(1):93-97.
1030. Brevetti G, Chiariello M, Ferulano G, Policicchio A, Nevola E; Rossini A; Attisano T; Ambrosio G; Siliprandi N; Angelini C. Increases in walking distance in patients with peripheral vascular disease treated with L-carnitine: a double-blind, cross-over study. *Circulation* 1988; 77(4):767-773.

1031. Bowyer BA, Fleming CR, Haymond MW, Miles JM. L-carnitine: effect of intravenous administration on fuel homeostasis in normal subjects and home-parenteral-nutrition patients with low plasma carnitine concentrations. *Am J Clin Nutr* 1989; 49(4):618-623.
1032. Arenas J, Ricoy JR, Encinas AR, Pola P, D'Iddio S, Zeviani M, Didonato S, Corsi M. Carnitine in muscle, serum, and urine of nonprofessional athletes: effects of physical exercise, training, and L-carnitine administration. *Muscle Nerve* Jul 1991, 14 (7) p598-604.
1033. Oyono-Enguelle S, Freund H, Ott C, Gartner M, Heitz A, Marbach J, Maccari F, Frey A, Bigot H, Bach AC. Prolonged submaximal exercise and L-carnitine in humans. *Eur J Appl Physiol* 1988; 58(1-2):53-61
1034. Marconi C, Sassi G, Carpinelli A, Cerretelli P. Effects of L-carnitine loading on the aerobic and anaerobic performance of endurance athletes. *Eur J Appl Physiol* 1985; 54(2):131-135.
1035. Gorostiaga EM, Maurer CA, Eclache JP. Decrease in respiratory quotient during exercise following L-carnitine supplementation. *Int J Sports Med* 1989; 10(3):169-174.
1036. Vecchiet L, Di Lisa F, Pieralisi G, Ripari P, Menabo R, Giamberardino MA, Siliprandi N. Influence of L-carnitine administration on maximal physical exercise. *Eur J Appl Physiol* 1990, 61 (5-6) p486-90.
1037. Siliprandi N, Di Lisa F, Pieralisi G, Ripari P, Maccari F, Menabo R, Giamberardino MA, Vecchiet L. Metabolic changes induced by maximal exercise in human subjects following L-carnitine administration. *Biochim Biophys Acta* 1990; 1034(1):17-21.
1038. Sahlin K. Muscle carnitine metabolism during incremental dynamic exercise in humans. Acta Physiol Scand 1990; 138(3):259-262.
1039. Dragan AM, Vasiliu D, Eremia NM, Georgescu E. Studies concerning some acute biological changes after endovenous administration of 1 g L-carnitine, in elite athletes. *Physiologie* 1987; 24(4):231-234.
1040. Huertas-R, Campos-Y, Diaz-E, Esteban-J, Vechietti-L, Montanari-G, D'Iddio-S, Corsi-M, Arenas-J. Respiratory chain enzymes in muscle of endurance athletes: Effect of L- carnitine. *Biochem Biophys Res Commun* 188/1 (102-107) 1992.
1041. Spagnoli LG, Palmieri G, Mauriello A, et al. Morphometric evidence of the trophic effect of L-carnitine on human skeletal muscle. *Nephron* 1990; 55(1): 16-23
1042. Cooper MB, Jones DA, Edwards RH, et al. The effect of marathon running on carnitine metabolism and on some aspects of muscle mitochondrial activities and antioxidant mechanisms. *J Sports Sci* 1986; 4(2):79-87.
1043. Lancha AH Jr, Recco MB, Abdalla DS, Curi R. Effect of aspartate, asparagine, and carnitine supplementation in the diet on metabolism of skeletal muscle during a moderate exercise. *Physiol Behav* 1995; 57(2):367-71.
1044. Minana MD, Felipo V, Wallace R, Grisolia S. Hyperammonemia decreases body fat content in rat. *FEBS Lett* 1989; 249(2):261-3.
1045. Matsuoka M, Igisu H. Comparison of the effects of L-carnitine, D-carnitine and acetyl-L-carnitine on the neurotoxicity of ammonia. *Biochem Pharmacol* 1993; 46(1):159-64.
1046. Soop M, Bjorkman O, Cederblad G, Hagenfeldt L, Wahren J. Influence of carnitine supplementation on muscle substrate and carnitine metabolism during exercise. *J Appl Physiol* 1988; 64(6):2394-2399.
1047. Greig C, Finch KM, Jones DA, Cooper M, Sargeant AJ, Forte CA. The effect of oral supplementation with L-carnitine on maximum and submaximum exercise capacity. *Eur J Appl Physiol* 1987; 56(4):457-460.
1048. Siliprandi N, Di Lisa F, Pieralisi G, Ripari P, Maccari F, Menabo R, Giamberardino MA, Vecchiet L. Metabolic changes induced by maximal exercise in human subjects following L-carnitine administration. *Biochim Biophys Acta* 1990; 1034(1):17-21.
1049. Rubaltelli FF, Orzali A, Rinaldo P, Donzelli F, Carnielli V. Carnitine and the premature. *Biol Neonate* 1987; 52(1):65-77.
1050. Stadler DD. Chenard CA. Rebouche CJ. Effect of dietary macronutrient content on carnitine excretion and efficiency of carnitine reabsorption. *Am J Clin Nutr.* 58(6):868-72, 1993.
1051. Rosenthal RE, Williams R, Bogaert YE, Getson PR, Fiskum G. Prevention of postischemic canine neurological injury through potentiation of brain energy metabolism by acetyl-L-carnitine. *Stroke* 1992; 23(9):1312-7; discussion 1317-8.
1052. Gasparetto A, Corbucci GG, De Blasi RA, et al. Influence of acetyl-L-carnitine infusion on haemodynamic parameters and survival of circulatory-shock patients. *Int J Clin Pharm Res* 1991; 11(2):83-92.
1053. Shug A, Paulson D, Subramanian R, Regitz V. Protective effects of propionyl-L-carnitine during ischemia and reperfusion. *Cardiovasc Drugs Ther* 1991; 5 Suppl 1:77-83.
1054. Castorina M, Ambrosini AM, Giuliani A, et al. A cluster analysis study of acetyl-L-carnitine effect on NMDA receptors in aging. *Exp Gerontol* 1993; 28(6):537-48.
1055. Castorina M, Ferraris L. Acetyl-L-carnitine affects aged brain receptorial system in rodents. *Life Sci.* 54(17):1205-14, 1994.
1056. Piovesan P, Pacifici L, Taglialatela G, Ramacci MT, Angelucci L. Acetyl-L-carnitine treatment increases choline acetyltransferase activity and NGF levels in the CNS of adult rats following total fimbria-fornix transection. *Brain Res* 633(1-2):77-82, 1994 Jan 7.
1057. Ruggiero FM, Cafagna F, Gadaleta MN, Quagliariello E. Effect of aging and acetyl-L-carnitine on the lipid composition of rat plasma and erythrocytes. *Biochem Biophys Res Commun* 1990; 170(2):621-6.

1058. Imperato A, Ramacci MT, Angelucci L. Acetyl L carnitine enhances acetylcholine release in the striatum and hippocampus of awake freely moving rats. *Neurosci Lett* 1989; 107(1-3):251-5.
1059. Sershen H, Harsing LG Jr, Banay-Schwartz M, Hashim A, Ramacci MT, Lajtha A. Effect of acetyl-L-carnitine on the dopaminergic system in aging brain. *J Neurosci Res* 1991; 30(3):555-9.
1060. Toth E, Harsing LG Jr, Sershen H, Ramacci MT, Lajtha A. Effect of acetyl-L-carnitine on extracellular amino acid levels in vivo in rat brain regions. *Neurochem Res* 1993; 18(5):573-8.
1061. Forloni G, Angeretti N, Smiroldo S. Neuroprotective activity of acetyl-L-carnitine: studies in vitro. *J Neurosci Res* 1994; 37(1):92-6.
1062. Aureli T, Miccheli A, Ricciolini R, et al. Aging brain: effect of acetyl-L-carnitine treatment on rat brain energy and phospholipid metabolism. A study by 31P and 1H NMR spectroscopy. *Brain Res* 1990; 526(1):108-12.
1063. Liu Y, Rosenthal RE, Starke-Reed P, Fiskum G. Inhibition of postcardiac arrest brain protein oxidation by acetyl-L-carnitine. *Free Radic Biol Med* 1993; 15(6):667-70.
1064. White HL, Scates PW. Acetyl-L-carnitine as a precursor of acetylcholine. *Neurochem Res* 1990; 15(6):597-601.
1065. Harman D. Free radical theory of aging: A hypothesis on pathogenesis of senile dementia of the Alzheimer's type. Age 1992; 16(1):23-30.
1066. Carta A, Calvani M, Bravi D, Bhuachalla SN. Acetyl-L-carnitine and Alzheimer's disease: pharmacological considerations beyond the cholinergic sphere. *Ann N Y Acad Sci* 1993; 695:324-6.
1067. Formenti A, Arrigoni E, Sansone V, Arrigoni Martelli E, Mancia M. Effects of acetyl-L-carnitine on the survival of adult rat sensory neurons in primary cultures. *Int J Dev Neurosci* 1992; 10(3):207-14.
1068. Rosenthal RE, Williams R, Bogaert YE, Getson PR, Fiskum G. Prevention of postischemic canine neurological injury through potentiation of brain energy metabolism by acetyl-L-carnitine. *Stroke* 1992; 23(9):1312-7; discussion 1317-8.
1069. Rampello L, Giammona G, Aleppo G, Favit A, Fiore L. Trophic action of acetyl-L-carnitine in neuronal cultures. *Acta Neurol* 1992; 14(1):15-21.
1070. Gasparetto A, Corbucci GG, De Blasi RA, et al. Influence of acetyl-L-carnitine infusion on haemodynamic parameters and survival of circulatory-shock patients. *Int J Clin Pharmacol Res* 1991; 11(2):83-92.
1071. Pettorossi VE, Brunetti O, Carobi C, Della Torre G, Grassi S. L-acetylcarnitine enhances functional muscle re-innervation. *Drugs Under Exp Clin Res* 1991; 17(2):119-25.
1072. Pettorossi VE, Draicchio F, Fernandez E, Pallini R. The influence of L-acetylcarnitine on reinnervation of the oculomotor nerve. *Int J Clin Pharmacol Res* 1993; 13(3):193-9.
1073. Formenti A, Arrigoni E, Sansone V, Arrigoni Martelli E, Mancia M. Effects of acetyl-L-carnitine on the survival of adult rat sensory neurons in primary cultures. *Int J Dev Neurosci* 1992; 10(3):207-14.
1074. Costell M, O'Connor JE, Grisolia S. Age-dependent decrease of carnitine content in muscle of mice and humans. *Biochem Biophys Res Commun* 1989; 161(3):1135-43.
1075. Ruggiero FM, Cafagna F, Gadaleta MN, Quagliariello E. Effect of aging and acetyl-L-carnitine on the lipid composition of rat plasma and erythrocytes. *Biochem Biophys Res Commun* 1990; 170(2):621-6.
1076. Pulvirenti G, Valerio C, Spadaro F, D'Agata V, Freni V, Nardo L, Drago F. Acetylcarnitine reduces the immobility of rats in a despair test (constrained swim). *Behav Neural Biol* 1990; 54(2):110-4.
1077. Garzya G, Corallo D, Fiore A, Lecciso G, Petrelli G, Zotti C. Evaluation of the effects of L-acetylcarnitine on senile patients suffering from depression. *Drugs Under Exp Clin Res* 1990; 16(2):101-6.
1078. Kim EK, Trevisani C, Trevisani M. [The action of carnitine-series preparations in experimental alloxan diabetes mellitus]. *Eksp Klin Farmakol* 1992; 55(4):35-6.
1079. Harris RC, Foster CV. Changes in muscle free carnitine and acetylcarnitine with increasing work intensity in the thoroughbred horse. *Eur J Appl Physiol Occup Physiol* 1990; 60(2):81-5.
1080. Harris RC, Foster CV, Hultman E. Acetylcarnitine formation during intense muscular contraction in humans. *J Appl Phys* 1987; 63(1):440-2.
1081. Ciman M, Caldesi Valeri V, Siliprandi N. Carnitine and acetylcarnitine in skeletal and cardiac muscle. *Int J Vitam Nutr Res* 1978; 48(2):177-81.
1082. Tanphaichitr V, Leelahagul P. Carnitine metabolism and human carnitine deficiency. *Nutrition* 1993; 9(3):246-54.
1083. Di Giacomo C, Latteri F, Fichera C, et al. Effect of acetyl-L-carnitine on lipid peroxidation and xanthine oxidase activity in rat skeletal muscle. *Neurochem Res* 1993; 18(11):1157-62.
1084. Boerrigter ME, Franceschi C, Arrigoni-Martelli E, Wei JY, Vijg J. The effect of L-carnitine and acetyl-L-carnitine on the disappearance of DNA single-strand breaks in human peripheral blood lymphocytes. *Carcinogenesis* 1993; 14(10):2131-6.
1085. Bidzinska B, Petraglia F, Angioni S, et al. Effect of different chronic intermittent stressors and acetyl-L-carnitine on hypothalamic beta-endorphin and GnRH and on plasma testosterone levels in male rats. *Neuroendocrinology* 1993; 57(6):985-90.

1086. Palmero S, Leone M, Prati M, Costa M, Messeni Leone M, Fugassa E, De Cecco L. The effect of L-acetylcarnitine on some reproductive functions in the oligoasthenospermic rat. *Horm Metabc Res* 1990; 22(12):622-6.
1087. Di Giacomo C, Latteri F, Fichera C, et al. Effect of acetyl-L-carnitine on lipid peroxidation and xanthine oxidase activity in rat skeletal muscle. *Neurochem Res* 1993; 18(11):1157-62.
1088. Moundras C, Remesy C, Levrat MA, Demigne C. Methionine deficiency in rats fed soy protein induces hypercholesterolemia and potentiates lipoprotein susceptibility to peroxidation. *Metab Clin Exp* 1995; 44(9):1146-52.
1089. Barak AJ, Beckenhauer HC, Junnila M, Tuma DJ. Dietary betaine promotes generation of hepatic S-adenosylmethionine and protects the liver from ethanol-induced fatty infiltration. *Alcoholism* 1993; 17(3):552-5.
1090. Trimble KC, Molloy AM, Scott JM, Weir DG. The effect of ethanol on one-carbon metabolism: increased methionine catabolism and lipotrope methyl-group wastage. *Hepatology* 1993; 18(4):984-9.
1091. Barak AJ, Beckenhauer HC, Junnila M, Tuma DJ. Dietary betaine promotes generation of hepatic S-adenosylmethionine and protects the liver from ethanol-induced fatty infiltration. *Alcoholism Clin Exp Res* 1993; 17(3):552-5.
1092. Storch KJ, Wagner DA, Burke JF, Young VR. (1-Carbon-13; methyl-Hydrogen-2 sub 3)-methionine kinetics in humans: methionine conservation and cystine sparing. *Am J Physiol* 1990; 258:E790-E798.
1093. Storch KJ, Wagner DA, Burke JF, et al. Quantitative study in vivo of methionine cycle in humans using (methyl-Hydrogen-2 sub 3)- and (1-Carbon-13)methionine. *Am J Physiol* 1988; 255:E322-31.
1094. Kien CL, Young VR, Rohrbaugh DK, et al. Increased rates of whole body protein synthesis and breakdown in children recovering from burns. *Ann Surg* 1978; 187:383-308.
1095. Yoshida A, Moritoki K. Nitrogen sparing action of methionine and threonine in rats receiving a protein-free diet. *Nutr Rep Int* 1974; 9:159-165.
1096. Millward DJ, Rivers JP. The need for indispensable amino acids: the concept of the anabolic drive. *Diabetes Metab Rev* 1989; 5(2):191-211.
1097. Yokogoshi H, Yoshida A. Some factors affecting the nitrogen sparing action of methionine and threonine in rats fed a protein free diet. *J Nutr* 1976; 106(1):48-57.
1098. Wolfe RR, Jahoor F, Hartl WH: Protein and amino acid metabolism after injury. *Diabetes Metab Rev* 1989; 5:149-154.
1099. Wolfe RR, Goodenough RD, Burke JF, et al. Response of protein and urea kinetics in burn patients to different levels of protein intake. *Ann Surg* 1983; 197:163-171.
1100. Young VR, Pellett PL. Some general considerations of amino acid and protein metabolism and nutrition. In Burke JF (ed), Surgical Physiology. Philadelphia, W.B. Saunders, 1983, pp 51-74.
1101. Yu, Yong-ming, Burke, John F. Young, Vernon R. A Kinetic Study of L-Hydrogen-2 sub 3-Methyl-1-Carbon-13-Methionine in Patients With Severe Burn Injury. *J Trauma* 1993; 35(1):1-7.
1102. Hiramatsu T, Fukagawa NK, Marchini JS, Cortiella J, Yu YM, Chapman TE, Young VR. Methionine and cysteine kinetics at different intakes of cystine in healthy adult men. *Am J Clin Nutr* 1994; 60(4):525-33.
1103. Hsu H, Yu YM, Babich JW, et al. Measurement of muscle protein synthesis by positron emission tomography with L-[methyl-11C]methionine. *Proc Natl Acad Sci U.S.A.* 1996; 93(5):1841-6.
1104. Krebs HA, Hems R, Tyler B. The regulation of folate and methionine metabolism. *Biochem J* 1976; 158:341-7.
1105. Zeisel SH, Costa K-AD, Franklin PD, et al. Choline, an essential nutrient for humans. *FASEB J* 1991; 5:2093-98.
1106. McGilvery RW, Goldsteine G (ed). *Biochemistry, A Functional Approach.* Philadelphia, W.B. Saunders, 1975, pp 589-615.
1107. Giulidori P, Galli Kienle M, Catto E, et al. Transmethylation, transsulfuration, and aminopropylation reactions of S-adenosyl-L-methionine in vivo. *J Biol Chem* 1984; 259:4205-11.
1108. Tabor CW, Tabor H. Polyamine. *Annu Rev Biochem* 1984; 53:749-57.
1109. Cederblad G, Larsson J, Nordstrom H, et al. Urinary excretion of carnitine in burned patients. *Burns* 1981; 8:102-108.
1110. Watson JD, Hopkins NH, Roberts JW, et al. (eds). The structures of DNA. In: *Molecular Biology of the Gene.* Menlo Park, Benjamin/Cummings 1987, pp 239-281.
1111. Iapichino G, Radrizzani D, Solca M, et al. Influence of total parenteral nutrition on protein metabolism following acute injury: Assessment by urinary 3-methylhistidine excretion and nitrogen balance. JPEN *J Parenteral Enteral Metab* 1985; 9:42.
1112. Juigens P, Dolif D. Nitrogen requirements in parenteral nutrition. *Nutr Metab* 1976; 20:34.
1113. Ingwall JS. Creatine and the control of muscle-specific protein synthesis in cardiac and skeletal muscle. *Circ Res* 1976; 38(5 Suppl 1):I115-23.
1114. Balsom PD, Soderlund K, Ekblom B. Creatine in humans with special reference to creatine supplementation. *Sports Med* 1994; 18(4):268-80.
1115. Harris RC, Soderlund K, Hultman E. Elevation of creatine in resting and exercised muscle of normal subjects by creatine supplementation. *Clin Sci* 1992; 83(3):367-374.

1116. Balsom PD, Harridge SD, Soderlund K, et al. Creatine supplementation and dynamic high-intensity intermittent exercise. *Scand J Med Sci Sport* 1993; 3:143-9.
1117. Greenhaff PL, Bodin K, Soderlund K, Hultman E. Effect of oral creatine supplementation on skeletal muscle phosphocreatine resynthesis. *Am J Physiol* 1994; 266(5 Pt 1):E725-30.
1118. Greenhaff PL, Casey A, Short AH, et al. Influence of oral creatine supplementation of muscle torque during repeated bouts of maximal voluntary exercise in man. *Clin Sci* 1993; 84(5):565-71.
1119. Birch R, Noble D, Greenhaff PL. The influence of dietary creatine supplementation on performance during repeated bouts of maximal isokinetic cycling in man. *Eur J Appl Physiol Occup Physiol* 1994; 69:268-70.
1120. Dawson B, Cutler M, Moody A, Lawrence S, Goodman C, Randall N. Effects of oral creatine loading on single and repeated maximal short sprints. *Aust J Sci Med Sport* 1995; 27(3):56-61.
1121. Balsom PD, Harridge SD, Soderlund K, Sjodin B, Ekblom B. Creatine supplementation per se does not enhance endurance exercise performance. *Acta Phys Scand* 1993; 149(4):521-3.
1122. Green AL, Simpson EJ, Littlewood JJ, et al. Carbohydrate ingestion augments creatine retention during creatine feeding in humans. *Acta Physiologica Scandinavica* 1996; 158(2):195-202.
1122a. Ferreira M, Kreider R, Wilson M, et al. Effects of Ingesting a supplement designed to enhance creatine uptake on strength and sprint capacity. Presneted May 30, 1997 at the American College of Sports Medicine Annual Meeting.
1123. Rossiter HB, Cannell ER, Jakeman PM. The effect of oral creatine supplementation on the 1000-m performance of competitive rowers. *J Sports Sci* 1996; 14(2):175-9.
1124. Casey A, Constantin-Teodosiu D, Howell S, et al. Creatine ingestion favorably affects performance and muscle metabolism during maximal exercise in humans. *Am J Physiol* 1996; 271(1 Pt 1):E31-7.
1125. Le Rumeur E, Le Moyec L, Toulouse P, et al. Muscle fatigue unrelated to phosphocreatine and pH: an 'in vivo' 31-P NMR spectroscopy study. *Muscle Nerve* 1990; 13(5):438-444.
1126. Barnett C, Hinds M, Jenkins DG. Effects of oral creatine supplementation on multiple sprint cycle performance. *Aust J Sci Med Sport* 1996; 28(1):35-9.
1127. Vandenberghe KN, Gillis M, Van Leemputte P, et al. Caffeine counteracts the ergogenic action of muscle creatine loading. *J Appl Physiol* 1996; in press.
1128. Fernstrom JD. Dietary effects on brain serotonin synthesis: relationship to appetite regulation. *Am J Clin Nutr.* 1985; 42(5 Suppl):1072-82.
1129. Kral' A. The role of pineal gland in circadian rhythms regulation. *Bratisl Lek Listy* 1994; 95(7):295-303.
1130. Huether G, Poeggeler B, Adler L, Ruther E. Effects of indirectly acting 5-HT receptor agonists on circulating melatonin levels in rats. *Eur J Pharmacol* 1993; 238(2-3):249-54.
1131. Heuther G, Hajak G, Reimer A, Poeggeler B, Blomer M. Rodenbeck A. Ruther E. The metabolic fate of infused L-tryptophan in men: possible clinical implications of the accumulation of circulating tryptophan and tryptophan metabolites. *Psychopharmacology* 1992; 109(4):422-32.
1132. Zimmermann RC, McDougle CJ, Schumacher M, Olcese J, Heninger GR, Price LH. Urinary 6-hydroxymelatonin sulfate as a measure of melatonin secretion during acute tryptophan depletion. *Psychoneuroendocrinology* 1993; 18(8):567-78.
1133. Zimmermann RC, McDougle CJ, Schumacher M, Olcese J, Mason JW, Heninger GR, Price LH. Effects of acute tryptophan depletion on nocturnal melatonin secretion in humans. *J Clin Endocrinol Metab* 1993; 76(5):1160-4.
1134. Muller EE, Branbilla F, Cavagnini F, et al. Slight effect of L-tryptophan on growth hormone release in normal human subjects. *J Clin Endocrinol Metab* 1974; 39:1-4.
1135. Segura, R, Ventura, J.L. Effect of L-tryptophan supplementation on exercise performance. *Int. J Sports Med* (Stuttgart) 9(5), Oct 1988.
1136. Stensrud T, Ingjer F, Holm H, Stromme SB. L-tryptophan supplementation does not improve running performance. *Int. J Sports Med* 1992; 13(6):481-485.
1137. Steinberg S, Annable L, Young SN, Belanger MC. Tryptophan in the treatment of late luteal phase dysphoric disorder: a pilot study. *J Psychiatry Neurosci* 1994; 19(2):114-9.
1138. Schneider-Helmert D, Spinweber CL. Evaluation of L-tryptophan for treatment of insomnia: a review. *Psychopharmacology* 1986; 89:1-7.
1139. Teman AJ, Hainline B. Eosinophilia-myalgia syndrome: athletes should discard dietary L-tryptophan. *Phys Sportsmed* 1991; 19(2):80-82; 84; 86.
1140. Centers for Disease Control. Eosinophilia-myalgia syndrome — New Mexico. MMWR. 1989; 38: 765-767.
1141. CDC Eosinophilia-myalgia syndrome and L-tryptophan-containing products — New Mexico, Minnesota, Oregon, and New York. MMWR 1989; 38:785.
1142. Swygert LA, Maes EF, Sewell LE, Miller L, Falk H, Kilbourne EM. Eosinophilia-myalgia syndrome: results of national surveillance. *J Am Med Assoc* 1990; 264:1698-1703.
1143. Centers for Disease Control. Update: eosinophilia-myalgia syndrome associated with ingestion of L-tryptophan — United States. MMWR 1989: 38:842.
1144. Centers for Disease Control. Update: analysis of L-tryptophan for the etiology of eosinophilia-myalgia syndrome. MMWR 1990; 39:789.

1145. Slutsker L, Hoesly FC, Miller L, Williams LP, Watson JC, Fleming DW. Eosinophilia-myalgia syndrome associated with exposure to tryptophan from a single manufacturer. *J Am Med Assoc* 1990; 264(2):213-7.
1146. Strongwater SL, Woda BA, Yood RA, et al. Eosinophilia-myalgia syndrome associated with L-tryptophan ingestion: analysis of four patients and implications for differential diagnosis and pathogenesis. *Arch Intern Med* 1990; 150:2178-85.
1147. Hertzman PA, Blevins WL, Mayer J, Greenfield B, Ting M, Gleich GJ. Association of the eosinophilia-myalgia syndrome with the ingestion of tryptophan. *N Engl J Med* 1990; 322:869-873.
1148. Eidson M, Philen RM, Sewell CM, Voorhees R, Kilbourne EM. L-Tryptophan and eosinophilia-myalgia syndrome in New Mexico. *Lancet* 1990; 335: 645-648.
1149. Kamb ML, Murphy JJ, Jones JL, et al. Eosinophilia-myalgia syndrome in L-tryptophan exposed patients. *J Am Med Assoc* 1992; 267:77-82.
1150. Sack KE, Criswell LA. Eosinophilia myalgia syndrome: The aftermath. *South Med J* 1992; 85(9):878-882.
1151. Campagna AC, Blanc PD, Criswell LA, et al. Pulmonary manifestations of the eosinophilia-myalgia syndrome associated with tryptophan ingestion. *Chest* 1992; 101(5):1274-81.
1152. Epstein SA, Krahn L, Clauw DJ, et al. Psychiatric aspects of the eosinophilia-myalgia syndrome. *Psychosomatics* 1995; 36(1):22-5.
1153. Campbell DS, Morris PD, Silver RM. Eosinophilia-myalgia syndrome: a long-term follow-up study. *South Med J* 1995; 88(9):953-8.
1154. Patmas MA. Eosinophilia-myalgia syndrome not associated with L-tryptophan. *N J Med* 1992; 89(4):285-6.
1155. Goda Y, Suzuki J, Maitani T, Yoshihira K, Takeda M, Uchiyama M. 3-Anilino-L-alanine, structural determination of UV-5, a contaminant in EMS-associated L-tryptophan samples. *Chem Pharm Bull* 1992; 40(8):2236-8.
1156. Zangrilli JG, Mayeno AN, Vining V, Varga J. 1,1′-Ethylidenebis[L-tryptophan], an impurity in L-tryptophan associated with eosinophilia-myalgia syndrome, stimulates type I collagen gene expression in human fibroblasts in vitro. *Biochem Mol Biol Int* 1995; 37(5):925-33.
1157. Adachi J, Gomez M, Smith CC, Sternberg EM. Accumulation of 3-(phenylamino)alanine, a constituent in L-tryptophan products implicated in eosinophilia-myalgia syndrome, in blood and organs of the Lewis rats. *Arch Toxicol* 1995; 69(4):266-70.
1158. Spitzer WO, Haggerty JL, Berkson L, et al. Continuing occurrence of eosinophilia myalgia syndrome in Canada. *Br J Rheumatol* 1995; 34(3):246-51.
1159. Clauw DJ, Flockhart DA, Mullins W, Katz P, Medsger TA Jr. Eosinophilia-myalgia syndrome not associated with the ingestion of nutritional supplements. *J Rheumatol* 1994; 21(12):2385-7.
1160. Daniels SR, Hudson JI, Horwitz RI. Epidemiology of potential association between L-tryptophan ingestion and eosinophilia-myalgia syndrome. *J Clin Epidemiol* 1995; 48(12):1413-27; discussion 1429-40.
1161. Hunnisett AG, Kars A, Howard JMH, Davies S. Changes in plasma amino acids during conditioning therapy prior to bone marrow transplantation. Their relevance to antioxidant status. *Amino Acids* 1993; 4(1-2):177-185.
1162. Soon Cho E, Krause GF, Anderson HL. Effects of dietary histidine and arginine on plasma amino acid and urea concentrations of men fed a low nitrogen diet. *J Nutr* 1977; 107(11):2078-89.
1163. Laidlaw SA, Kopple JD. Newer concepts of the indispensable amino acids. *Am J Clin Nutr* 1987; 46(4):593-605.
1164. Harper AE, Yoshimura NN. Protein quality, amino acid balance, utilization, and evaluation of diets containing amino acids as therapeutic agents. *Nutrition* 1993; 9(5):460-9.
1165. Kihlberg R, Bark S, Hallberg D. An oral amino acid loading test before and after intestinal bypass operation for morbid obesity. *Acta Chir Scand* 1982; 148(1):73-86.
1166. Zieve, L. Conditional deficiencies of ornithine or arginine. *J Am Coll Nutr* 1986; 5:167-176.
1167. Espat NJ, Watkins KT, Lind DS, Weis JK, Copeland EM, Souba WW. Dietary modulation of amino acid transport in rat and human liver. *J Surg Res* 1996; 63(1):263-8.
1168. Visek WJ, Shoemaker JD. Orotic acid, arginine, and hepatotoxicity. *J Am Coll Nutr* 1986; 5(2):153-66.
1169. Ziegler TR, Gatzen C, Wilmore DW. Strategies for attenuating protein-catabolic responses in the critically ill. *Annu Rev Med* 45:459-80, 1994.
1170. Barbul A. Arginine: biochemistry, physiology, and therapeutic implications. *J Parenteral Enteral Nutr* 1986; 10:227-238.
1171. Alexander JW, Peck MD. Future prospects for adjunctive therapy: pharmacologic and nutritional approaches to immune system modulation. *Crit Care Med* 1990; 18(2 Suppl):S159-64.
1172. Senkal M, Kemen M, Homann HH, Eickhoff U, Baier J, Zumtobel V. Modulation of postoperative immune response by enteral nutrition with a diet enriched with arginine, RNA, and omega-3 fatty acids in patients with upper gastrointestinal cancer. *Eur J Surg* 1995; 161(2):115-22.
1173. Bower RH, Cerra FB, Bershadsky B, et al. Early enteral administration of a formula (Impact) supplemented with arginine, nucleotides, and fish oil in intensive care unit patients: results of a multicenter, prospective, randomized, clinical trial. *Crit Care Med* 1995; 23(3):436-49.

1174. Kemen M, Senkal M, Homann HH, et al. Early postoperative enteral nutrition with arginine-omega-3 fatty acids and ribonucleic acid-supplemented diet vs. placebo in cancer patients: an immunologic evaluation of Impact. *Crit Care Med* 1995; 23(4):652-9.
1175. Lowell JA, Parnes HL, Blackburn GL. Dietary immunomodulation: beneficial effects on oncogenesis and tumor growth. *Crit Care Med* 1990; 18(2 Suppl):S145-8.
1176. Park KG, Hayes PD, Garlick PJ, et al. Stimulation of lymphocyte natural cytotoxicity by L-arginine. *Lancet* 1991; 337:645.
1177. Daly JM, Reynolds J, Sigal RK, et al. Effect of dietary protein and amino acids on immune function. *Crit Care Med* 1990; 18(2 Suppl):S86-93.
1178. Daly JM, Reynolds J, Sigal RK, et al. Effect of dietary protein and amino acids on immune function. *Crit Care Med* 1990; 18(2 Suppl):S86-93.
1179. Tyson, JE, Friedler, A. Hyperglycemia and arginine initiated growth hormone release during pregnancy. *Obstet Gynecol* 1969; 34:319-321.
1180. Merimee TJ, Lillicrap DA, Rabinowitz D. Effect of arginine on serum-levels of growth-hormone. *Lancet* 1965; 2:668.
1181. Floyd JC, Fajans SS, Conn JW, et al. Stimulation of insulin secretion by amino acids. *J Clin Invest* 1966; 45:1487.
1182. Isidori A, Lo Monaco A, Cappa M: A study of growth hormone release in man after oral administration of amino acids. *Curr Med Res Opin* 1981; 7:475.
1183. Maccario M, Procopio M, Loche S, Cappa M, Martina V, Camanni F, Ghigo E. Interaction of free fatty acids and arginine on growth hormone secretion in man. *Metab Clin Exp* 1994; 43(2):223-6.
1184. Cynober L. Can arginine and ornithine support gut functions?. *Gut* 1994; 35(1 Suppl):S42-5.
1185. Iwasaki K, Mano K, Ishihara M, Yugari Y, Matsuzawa T. Effects of ornithine or arginine administration on serum amino acid levels. *Biochem Int* May 1987 14 (5) p971-6.
1185a. Suminski RR, Robertson RJ, Goss FL, Arslanian S, Kang J, DaSilva S, Utter AC, Metz KF. Acute effect of amino acid ingestion and resistance exercise on plasma growth hormone concentration in young men. *Int J Sport Nutr* 1997; 7(1):48-60.
1186. Minuskin ML, Lavine ME, Ulman EA, Fisher H. Nitrogen retention, muscle creatine and orotic acid excretion in traumatized rats fed arginine and glycine enriched diets. *J Nutr* 1981; 111(7):1265-74.
1187. Ketteler M, Border WA, Noble NA. Cytokines and L-arginine in renal injury and repair. *Am J Physiol* 1994; 267(2 Pt 2):F197-207.
1188. Reyes AA, Karl IE, Klahr S. Role of arginine in health and in renal disease. *Am J Physiol* 1994; 267(3 Pt 2):F331-46.
1189. Berdeaux A. Nitric oxide: an ubiquitous messenger. *Fundam Clin Pharmacol* 1993; 7(8):401-11.
1190. Morikawa E, Huang Z, Moskowitz MA. L-arginine decreases infarct size caused by middle cerebral arterial occlusion in SHR. *Am J Physiol* 1992; 263(5 Pt 2):H1632-5.
1191. Moncada S, Higgs A. The L-arginine-nitric oxide pathway. *N Engl J Med* 1993; 329:2002-12.
1192. Marin J, Govantes C. Angiotensin-converting enzyme inhibitors and the role of nitric oxide and excitatory amino acids in improvement of cognition and memory. *J Autonom Pharmacol* 1995; 15(2):129-49.
1193. Albina JE, Reichner JS. Nitric oxide in inflammation and immunity. *New Horizons* 1995; 3(1):46-64.
1194. Guyton AC, Hall JE. *Textbook of Medical Physiology,* ed 9. Philadelphia, PA, W B Saunders Co, 1995, chaps 17,45.
1195. Reyes AA, Karl IE, Klahr S. Role of arginine in health and in renal disease. *Am J Physiol* 1994; 267(3 Pt 2):F331-46.
1196. Cooke JP, Singer AH, Tsao P, Zera P, Rowan RA, Billingham ME. Antiatherogenic effects of L-arginine in the hypercholesterolemic rabbit. *J Clin Invest* 1992; 90:1168-72.
1197. Fraser GE. Diet and coronary heart disease: beyond dietary fats and low-density-lipoprotein cholesterol. *Am J Clin Nutr* 1994; 59(5 Suppl):1117S-1123S.
1198. Ignarro LJ, Bush PA, Buga GM, Wood KS, Fukuto JM, Rajfer J. Nitric oxide and cyclic GMP formation upon electrical field stimulation cause relaxation of corpus cavernosum smooth muscle. *Biochem Biophys Res Commun* 1990; 170:843-50.
1199. Burnett AL, Lowenstein CJ, Bredt DS, Chang TSK, Snyder SH. Nitric oxide: a physiologic mediator of penile erection. *Science* 1992; 257:401-3.
1200. Lugg JA, Rajfer J, Gonzalez-Cadavid NF. Dihydrotestosterone is the active androgen in the maintenance of nitric oxide-mediated penile erection in the rat. *Endocrinology* 1995; 136(4):1495-501.
1201. Fryburg DA. NG-monomethyl-L-arginine inhibits the blood flow but not the insulin-like response of forearm muscle to IGF- I: possible role of nitric oxide in muscle protein synthesis. *J Clin Invest* 1996; 97(5):1319-28.
1202. Sandi C, Venero C, Guaza C. Nitric oxide synthesis inhibitors prevent rapid behavioral effects of corticosterone in rats. *Neuroendocrinology* 1996; 63(5):446-53.
1203. Balfagon G, Ferrer M, Encabo A, Regadera J, Marin J. Changes in reactivity of rabbit aorta induced by chronic treatment with the anabolic steroid nandrolone. In: Moncada S, Marletta MA, Hibbs JB, Higgs EA, eds. *The Biology of Nitric Oxide: Physiological and Clinical Aspects.* London: Portland Press, 1992: 118-22.

1204. Petros AJ, Hewlett AM, Bogle RG, Pearson JD. L-arginine-induced hypotension. *Lancet* 1991; 337:1044-5.
1205. Reibe D, Fernhall B, Thompson PD. The blood pressure response to exercise in anabolic steroid users. *Med Sci Sports Exerc* 1992; 24: 633-37.
1206. Glazer G. Atherogenic effects of anabolic steroids on serum lipid levels. *Arch Intern Med* 1991; 151: 1925-33.
1207. Lowell JA, Parnes HL, Blackburn GL. Dietary immunomodulation: beneficial effects on oncogenesis and tumor growth. *Crit Care Med* 1990; 18(2 Suppl):S145-8.
1208. Kemen M, Senkal M, Homann HH, et al. Early postoperative enteral nutrition with arginine-omega-3 fatty acids and ribonucleic acid-supplemented diet vs. placebo in cancer patients: an immunologic evaluation of Impact. *Crit Care Med* 1995; 23(4):652-9.
1209. Senkal M, Kemen M, Homann HH, et al. Modulation of postoperative immune response by enteral nutrition with a diet enriched with arginine, RNA, and omega-3 fatty acids in patients with upper gastrointestinal cancer. *Eur J Surg* 1995; 161(2):115-22.
1210. Bower RH, Cerra FB, Bershadsky B, et al. Early enteral administration of a formula (Impact) supplemented with arginine, nucleotides, and fish oil in intensive care unit patients: results of a multicenter, prospective, randomized, clinical trial. *Crit Care Med* 1995; 23(3):436-49.
1211. Elam RP. Morphological changes in adult males from resistance exercise and amino acid supplementation. *J Sports Med Phys Fitness* 1988; 28(1):35-9.
1212. Elam RP, Hardin DH, Sutton RA, Hagen L. Effects of arginine and ornithine on strength, lean body mass and urinary hydroxyproline in adult males. *J Sports Med Phys Fitness* 1989; 29(1):52-6.
1213. Kikuchi K, Kadono T, Ihn H, Sato S. Igarashi A. Nakagawa H. Tamaki K. Takehara K. Growth regulation in scleroderma fibroblasts: increased response to transforming growth factor-beta 1. *J. Invest Dermatol* 1995; 105(1):128-32.
1214. Igarashi A, Okochi H, Bradham DM, Grotendorst GR. Regulation of connective tissue growth factor gene expression in human skin fibroblasts and during wound repair. *Mol Biol Cell* 1993; 4(6):637-45.
1215. Olney J. Cysteine-induced brain damage in infant and fetal rodents. *Brain Res* 1972; 45:309-313.
1216. Meister A. Intracellular cysteine and glutathione delivery systems. *J Am Coll Nutr* 1986; 5:137-151, .
1217. Izzotti A, D'Agostini F, Bagnasco M, Scatolini L, Rovida A. Balansky RM, Cesarone CF, De Flora S. Chemoprevention of carcinogen-DNA adducts and chronic degenerative diseases. *Cancer Res* 1994; 54(7 Suppl):1994s-1998s.
1218. Bongers V, de Jong J, Steen I, et al. Antioxidant-related parameters in patients treated for cancer chemoprevention with N-acetylcysteine. *Eur J Cancer* 1995; 31A(6):921-3.
1219. Ziment I. Acetyl cysteine: a drug with an interesting past and a fascinating future. *Respiration* 1986; 50(suppl):26-30.
1220. Konrad F, Schoenberg MH, Wiedmann H, Kilian J, Georgieff M. [The application of n-acetylcysteine as an antioxidant and mucolytic in mechanical ventilation in intensive care patients. A prospective, randomized, placebo-controlled, double-blind study]. *Anaesthesist* 1995; 44(9):651-8.
1221. Smilkstein M, Knapp GL, Kulig KW, et al. Efficacy of oral N-acetyl cysteine in the treatment of acetaminophen overdose. *N Engl J Med* 1988; 319:1557-1562.
1222. Roederer M, Ela SW, Staal FJ, Herzenberg LA, Herzenberg LA. N-acetylcysteine: a new approach to anti-HIV therapy. *AIDS Res Hum Retroviruses* 1992; 8(2):209-17.
1223. Kalebic T, Schein PS. Organic thiophosphate WR-151327 suppresses expression of HIV in chronically infected cells. *AIDS Res Hum Retroviruses* 1994; 10(6):727-33.
1224. Sen CK, Rankinen T, Vaisanen S, Rauramaa R. Oxidative stress after human exercise: effect of N-acetylcysteine supplementation. *J Appl Physiol* 1994; 76(6):2570-7.
1225. Kapadia CR, Colpoys MF, Jiang ZM, et al. Maintenance of skeletal muscle intracellular glutamine during standard surgical trauma. *J Parenteral Enteral Nutr* 1985; 9:583-589.
1226. Wasa M, Bode BP, Abcouwer SF, Collins CL, Tanabe KK, Souba WW. Glutamine as a regulator of DNA and protein biosynthesis in human solid tumor cell lines. *Ann Surg* 1996; 224(2):189-97.
1227. Hall JC, Heel K, McCauley R. Glutamine. *Br J Surg* 1996; 83(3):305-12.
1228. Neu J, Shenoy V, Chakrabarti R. Glutamine nutrition and metabolism: where do we go from here ?. *FASEB J* 1996; 10(8):829-37.
1229. Rennie MJ, Ahmed A, Khogali SE, Low SY, Hundal HS, Taylor PM. Glutamine metabolism and transport in skeletal muscle and heart and their clinical relevance. *J Nutr* 1996; 126(4 Suppl):1142S-9S.
1230. Anderson KE, Hormones and Liver Function: Peptide Hormones and Catecholamines. Schiff, Leon, Ed.; Schiff, Eugene R., Ed. *Diseases of the Liver,* Philadelphia: Lippincott, 1982. 6B. pp 199-211.
1231. Newsholme EA, Newsholme P, Curi R, Challoner E, Ardawi S. A role for muscle in the immune system and its importance in surgery, trauma, sepsis and burns. *Nutrition* 1988; 4:261-8.
1232. Wernerman J, Vinnars E. The effect of trauma and surgery on inter-organ fluxes of amino acids in man. *Clin Sci* 1987; 73:129-133.
1233. Rennie MJ. Muscle protein turnover and the wasting due to injury and disease. *Br Med Bull* 1985; 41(3):257-64.

1234. Bulus N, Cersosimo E, Ghishan F, Abumrad NN. Physiologic importance of glutamine. *Metab Clin Exp* 1989; 38(8 Suppl 1):1-5.
1235. Furst P, Albers S, Stehle P. Evidence for a nutritional need for glutamine in catabolic patients. *Kidney Int* Suppl 1989; 27:S287-92.
1236. Rennie MJ, Hundal H, Babij P, et al. Characteristics of a glutamine carrier in skeletal muscle have important consequences for nitrogen loss in injury, infection and chronic disease. *Lancet* 1986; 2:1008-1012.
1237. Golden MN, Jahoor P, Jackson AA. Glutamine production rate and its contribution to urinary ammonia in normal man. *Clin Sci* 1982; 62:299-305.
1238. Rose WC. Amino acid requirements of man. *Fed Proc* 1949; 8:546-52.
1239. Lacey JM, Wilmore DW. Is glutamine a conditionally essential amino acid?. *Nutr Rev* 1990; 48(8):297-309.
1240. Smith RJ. Glutamine metabolism and its physiologic importance. *J Parenteral Enteral Nutr* 1990; 14(4 Suppl):40S-44S.
1241. Rowbottom DG, Keast D, Goodman C, Morton AR. The haematological, biochemical and immunological profile of athletes suffering from the overtraining syndrome. *Eur J Appl Physiol Occup Physiol* 1995; 70(6):502-9.
1242. Curthoys NP, Watford M. Regulation of glutaminase activity and glutamine metabolism. *Annu Rev Nutr* 1995; 15:133-59.
1243. Yaqoob P, Calder PC. Glutamine requirement of proliferating T lymphocytes. *Biochem Soc Trans* 1996; 24(1):78S.
1244. Okawa Y. [Influence of total parenteral nutrition in immature rats: effect of glutamine infusion on bowel integrity]. Hokkaido Igaku Zasshi — *Hokkaido J Med Sci* 1996; 71(1):55-68.
1245. Newsholme EA, Crabtree B, Ardawi MSM. Glutamine metabolism in lymphocytes: its biochemical, physiological and clinical importance. *Q J Exp Physiol* 1985; 70:473-89.
1246. Yu B, Wang S, You Z. [Influences of early enteral feeding enriched with glutamine on the gut blood flow and oxygen consumption in severely burned mini-swines]. Chung-Hua Cheng Hsing Shao Shang Wai Ko Tsa Chih — *Chin J Plastic Surg Burns* 1996; 12(1):37-40.
1247. Newsholme EA, Parry-Billings M. Properties of glutamine release from muscle and its importance for the immune system. *J Parenteral Enteral Nutr* 1990; 14:635-75.
1248. MacLennan PA, Smith K, Weryk B, Watt PW, Rennie MJ. Inhibition of protein breakdown by glutamine in profused rat skeletal muscle. *FEBS Lett* 1988; 237:133-6.
1249. MacLennan PA, Braun RA, Rennie MJ. A positive relationship between protein synthetic rate and intracellular glutamine concentration in perfused rat skeletal muscle. *FEBS Lett* 1987; 215:187-91.
1250. Jepson MM, Boles PC, Broadbent P, Pell JM, Millward DJ. Relationship between glutamine concentration and protein synthesis in rat skeletal muscle. *Am J Physiol* 1988; 255:E166-72.
1251. Wusteman M, Wight DGD, and Elia M. Protein metabolism after injury with turpentine: a rat model for clinical trauma. *Am J Physiol* 1990; 259:E763-E769.
1252. MacLennan PA, Brown RA, Rennie MJ. A positive relationship between protein synthetic rate and intracellular glutamine concentration in perfused rat skeletal muscle. *FEBS Lett* 1987; 215:187-191.
1253. Darmaun D. [In vivo exploration of glutamine metabolism in man] L'exploration du metabolisme de la glutamine in vivo chez l'homme. *Diabete Metab* 1992; 18 1 Pt 2):117-121.
1254. Rennie MJ, MacLennan PA, Hundal HS, et al. Skeletal muscle glutamine transport, intramuscular glutamine concentration, and muscle-protein turnover. *Metabolism* 1989; 38(8 Suppl 1):47-51.
1255. Rennie MJ, Hundal HS, Babij P, et al. Characteristics of a glutamine carrier in skeletal muscle have important consequences for nitrogen loss in injury, infection, and chronic disease. *Lancet* 1986; 2:1008-1012.
1256. Jepson MM, Bates PC, Broadbent P, et al. Relationship between glutamine concentration and protein synthesis in rat skeletal muscle. *Am J Physiol* 1988; 255:E166-E172.
1257. Parry-Billings M, Leighton B, Dimitriadis G, et al. Skeletal muscle glutamine metabolism during sepsis in the rat. *Int J Biochem* 1989; 21:419-423.
1258. Jepson MM, Bates PC, Broadbent P, et al. Relationship between glutamine concentration and protein synthesis in rat skeletal muscle. *Am J Physiol* 1988; 255:E166-E172.
1259. Hasselgren PO, Talamini M, James H, Fischer JE. Protein metabolism in different types of skeletal muscle during early and late sepsis in rats. *Arch Surg* 1986; 121:918-923.
1260. Christensen HN. Interorgan amino acid nutrition. *Physiol Rev* 1982; 62:1193-1233.
1261. Tamarappoo BK, Nam M, Kilberg MS, et al. Glucocorticoid regulation of splanchnic glutamine, alanine, ammonia, and glutathione fluxes. *Am J Physiol* 1993; 264:E526-E533.
1262. Muhlbacker F, Capodia CR, Colpoys MF, et al. Effects of glucocorticoids on glutamine metabolism in skeletal muscle. *Am J Physiol* 1984; 247:E75-E88.
1263. Jungas RL, Halperin ML, Brosnan JT. Quantitative analysis of amino acid oxidation and related gluconeogenesis in humans. *Physiol Rev* 1992; 72:419-448.
1264. Remesy C, Demigne C, Aufrere J. Inter-organ relationship between glucose, lactate, and amino acids in rats fed on high-carbohydrate or high-protein diets. *Biochem J* 1978; 170:321-329.

1265. Katz A, Broberg S, Sahlin K, Wahren J. Muscle ammonia and amino acid metabolism during dynamic exercise in man. *Clin Physiol* 1986; 6(4):365-79.

1266. Jepson MM, Boles PC, Broadbent P, Pell JM, Millward DJ. Relationship between glutamine concentration and protein synthesis in rat skeletal muscle. *Am J Physiol* 1988; 255:E166-72.

1267. Rennie MJ, Hundal HS, Babij P, et al. Characteristics of a glutamine carrier in skeletal muscle have important consequences for nitrogen loss in injury, infection, and chronic disease. *Lancet* 1986; 2:1008-1012.

1268. Askanazi JYA, Carpentier CB, Michelson CB, et al. Muscle and plasma amino acids following injury: influence of intercurrent infection. *Ann Surg* 1980; 192:78-85.

1269. Haussinger D, Roth E, Lang F, et al. Cellular hydration state: an important determinant of protein catabolism in health and disease. *Lancet* 1993; 341:1330-1332.

1270. Wusteman M, Wight DGD, Elia M. Protein metabolism after injury with turpentine: a rat model for clinical trauma. *Am J Physiol* 1990; 259:E763-E769.

1271. Roth E, Funovics J, Muhlbacher F, et al. Metabolic disorders in severe abdominal sepsis: glutamine deficiency in skeletal muscle. *Clin Nutr* 1982; 1:25-41.

1272. Wilmore DW, Smith RJ, O'Dwyer ST, Jacobs DO, Ziegler TR, Wang XD. The gut: a central organ after surgical stress. *Surgery* 1988; 104(5):917-23.

1273. Haque SM, Chen K, Usui N, Iiboshi Y, Okuyama H, Masunari A. Cui L. Nezu R. Takagi Y. Okada A. Alanyl-glutamine dipeptide-supplemented parenteral nutrition improves intestinal metabolism and prevents increased permeability in rats. *Ann Surg* 1996; 223(3):334-41.

1274. Souba WW, Smith RJ, Wilmore DW. Glutamine metabolism by the intestinal tract. *JPEN* 1985; 9:608-617.

1275. Byrne TA, Morrissey T, Zeigler TR, Gatzen C, Young VL, Wilmore DW. Growth hormone, glutamine and fiber enhance adaptation of remnant bowel following massive intestinal resection. *Surg Forum* 1992; 43:151-53.

1276. Wusteman M, Tate H, Weaver L, Austin S, Neale G, Elia M. The effect of enteral glutamine deprivation and supplementation on the structure of rat small-intestine mucosa during a systemic injury response. *J Parenteral Enteral Nutr* 1995; 19(1):22-7.

1277. Harper AE, Yoshimura NN. Protein quality, amino acid balance, utilization, and evaluation of diets containing amino acids as therapeutic agents. *Nutrition* 1993; 9(5):460-9.

1278. Mainous MR, Deitch EA. Nutrition and infection. *Surg Clin North Am* 1994; 74(3):659-76.

1279. Grant JP. Nutritional support in critically ill patients. *Ann Surg* 1994; 220(5):610-6.

1280. Legaspi A. Adjunctive therapy for nutritional support in hospitalized patients. *Nutr Clin Pract* 1989; 4(3):95-100.

1281. Caldwell MD. Local glutamine metabolism in wounds and inflammation. *Metabolism* 1989; 38(Suppl 1):34-9.

1282. Windmueller HG. Glutamine utilization by the small intestine. *Adv Enzymol Relat Areas Mol Biol* 1982; 53:201-37.

1283. Elia, Marinos. Review Article: Changing concepts of nutrient requirements in disease: implications for artificial nutritional support. *Lancet* 1995; 345(8960):1279-1284.

1284. Hwang TL, O'Dwyer ST, Smith RJ, et al. Preservation of small bowel mucosa using glutamine-enriched parenteral nutrition. *Surg Forum* 1986; 37:56-61.

1285. Grant JP, Snyder PJ: Use of L-glutamine in total parenteral nutrition. *J Surg Res* 1988; 44:506-511.

1286. Stehle P, Zander J, Mertes N, et al. Effect of parenteral glutamine peptide supplements on muscle glutamine loss and nitrogen balance after major surgery. *Lancet* 1989; 1:231-233.

1287. Zeigler TR, Young LS, Benfell K, et al. Clinical and metabolic efficacy of glutamine-supplemented parenteral nutrition after bone marrow transplantation. A randomized, double blind, controlled study. *Ann Intern Med* 1992; 116:821-28.

1288. Elia M. Artificial feeding: requirements and complications. *Med Int* 1994; 22:411-15.

1289. Elia M. Glutamine in parenteral nutrition. *Int J Food Sci Nutr* 1992; 43:47-59.

1290. Jiang ZM, Wang LJ, Qi Y, et al. Comparison of parenteral nutrition supplemented with L-glutamine or glutamine dipeptides. *J Parenteral Enteral Nutr* 1993; 17(2):134-41.

1291. Furst P. New strategies in clinical nutrition. *Peritoneal Dialysis Int* 1996; 16 Suppl 1:S28-35.

1292. Hammarqvist F, Wernerman J, Ali R, von der Decken A, Vinnars E. Addition of glutamine to total parenteral nutrition after elective abdominal surgery spares free glutamine in muscle, counteracts the fall in muscle protein synthesis, and improves nitrogen balance. *Ann Surg* 1989; 209(4):455-461.

1293. Wernerman J, Hammarkvist F, Ali MR, Vinnars E. Glutamine and ornithine-alpha-ketoglutarate but not branched-chain amino acids reduce the loss of muscle glutamine after surgical trauma. *Metabolism* 1989; 38(8 Suppl 1):63-66.

1294. Blomqvist BI, Hammarqvist F, von der Decken A, Wernerman J. Glutamine and alpha-ketoglutarate prevent the decrease in muscle free glutamine concentration and influence protein synthesis after total hip replacement. *Metab Clin Exp* 1995; 44(9):1215-22.

1295. Vinnars E, Hammarqvist F, von der Decken A, Wernerman J. Role of glutamine and its analogs in posttraumatic muscle protein and amino acid metabolism. *J Parenteral Enteral Nutr* 1990; 14(4 Suppl):125S-129S.

1295a. Perriello G, Nurjhan N, Stumvoll M, et al. Regulation of gluconeogenesis by glutamine in normal postabsorptive humans. *Am J Physiol* 1997; 272(3 Pt 1):E437-E445.
1296. Brillon DJ, Zheng B, Campbell RG, Matthews DE. Effect of cortisol on energy expenditure and amino acid metabolism in humans. *Am J Physiol* 1995; 268(3 Pt 1):E501-13.
1297. Wing SS, Goldberg AL. Glucocorticoids activate the ATP-ubiquitin-dependent proteolytic system in skeletal muscle during fasting. *Am J Physiol* 1993; 264:E668-E676.
1298. Hundal HS, Babij P, Taylor PM, et al. Effects of corticosterone on the transport and metabolism of glutamine in rat skeletal muscle. *Biochim Biophys Acta* 1991; 1092:376-383.
1299. Heitman RN, Bergman EN. Glutamine metabolism, interorgan transport and glucogenicity in the sheep. *Am J Physiol* 234 *Endocrinol Metab Gastrointest Physiol* 1978; 3:E197-E203.
1300. Muhlbacher F, Capodia CR, Colpoys MF, et al. Effects of glucocorticoids on glutamine metabolism in skeletal muscle. *Am J Physiol* 1984; 247:E75-E88.
1301. Ardawi MSM, Jamal YS. Glutamine metabolism in skeletal muscle of gludcocorticoid treated rats. *Cin. Sci* 1990; 79:139-147.
1302. Babij P, Hundal HS, Rennie MJ, et al. Effects of corticosteroids on glutamine tarnsport in rat skeletal muscle. *J Physiol* 1986; 374:35P.
1303. Rennie MJ, MacLennan PA, Hundal HS, et al. Skeletal muscle glutamine transport, intramuscular glutamine concentration, and muscle-protein turnover. *Metabolism* 1989; 38(8 Suppl 1):47-51.
1304. Parry-Billings M, Leighton B, Dimitriadis G, et al. Effects of physiological and pathological levels of glucocorticoids on skeletal muscle glutamine metabolism in the rat. *Biochem Pharmacol* 1990; 40:1145-1148.
1305. Hickson, RC and Marone, JR. Exercise and inhibition of glucocorticoid-induced muscle atrophy. *Exerc Sports Sci Rev* 1993; 17:135-167.
1306. Rowbottom DG, Keast D, Morton AR. The emerging role of glutamine as an indicator of exercise stress and overtraining. *Sports Med* 1996; 21(2):80-91.
1307. Hickson RC, Czerwinski SM, Wegrzyn LE. Glutamine prevents downregulation of myosin heavy chain synthesis and muscle atrophy from glucocorticoids. *Am J Physiol* 1995; 268(4 Pt 1):E730-4.
1308. Max SR. Glucocorticoid-mediated induction of glutamine synthetase in skeletal muscle. *Med Sci Sports Exerc* 1990; 22(3):325-30.
1309. Hickson RC, Wegrzyn LE, Osborne DF, Karl IE. Alanyl-glutamine prevents muscle atrophy and glutamine synthetase induction by glucocorticoids. *Am J Physiol* 1996; 271(5 Pt 2):R1165-72.
1310. Hammarqvist F, Wernerman J, Ali R, et al. Addition of glutamine to total parenteral nutrition after elective abdominal surgery spares free glutamine in muscle, counteracts the fall in muscle protein synthesis, and improves nitrogen balance. *Ann Surg* 1989; 209:455-61.
1311. Hankard RG, Haymond MW, Darmaun D. Effect of glutamine on leucine metabolism in humans. *Am J Physiol* 1996; 271(4 Pt 1):E748-54.
1312. Haussinger D, Roth E, Lang F, et al. Cellular hydration state: an important determinant of protein catabolism in health and disease. *Lancet* 1993; 341:1330-1332.
1313. Bevan SJ, Parry-Billings M, Opara E, et al. The effect of cell volume on the rate of lactate release from rat skeletal muscle. *Biochem Soc Trans* 1991; 19:198S.
1314. Low SY, Taylor PM, Rennie MJ. Responses of glutamine transport in cultured rat skeletal muscle to osmotically induced changes in cell volume. *J Physiol* 1996; 492(Pt 3):877-85.
1315. Haussinger D, Lang F, Bauers K, et al. Interactions between glutamine metabolism and cell volume regulation in perfused rat liver. *Eur J Biochem* 1990; 188:689-95.
1316. Haussinger D, et al. Cell volume and hormone action. *Trends Pharmacol Sci* 1992; 13:371-73.
1317. Hallbrucker C, et al. Control of hepatic proteolysis by amino acids — the role of cell volume. *Eur J Biochem* 1991; 197:717-24.
1318. Varnier M, Leese GP, Thompson J, Rennie MJ. Stimulatory effect of glutamine on glycogen accumulation in human skeletal muscle. *Am J Physiol* 1995; 269(2pt1);E309-E315.
1319. Varnier M, Leese GP, Thompson J, Rennie MJ. Stimulatory effect of glutamine on glycogen accumulation in human skeletal muscle. *Am J Physiol* 1995; 269(2 Pt 1):E309-15.
1320. Nurjhan N, Bucci A, Perriello G, et al. Glutamine: a major gluconeogenic precursor and vehicle for interorgan carbon transport in man. *J Clin Invest* 1995; 95(1):272-7.
1321. Rouse K, Nwokedi E, Woodliff JE, Epstein J, Klimberg VS. Glutamine enhances selectivity of chemotherapy through changes in glutathione metabolism. *Ann Surg* 1995; 221(4):420-6.
1322. Nattakom TV, Charlton A, Wilmore DW. Use of vitamin E and glutamine in the successful treatment of severe veno-occlusive disease following bone marrow transplantation. *Nutr Clin Pract* 1995; 10(1):16-8.
1323. Carlson HE, Miglietta JT, Roginsky MS, Stegink LD. Stimulation of pituitary hormone secretion by neurotransmitter amino acids in humans. *Metab Clin Exp* 1989; 38(12):1179-1182.
1324. Welbourne TC. Increased plasma bicarbonate and growth hormone after an oral glutamine load. *Am J Clin Nutr* 1995; 61:1058-61.

1325. Bourguignon JP, Gerard A, Alvarez Gonzalez ML, Purnelle G, Franchimont P. Endogenous glutamate involvement in pulsatile secretion of gonadotropin-releasing hormone: evidence from effect of glutamine and developmental changes. *Endocrinology* 1995; 136(3):911-6.
1326. Rennie MJ, Tadros L, Khogali S, Ahmed A, Taylor PM. Glutamine transport and its metabolic effects. *J Nutr* 1994; 124(8 Suppl):1503S-1508S.
1327. Hickson RC, Marone JR. Exercise and inhibition of glucocorticoid-induced muscle atrophy. *Exerc Sport Sci Rev* 1993; 21:135-67.
1328. Falduto MT, Young AP, Hickson RC. Exercise interrupts ongoing glucocorticoid-induced muscle atrophy and glutamine synthetase induction. *Am J Physiol* 1992; 263(6 Pt 1):E1157-63.
1329. Yaqoob P, Calder PC. Glutamine requirement of proliferating T lymphocytes. *Biochem Soc Trans* 1996; 24(1):78S.
1330. Newsholme P, Gordon S, and Newsholme EA. Rates of utilization and fates of glucose, glutamine, pyruvate, fatty acids and ketone bodies by mouse macrophages. *Biochem J* 1987: 242:631-636.
1331. Newsholme EA, Crabtree B, Ardawi MSM. Glutamine metabolism in lymphocytes: its biochemical, physiological and clinical importance. *Q J Exp Physiol* 1985; 70:473-89.
1332. Ogle CK, Ogle JD, Mao JX, et al. Effect of glutamine on phagocytosis and bacterial killing by normal and pediatric burn patient neutrophils. *J Parenteral Enteral Nutr* 1994; 18(2):128-33.
1333. Pederson BK, Bruunsgaard H. How physical exercise influences the establishment of infections. *Sports Med* 1995; 19(6):393-400.
1334. Frisina JP, Gaudieri S, Cable T, Keast D, Palmer TN. Effects of acute exercise on lymphocyte subsets and metabolic activity. *Int J Sports Med* 1994; 15(1):36-41.
1335. Parry Billings M, Blomstrand E, McAndrew N, Newsholme EA. A communicational link between skeletal muscle, brain, and cells of the immune system. *Int J Sports Med* 1990; 11(Suppl 2):S122-8.
1336. Rowbottom DG, Keast D, Goodman C, Morton AR. The haematological, biochemical and immunological profile of athletes suffering from the overtraining syndrome. *Eur J Appl Physiol Occup Physiol* 1995; 70(6):502-9.
1337. Sharp NC, Koutedakis Y. Sport and the overtraining syndrome: immunological aspects. *Br Med Bull* 1992; 48(3):518-33.
1338. Keast D, Arstein D, Harper W, Fry RW, Morton AR. Depression of plasma glutamine concentration after exercise stress and its possible influence on the immune system. *Med J Aust* 1995; 162(1):15-8.
1339. Nieman DC. Exercise, infection, and immunity. *Int J Sports Med* 1994; 15(Suppl 3):S131-41.
1340. Peters E, Bateman ED. Ultramarathon running and upper respiratory tract infections: an epidemiological survey. *S Afr Med J* 1983; 64:583-4.
1341. Newsholme EA. Biochemical mechanisms to explain immunosuppression in well-trained and overtrained athletes. *Int J Sports Med* 1994; 15 Suppl 3:S142-7.
1342. Keast D, Arstein D, Harper W, Fry RW, Morton AR. Depression of plasma glutamine concentration after exercise stress and its possible influence on the immune system. *Med J Aust* 1995; 162(1):15-8.
1343. Rowbottom DG, Keast D, Morton AR. The emerging role of glutamine as an indicator of exercise stress and overtraining. *Sports Med* 1996; 21(2):80-91.
1344. Moriguchi S, Miwa H, Kishino Y. Glutamine supplementation prevents the decrease of mitogen response after a treadmill exercise in rats. *J Nutr Sci Vitam* 1995; 41(1):115-25.
1345. Parry-Billings M, Budgett R, Koutedakis Y, et al. Plasma amino acid concentrations in the overtraining syndrome: possible effects on the immune system. *Med Sci Sports Exerc* 1992; 24(12):1353-8.
1346. Jungas RL, Halperin ML, Brosnan JT. Quantitative analysis of amino acid oxidation and related gluconeogenesis in humans. *Physiol Rev* 1992; 72(2):419-448.
1347. Byrne TA, Persinger RL, Young LS, Ziegler TR, Wilmore DW. A new treatment for patients with short-bowel syndrome. Growth hormone, glutamine, and a modified diet. *Ann Surg* 1995; 222(3):243-54; discussion 254-5.
1348. Klimberg VS, Salloum RM, Kasper M, et al. Oral glutamine accelerates healing of the small intestine and improves outcome after whole abdominal radiation. *Arch Surg* 1990; 125(8):1040-5.
1349. Gianotti L, Alexander JW, Gennari R, Pyles T, Babcock GF. Oral glutamine decreases bacterial translocation and improves survival in experimental gut-origin sepsis. Jpen: *J Parenteral Enteral Nutr* 1995; 19(1):69-74.
1350. Ito A, Higashiguchi T, Kitagawa M, Yokoi H, Noguchi T, Kawarada Y. Effect of luminal administration of glutamine to suppress preservation graft injury in small bowel transplants. *Transplant Proc* 1995; 27(1):780-2.
1351. Zhang W, Frankel WL, Bain A, Choi D, Klurfeld DM, Rombeau JL. Glutamine reduces bacterial translocation after small bowel transplantation in cyclosporine-treated rats. *J Surg Res* 1995; 58(2):159-64.
1352. Windmueller HG, Spaeth AE. Intestinal metabolism of glutamine and glutamate from the lumen as compared to glutamine from the blood. *Arch Biochem Biophys* 1975; 171:662-672.
1353. Windmueller HG, Spaeth AE. Respiratory fuels and nitrogen metabolism in vivo in small intestine of fed rats. *J Biol Chem* 1980; 255:107-112.
1354. Jungas RL, Halperin ML, Brosnan JT. Quantitative analysis of amino acid oxidation and related gluconeogenesis in humans. *Physiol Rev* 1992; 72:419-448.

1355. Moriguchi, Miwa H, Kishino Y. Glutamine supplementation prevents the decrease of mitogen response after a treadmill exercise in rats. *J Nutr Sci Vitam* 1995; 41(1):115-25.

1356. Welbourne TC, Joshi S. Enteral glutamine spares endogenous glutamine in chronic acidosis. *J Parenteral Enteral Nutr* 1994; 18(3):243-7.

1357. Fahr MJ, Kornbluth J, Blossom S, Schaeffer R, Klimberg VS, Harry M. Vars Research Award. Glutamine enhances immunoregulation of tumor growth. *J Parenteral Enteral Nutr* 1994; 18(6):471-6.

1358. Newsholme P, Gordon S, Newsholme EA. Rates of utilization and fates of glucose, glutamine, pyruvate, fatty acids and ketone bodies by mouse macrophages. *Biochem J* 1987; 242:631-636.

1359. Newsholme EA, Newsholme P, Curi R, et al. A role for muscle in the immune system and its importance in *surgery*, trauma, sepsis, and burns. *Nutrition* 1988; 4:261-268.

1360. Roth E, Karner J, Ollenschlager G. Glutamine: An Anabolic Effector? *J Parenteral Enteral Nutr* 1990: 14:130S-136S.

1361. Roth E, Funovics J, Muhlbacher F, et al. Metabolic disorders in severe abdominal sepsis: glutamine deficiency in skeletal muscle. *Clin Nutr* 1982; 1:25-41.

1362. Calder PC, Newsholme EA. Glutamine promotes interleukin-2 production by concanavalin A-stimulated lymphocytes. *Proc Nutr Soc* 1992; 51:105A.

1363. Shabert JK, Wilmore DW. Glutamine deficiency as a cause of human immunodeficiency virus wasting. *Med Hypotheses* 1996; 46(3):252-6.

1364. Dechelotte P, Darmaun D, Rongier M, Hecketsweiler B, Rigal O, Desjeux JF. Absorption and metabolic effects of enterally administered glutamine in humans. *Am J Physiol* 1991; 260(5 Pt 1):G677-G682.

1365. Jungas RL, Halperin ML, Brosnan JT. Quantitative analysis of amino acid oxidation and related gluconeogenesis in humans. *Physiol Rev* 1992; 72(2):419-448.

1366. Tadros LB, Taylor PM, Rennie MJ. Characteristics of glutamine transport in primary tissue culture of rat skeletal muscle. *Am J Physiol* 1993; 265:E135-E144.

1367. Jungas RL, Halperin ML, Brosnan JT. Quantitative analysis of amino acid oxidation and related gluconeogenesis in humans. *Physiol Rev* 1992; 72(2):419-448.

1368. Newsholme EA, Newsholme P, Curi R, Challoner E, Ardawi S. A role for muscle in the immune system and its importance in surgery, trauma, sepsis and burns. *Nutrition* 1988; 4:261-8.

1369. Wagenmakers AJ, Salden HJ, Veerkamp JH. The metabolic fate of branched-chain amino acids and 2-oxo acids in rat muscle homogenates and diaphragms. *Int J Biochem* 1985; 17(9):957-65.

1370. A White, P Handler, Smith E., *Principles of Biochemistry*, Third Edition, McGraw-Hill, New York (1964): 945.Supplement Update.

1371. Hammarqvist F, Wernerman J, von der Decken A, Vinnars E. Alpha-ketoglutarate preserves protein synthesis and free glutamine in skeletal muscle after surgery. *Surgery* 1991; 109(1):28-36.

1372. Roth E, Karner J, Roth-Merten A, Winkler S; Valentini L; Schaupp K. Effect of alpha-ketoglutarate infusions on organ balances of glutamine and glutamate in anaesthetized dogs in the catabolic state. *Clin Sci* 1991; 80(6):625-631.

1373. Wernerman J, Hammarqvist F, Vinnars E. Alpha-ketoglutarate and postoperative muscle catabolism. *Lancet* 1990; 335(8691):701-703.

1374. Marconi C, Sassi G, Cerretelli P. The effect of an alpha-ketoglutarate-pyridoxine complex on human maximal aerobic and anaerobic performance. *Eur J Appl Physiol* 1982; 49(3):307-17.

1375. Hammarqvist F, Wernerman J, Ali R, Vinnars E. Effect of an amino acid solution enriched with branched chain amino acid or ornithine-ketoglutarate on the post-operative intracellular amino acid concentration of muscle. *Br J Surg* 1990; 77(2):214-218.

1376. Wernerman J, Hammarqvist F, Vinnars E. Alpha-ketoglutarate and postoperative muscle catabolism. *Lancet* 1980; 335:701.

1377. Blomqvist BI, Hammarqvist F, von der Decken A, et al. Glutamine and alpha-ketoglutarate prevent the decrease in muscle free glutamine concentration and influence protein synthesis after total hip replacement. *Metabolism* 1995; 44:1215-1222.

1378. Shurtleff D, Thomas JR, Shlers ST, et al. Tyrosine ameliorates a cold-induced delayed matching to sample performance decrements in rats. *Psychopharmacology* 1993; 112:228-232.

1379. Owasoyo JO, Neri DF, Lamberth JG. Tyrosine and its potential use as a countermeasure to performance decrement in military sustained operations. *Aviat Space Environ Med* 1992; 63:364-369.

1380. Huq F, Thompson M, Ruell P. Changes in serum amino acid concentrations during prolonged endurance running. *J Physiol* 1993; 43(6):797-807.

1381. Silbermann M, Bar-Shira-Maymon B, Coleman R, et al. Long-term physical exercise retards trabecular bone loss in lumbar vertebrae of aging female mice. *Calcif Tissue Int* 1990; 46(2):80-93.

1382. Moyes CD, Buck LT, Hochachka PW, Suarez RK. Oxidative properties of carp red and white muscle. *J Exp Biol* 1989; 143:321-31.

1383. Jaksic T, Wagner DA, Burke JF, Young VR. Proline metabolism in adult male burned patients and healthy control subjects. *Am J Clin Nutr* 1991; 54(2):408-13.

1384. Askanazi J, Furst P, Michelsen CB, et al. Muscel and plasma amino acids after injury: hypocaloric glucose vs. amino acid infusion. *Ann Surg* 1980; 191:465-472.
1385. Sitren HS, Fisher H. Nitrogen retention in rats feed on diets enriched with arginine and glycine. *Br J Nutr* 1977; 37:195-208.
1386. Motil KJ, Thotathuchery M, Montandon CM, Hachey DL, Boutton TW, Klein PD, Garza C. Insulin, cortisol and thyroid hormones modulate maternal protein status and milk production and composition in humans. *J Nutr* 1994; 124(8):1248-57.
1387. Miller RG, Keshen TH, Jahoor F, et al. Compartmentation of endogenously synthesized amino acids in neonates. *J Surg Res* 1996; 63(1):199-203.
1388. Hiramatsu T, Cortiella J, Marchini JS, Chapman TE, Young VR. Plasma proline and leucine kinetics: response to 4 wk with proline-free diets in young adults. *Am J Clin Nutr* 1994; 60(2):207-15.
1389. Jaksic T, Wagner DA, Young VR. Plasma proline kinetics and concentrations in young men in response to dietary proline deprivation. *Am J Clin Nutr* 1990; 52(2):307-12.
1390. Tischler ME, Goldberg AL. Production of alanine and glutamine by atrial muscle from fed and fasted rats. *Am J Physiol* 1980; 238(5):E487-93.
1391. Wesson M, McNaughton L, Davies P, Tristram S. Effects of oral administration of aspartic acid salts on the endurance capacity of trained athletes. *Res Q Exerc Sport* 1988; 59(3):234-239.
1392. Besset L. Increase in sleep related growth hormone and prolactin secretion after chronic arginine aspartate administration. *Acta Endocrinol* 1982; 99:18-23.
1393. Tuttle JL, Potteiger JA, Evans BW, et al. Effect of acute potassium-magnesium aspartate supplementation on ammonia concentrations during and after resistance training. *Int J Sport Nutr* 1995; 5:102-109.
1394. D'Aniello A, Di Cosmo A, Di Cristo C, Annunziato L, Petrucelli L, Fisher G. Involvement of D-aspartic acid in the synthesis of testosterone in rat testes. *Life Sci* 1996; 59(2):97-104.
1395. Bucci L. Aspartic Acid. In: *Nutrients as Ergogenic Aids for Sports and Exercise* 1993. CRC Press. Boca Raton. FL, 71.
1396. Bucci LR. Micronutrient supplementation and ergogenesis — amino acids. In: *Nutrients as Ergogenic Aids for Sports and Exercise* 1993. CRC Press. Boca Raton. FL, 72-73.
1397. Brodan V, Kuhn E, Pechar J, Slabochova Z. Effects of sodium glutamate infusion on ammonia formation during intense physical exercise in man. *Nutr Rep Int* 1994; 9:223-226.
1398. Bucci LR, Hickson JF Jr, Pivarnik JM, et al. Ornithine ingestion and growth hormone release in bodybuilders. *Nutr Res* 1990; 10(3):239-245.
1399. Banister EW, Rajendra W, Mutch BJ. Ammonia as an indicator of exercise stress implications of recent findings to sports medicine. *Sports Med* 1985; 2(1):34-46.
1400. Cynober L, Coudray LC, de Bandt JP, et al. Action of ornithine alpha-ketoglutarate, ornithine hydrochloride, and calcium alpha-ketoglutarate on plasma amino acid and hormonal patterns in healthy subjects. *J Am Coll Nutr* 1990; 9(1):2-12.
1401. Hammarqvist F, Wernerman J, Ali R, Vinnars E. Effects of an amino acid solution enriched with either branched chain amino acids or ornithine-alpha-ketoglutarate on the postoperative intracellular amino acid concentration of skeletal muscle. *Br J Surg* 1990; 77(2):214-218.
1402. Le Bricon T, Cynober L, Baracos VE. Ornithine alpha-ketoglutarate limits muscle protein breakdown without stimulating tumor growth in rats bearing Yoshida ascites hepatoma. *Metab Clin Exp* 1994; 43(7):899-905.
1403. Jeevanandam M. Ornithine alpha-ketoglutarate in trauma situations. *Clin Nutr* 1993; 312:61-65.
1404. Wernerman J, Hammarqvist F, von der Decken A, et al. Ornithine alpha ketoglutarate improves skeletal muscle protein synthesis as assessed by ribosome analysis and nitrogen use after surgery. *Ann Surg* 1987; 206:674-8.
1405. Moukarzel A, Goulet O, Cynober L, Ricour C. Positive effects of ornithine alpha-ketoglutarate in paediatric patients on parenteral nutrition with failure to thrive. *Clin Nutr* 1993; 12: 59-60.
1406. Wernerman J, Vinnars E. The effect of trauma and surgery on inter-organ fluxes of amino acids in man. *Clin Sci* 1987; 73:129-133.
1407. Grimble GK. Augmentation of plasma arginine and glutamine by ornithine alpha-ketoglutarate in healthy, enterally-fed volunteers. *Proc Nutr Soc* 1992; 51:119A.
1408. Roch-Arveiller M, Tissot M, Coudray-Lucas C, et al. Immunomodulatory effects of ornithine alpha-ketoglutarate in rats with burn injuries. *Arch Surg* 1996; 131(7):718-23.
1409. Moukarzel AA, Goulet O, Salas JS, et al. Growth retardation in children receiving long-term total parenteral nutrition: effects of ornithine alpha-ketoglutarate. *Am J Clin Nutr* 1994; 60(3):408-13.
1410. Roch-Arveiller M, Tissot M, Coudray-Lucas C, et al. Immunomodulatory effects of ornithine alpha-ketoglutarate in rats with burn injuries. *Arch Surg* 1996; 131(7):718-23.
1411. Jeevanandam M, Holaday NJ, Ali MR. Altered tissue polyamine levels due to ornithine-alpha-ketoglutarate in traumatized growing rats. *Metab Clin Exp* 1992; 41(11):1204-9.
1412. Cynober L. Ornithine alpha-ketoglutarate in nutritional support. *Nutrition* 1991; 7(5):313-322.

1413. Vaubourdolle M, Coudray-Lucas C, Jardel A, et al. Action of enterally administered ornithine alpha-ketoglutarate on protein breakdown in skeletal muscle and liver of the burned rat. *J Parenteral Enteral Nutr* 1991; 15(5):517-20.

1414. Roch-Arveiller M, Tissot M, Coudray-Lucas C, et al. Immunomodulatory effects of ornithine alpha-ketoglutarate in rats with burn injuries. *Arch Surg* 1996; 131(7):718-23.

1415. Vauboudolle M, Salvucci M, Coudray-Lucas C, et al. Action of ornithine alpha ketoglutarate on DNA synthesis by human fibroblasts. *In Vitro Cell Dev Biol Anim* 1990; 26(2):187-92.

1416. Vauboudolle M, Cynober L, Lioret N, Coudray-Lucas C; Aussel C; Saizy R; Giboudeau J. Influence of enterally administered ornithine alpha-ketoglutarate on hormonal patterns in burn patients. *Burns Therm Inj* 1987; 13(5):349-356.

1416a. Le Boucher J, Coudray-Lucas C, Lasnier E, et al. Enteral administration of ornithine alpha-ketoglutarate or arginine alpha-ketoglutarate: a comparative study of their effects on glutamine pools in burn-injured rats. *Critical Care Medicine* 1997; 25(2):293-8.

1416b. Le Bricon T, Coudray-Lucas C, Lioret N, et al. Ornithine alpha-ketoglutarate metabolism after enteral administration in burn patients: bolus compared with continuous infusion. *Am. J. Clin. Nutr.* 1997; 65(2):512-8.

1417. Remesy C, Fafournoux P, Demigne C. Control of hepatic utilization of serine, glycine and threonine in fed and starved rats. *J Nutr* 1983; 113(1):28-39.

1418. Bjerve KS. The biosynthesis of phosphatidylserine and phosphatidylethanolamine from L-[3-^{14}C]serine in isolated rat hepatocytes. *Biochim Biophys Acta* 1985; 833(3):396-405.

1419. Henzi V, MacDermott AB. Characteristics and function of Ca sup 2+ and inositol 1,4,5-trisphosphate-releasable stores of Ca sup 2+ in neurons. *Neuroscience* 1992; 46: 251-73.

1420. Araki T, Kato H, Hara H, Kogure K. Postischemic binding of (Hydrogen-3) phorbol 12,13 dibutyrate and (Hydrogen-3) inositol 1,4,5-trisphosphate in the gerbil brain: an autoradiographic study. *Neuroscience* 1992; 46: 973-80.

1421. Fisher SK, Agranoff BW. Receptor activation and inositol lipid hydrolysis in neural tissues. *J Neurochem* 1987; 48: 999-1017.

1422. Cullis PR, De Kruijff B. Lipid polymorphism and the functional roles of lipids in biological membranes. *Biochim Biophys Acta* 1979; 559: 399-420.

1423. Cook AM, Low E, Ishijimi M. Effect of phosphatidylserine decarboxylase on neural excitation. *Nat New Biol* 1972; 239: 150-1.

1424. Fenske DB, Jarrell HC, Guo Y, Hui SW. Effect of unsaturated phosphatidylethanolamine on the chain order profile of bilayers at the onset of the hexagonal phase transition. A Hydrogen-2 NMR study. *Biochemistry* 1990; 29: 11222-9.

1425. Tanaka R. Comparison of lipid effects on K sup +-Mg sup 2+ activated p-nitrophenyl phosphatase and Na sup +-K sup +-Mg sup 2+ activated adenosine triphosphatase of membrane. *J Neurochem* 1969; 16:1301-7.

1426. Orlacchio A, Maffei C, Binaglia L, Porcellati G. The effect of membrane phospholipid acyl-chain composition on the activity of brain beta-N-acetyl-D-glucosaminidase. *Biochem J* 1981; 195: 383-8.

1427. Porcellati G, Arienti G, Pirotta M, Giorgini D. Base-exchange reactions for the synthesis of phospholipids in nervous tissue: the incorporation of serine and ethanolamine into the phospholipids of isolated brain microsomes. *J Neurochem* 1970; 18: 1395-417.

1428. Slaughter MM, Miller RF. 2-Amino-4-phosphonobutyric acid: a new pharmacological tool for retinal research. *Science* 1981; 211: 182-5.

1429. Nawy S, Jahr CE. Suppression by glutamate of cGMP- activated conductance in retinal bipolar cells. *Nature* 1990; 346: 269-71.

1430. Forsythe ID, Clements JD. Presynaptic glutamate receptors depress excitatory monosynaptic transmission between mouse hippocampal neurones. *J Physiol* 1990; 429: 1-16.

1431. Nunzi MG, Milan F, Guidolin D, Polato P, Toffano G. Effects of phosphatidylserine administration of aged-related structural changes in the rat hippocampus and septal complex. *Pharmacopsychiatry* 1989; 22(Suppl 2):125-8.

1432. Valzelli L, Kozak W, Zanotti A, Toffano G. Activity of phosphatidylserine on memory retrieval and on exploration in mice. *Methods Findings Exp Clin Pharmacol* 1987; 9(10):657-60.

1433. Calderini G, Aporti F, Bellini F, Bonetti AC, Teolato S, Zanotti A, Toffano G. Pharmacological effect of phosphatidylserine on age-dependent memory dysfunction. *Ann N Y Acad Sci* 1985; 444:504-6.

1434. Gianotti C, Porta A, De Graan PN, Oestreicher AB, Nunzi MG. B-50/GAP-43 phosphorylation in hippocampal slices from aged rats: effects of phosphatidylserine administration. *Neurobiol Aging* 1993; 14(5):401-6.

1435. Crook TH, Tinklenberg J, Yesavage J, et al. Effects of phosphatidylserine in age-associated memory impairment. *Neurology* 1991; 41(5):644-9.

1436. Maggioni M, Picotti GB, Bondiolotti GP, Panerai A. Cenacchi T. Nobile P. Brambilla F. Effects of phosphatidylserine therapy in geriatric patients with depressive disorders. *Acta Psychiatr Scand* 1990; 81(3):265-70.

1437. Scapagnini U, Guarcello V, Triolo G, Cioni M, Morale MC, Farinella Z, Marchetti B. Therapeutic perspectives in psychoneuroendocrinimmunology (PNEI): potential role of phosphatidylserine in neuroendocrine-immune communications. *Int J Neurosci* 1990; 51(3-4):299-301.
1438. Amaducci L, Crook TH, Lippi A, et al. Use of phosphatidylserine in Alzheimer's disease. *Ann N Y Acad Sci* 1991; 640:245-9.
1439. Soares JC, Gershon S. Advances in the pharmacotherapy of Alzheimer's disease [published erratum appears in Eur Arch Psychiatry Clin Neurosci 1995; 245(2):128]. *Eur Arch Psychiatry Clin Neurosci* 1994. 244(5):261-71.
1440. Guarcello V, Triolo G, Cioni M, Morale MC. Farinella Z. Scapagnini U. Marchetti B. Phosphatidylserine counteracts physiological and pharmacological suppression of humoral immune response. *Immunopharmacology* 1990; 19(3):185-95.
1441. Monteleone P, Beinat L, Tanzillo C, et al. Effects of phosphatidylserine on the neuroendocrine response to physical stress in humans. *Neuroendocrinology* 1990; 52:243-248.
1442. Monteleone P, Maj M, Beinat L, et al. Blunting by chronic phosphatidylserine administration of the stress-induced activation of the hypothalamo-pituitary-adrenal axis in healthy men. *Eur J Clin Pharmacol* 1992; 41:385-388.
1443. Hahn R, Essen P, Wernerman J. Amino acid concentrations in plasma and skeletal muscle after transurethral resection syndrome. *Scand J Urol Nephrol* 1992; 26(3):235-9.
1444. Brand E, Harris M, Sandberg W, et al. Studies on the origin of creatine. *Am J Physiol* 1929; 90:296-301.
1445. Crim MC, Calloway DH, Margen S. Creatine metabolism in men: urinary creatine and creatinine excretions with creatine feeding. *J Nutr* 1975; 105(4):428-38.
1446. Crim MC, Calloway DH, Margen S. Creatine metabolism in men: creatine pool size and turnover in relation to createine intake. *J Nutr* 1976; 106:371-375.
1447. Bucci L. Glycine. In: *Nutrients as Ergogenic Aids for Sports and Exercise* 1993. CRC Press. Boca Raton. pg. 74.
1448. Fernstrom JD. Dietary precursors and brain neurotransmitter formation. *Annu Rev Med* 1981. 32:413-25.
1449. Banay-Schwartz M, Palkovits M, Lajtha A. Heterogeneous distribution of functionally important amino acids in brain areas of adult and aging humans. *Neurochem Res* 1993; 18(4):417-23.
1450. Nakamura S. [Amino acid metabolism in neurodegenerative diseases]. Nippon Rinsho. *Jpn J Clin Med* 1992; 50(7):1637-42.
1451. Kasai K, Kobayashi M, Shimoda S. Stimulatory effect of glycine on human growth hormone secretion. *Metabolism* 1978; 27:201-204.
1452. Kasai K, Suzuki H, Nakamura T, Shiina H, Shimoda SI. Glycine stimulated growth hormone release in man. *Acta Endocrinol* 1980; 93(3):283-6.
1453. Hankard RG, Haymond MW, Darmaun D. Effect of glutamine on leucine metabolism in humans. *Am J Physiol* 1996; 271(4 Pt 1):E748-54.
1454. Pozefsky T, Tancredi RG, Moxley RT, Dupre J, Tobin JD. Effects of brief starvation on muscle amino acid metabolism in nonobese man. *J Clin Invest* 1976; 57(2):444-9.
1455. Hayes KC. Taurine nutrition. *Nutr Res* 1988; Rev 5:99-113.
1456. Lehmann A. Effects of microdialysis-perfusion with anisoosmotic media on extracellular amino acids in the rat hippocampus and skeletal muscle. *J Neurochem* 1989; 53(2):525-35.
1457. Kendler BS. Taurine: an overview of its role in preventive medicine. *Prev Med* 1989; 18(1):79-100.
1458. Lee CS, Lee KY, Lee KS. Inhibitory effect of taurine on $HOCl^-$ and NH-2Cl-induced degradation of hyaluronic acid. *Korean J Pharmacol* 1992; 28(2):201-212.
1459. Tanabe Y, Urata H, Kiyonaga A, Ikeda M, Tanaka H, Shindo M, Arakawa K. Changes in serum concentrations of taurine and other amino acids in clinical antihypertensive exercise therapy. *Clin Exp Hypertens* 1989; 11(1):149-65.
1460. Ikuyama S, Okajima T, Kato KI, Ibayashi H. Effect of taurine on growth hormone and prolactin secretion in rats: Possible interaction with opioid peptidergic system. *Life Sci* 1988; 43(10):807-812.
1461. Galler S, Hutzler C, Haller T. Effects of taurine on Ca2(+)-dependent force development of skinned muscle fiber preparations. *J Exp Biol* 1990; 152:255-64.
1462. Timbrell JA, Seabra V, Waterfield CJ. The in vivo and in vitro protective properties of taurine. *Gen Pharmacol* 1995; 26(3):453-62.
1463. Grinde B. Seglen PO. Effects of amino acid analogues on protein degradation in isolated rat hepatocytes. *Biochim Biophys Acta* 1981; 676(1):43-50.
1464. Chandler RM, Byrne HK, Patterson JG, Ivy JL. Dietary supplements affect the anabolic hormones after weight-training exercise. *J Appl Physiol* 1994; 76(2):839-45.
1465. Carli G, Bonifazi M, Lodi L, et al. Changes in the exercise-induced hormone response to branched chain amino acid administration. *Eur J Appl Physiol* 1992; 64:272-277.
1466. Leung K, Rajkovic IA, Peters E, Markus I, Van Wyk JJ, Ho KK. Insulin-like growth factor-1 and insulin down-regulate growth hormone (GH) receptors in rat osteoblasts: evidence for a peripheral feedback loop regulating GH action. *Endocrinology* 1996; 137(7):2694-702.

1467. Hakkinen K. Neuromuscular and hormonal adaptations during strength and power training. A review. *J Sports Med Phys Fitness* 1989; 29(1):9-26.

1468. Eichner ER. Ergolytic Drugs in Medicine and Sports. Am. J. Med. 1993; 94(2):205-211.

1469. Spence JC, Gauvin L. Drug and alcohol use by Canadian university athletes: a national survey. *J. Drug Ed.* 1996; 26(3):275-87.

1470. Tentler JJ, LaPaglia N, Steiner J, Williams D, Castelli M, Kelley MR, Emanuele NV, Emanuele MA. Ethanol, growth hormone and testosterone in peripubertal rats. *J Endocrinol* 1997; 152 (3): 477-487.

1471. Opstad PK, Aakvaag A. The effect of sleep deprivation on the plasma levels of hormones during prolonged physical strain and calorie deficiency. *Eur. J. Appl. Physiol. Occup. Physiol.* 1983; 51(1):97-107.

1472. Noth RH, Walter RM Jr. The effects of alcohol on the endocrine system. *Med. Clin. North Am.* 1984; 68(1):133- 146.

1473. Babichev VN, Peryshkova TA, Aivazashvili NI, Shishkina IV. [Effect of alcohol on the content of sex steroid receptors in the hypothalamus and hypophysis of male rats] *Biull Eksp Biol Med* 1989, 107 (2) p204-7.

1474. Chung KW. Effect of ethanol on androgen receptors in the anterior pituitary, hypothalamus and brain cortex in rats. *Life Sci* 1989, 44 (4) p273-80.

1475. Steiner JC, Holloran MM, Jabamoni K, Emanuele NV, Emanuele MA. Sustained effects of a single injection of ethanol on the hypothalamic-pituitary-gonadal axis in the male rat. *Alcohol Clin Exp Res* 1996; 20(8):1368-1374.

1475a. Chesley A, MacDougall JD, Tarnopolsky MA, et al. Changes in human muscle protein synthesis after resistance exercise. *J Appl Physiol* 1992; 73:1383-1388.

1476. Viru A. *Adaptation in Sports Training*. CRC Press, Boca Raton, FL. 1995.

1477. Hartley LH, Mason JW. Multiple hormonal responses to graded exercise in relation to physical training. *J Appl Physiol* 1972; 33:602-606.

1478. Viru A, Karelson K, Smirnova T. Stability and variability in hormonal responses to prolonged exercise. J *Sports Med* 1992; 13:230-235.

1479. Hakkinen K, Pakarinen A, Alen M, et al. Relationships between training volume, physical performance capacity, and serum hormone concentrations during prolonged training in elite weight lifters. *Int J Sports Med* 1987; 8:61-65.

1480. Kraemer WJ, Marchitelli L, Gordon SE, et al. Hormonal and growth factor responses to heavy resistance exercise protocols. *J Appl Physiol* 1990; 69(4):1442-50.

1481. Kraemer WJ, Gordon SE, Fleck SJ, et al. Endogenous anabolic hormonal and growth factor responses to heavy resistance exercise in males and females. *Int J Sports Med* 1991; 12(2):228-35.

1482. Stone MH. Periodization muscle conditioning and muscle injuries — a method of increasing performance to maximum or optimal values while reducing overtraining and injury potential. *Med Sci Sports Exerc* 1990; 22(4):457-62.

1483. Bompa TO. *Theory and Methodology of Training,* Kendall/Hunt; Dubuque, Indiana. 1983.

1484. Bompa TO. *Periodization of Strength: The New Wave in Strength Training.* Veritas Publishing; Toronto, Canada. 1993.

1485. Hakkinen K, Kallinen M, Komi PV, Kauhanen H. Neuromuscular adaptations during short-term "normal" and reduced training periods in strength athletes. *Electromyogr Clin Neurophysiol* 1991; 31(1):35-42.

1486. Hortobgyi T, Hill JP, Houmard JA, et al. Adaptive responses to muscle lengthening and shortening in humans. *J Appl Physiol* 1996; 80:765-772.

1487. Benson DW, Foley-Nelson T, Chance WT, et al. Decreased myofibrillar protein breakdown following treatment with clenbuterol. *J Surg Res* 1991; 50(1):1-5.

1488. Sharman I. Nutrition and athletic performance. *Nutr Food Sci* 1980; 67:5-9.

1489. Nelson RA. Nutrition and physical performance. *Phys Sportsmed* 1982; 10(4):54-59; 62-63.

1490. Donagelo CM. Nutrition, diet and physical activity. *Bol Fed Int Educacao Fisica* 1984; 54(2):51-60.

1491. Brotherhood JR. Nutrition and sports performance. *Sports Med* 1984; 1(5):350-389.

1492. Hanne N. Tezuna wehesegim seportiviim. (Nutrition and physical performance.). Publisher Information: Netanya, Israel: Wingate Institute, 1984, 21 pages.

1493. Grandjean AC. Vitamins, diet, and the athlete. *Clin Sports Med* 1983; 2(1):105-114.

1494. Summer J, Mobley M. Training and dietary correlates of marathon performance in men and women. *Aust J Sports Med* 1981; 13(2):37-42.

1495. Durnin JV. Muscle in sports medicine — nutrition and muscular performance. *Int J Sports Med* 1982; 3(Suppl 1):52-57.

1496. Malomsoki J. The improvement of sports performance by means of complementary nutrition) *Sportorvosi szemle/Hung Rev Sports Med* 1983; 24(4):269-282.

1497. Borer KT. Neurohumoral mediation of exercise-induced growth. *Med Sci Sports Exerc* 1994; 26(6):741-54.

1498. Darden E. Protein. *Nautilus Mag* 1981; 3(1):12-17.

1499. Grunewald KK, Bailey RS. Commercially marketed supplements for bodybuilding athletes. *Sports Med* 1993; 15(2):90-103.

1500. Nielsen FH, Hunt CD, Mullen LM, Hunt Jr.Effect of dietary boron on mineral, estrogen, and testosterone metabolism in postmenopausal women. *FASEB J* 1987; 1(5):394-7.
1501. Ferrando AA, Green NR. The effect of boron supplementation on lean body mass, plasma testosterone levels, and strength in male bodybuilders. *Int J Sport Nutr* 1993; 3(2):140-9.
1502. Beattie JH, Peace HS. The influence of a low-boron diet and boron supplementation on bone, major mineral and sex steroid metabolism in postmenopausal women. *Br J Nutr* 1993; 69(3):871-84.
1503. Lee IP, Sherins RJ, Dixon RL. Evidence for induction of germinal aplasia in male rats by environmental exposure to boron. *Toxicol Appl Pharmacol* 1978; 45(2):577-90.
1504. Jobin C, Duhamel JF, Sesboue B, et al. Nutrition of children and adolescents engaged in high-level sports activities. *Pediatrie* 1993; 48(2):109-17.
1505. Risser WL, Lee EJ, Poindexter HBW, West MS, Pivarnik JM, Risser JMH, Hickson JF. Iron deficiency in female atheltes: its prevalence and impact on performance. *Med Sci Sports Exerc* 1988; 20(2):116-121.
1506. Eichner ER. The anemias of athletes. *Phys Sportsmed* 1986; 14(9):122-125; 129-130.
1507. Van-Swearingen J. Iron deficiency in athletes: consequence or adaption in strenuous activity. *J Orthopaed Sports Phys Ther* 1986; 7(4):192-195.
1508. Clement DB, Sawchuk LL. Iron status and sports performance. *Sports Med* 1984; 1(1):65-74.
1509. Keul J, Jakob E, Berg A, Dickhuth HH, Lehmann M. Effect of vitamins and iron on performance and recovery in humans and in sports anemia. *Z Ernahrungswiss* 1987; 26(1):21-42.
1510. Haralambie G. Electrolytes, trace elements and vitamins in exercise. *Int Course Physiol Chem Exerc Training* 1979; (1st).
1511. Suzuki M, Itokawa Y. Effects of thiamine supplementation on exercise-induced fatigue. *Metab Brain Dis* 1996; 11(1):95-106.
1512. Sjodin B, Hellsten Westing Y, Apple FS. Biochemical mechanisms for oxygen free radical formation during exercise. *Sports Med* Oct 1990; 10(4):236-54.
1513. Gohil K, Rothfuss L, Lang J, Packer L. Effect of exercise training on tissue vitamin E and ubiquinone content. *J Appl Physiol* 1987; 63(4):1638-41.
1514. Bushell A, Klenerman L, Davies H, Grierson I, Jackson MJ. Ischemia-reperfusion-induced muscle damage. Protective effect of corticosteroids and antioxidants in rabbits. *Acta Orthopaed Scand* 1996; 67(4):393-8.
1515. Mortensen SA. Perspectives on therapy of cardiovascular diseases with coenzyme Q10 (ubiquinone). [Review] *Clin Invest* 1993; 71(8 Suppl):S116-23.
1516. Beyer RE. An analysis of the role of coenzyme Q in free radical generation and as an antioxidant. *Biochem Cell Biol* 1992; 70(6):390-403.
1517. Borisova IG, Seifulla RD, Zhuravlev AI. [Action of antioxidants on physical work capacity and lipid peroxidation in the body]. *Farmakol Toksikol* 1989; 52(4):89-92.
1518. Lemke M, Frei B, Ames BN, Faden AI. Decreases in tissue levels of ubiquinol 9 and 10, ascorbate and alpha tocopherol following spinal cord impact trauma in rats. *Neurosci Lett* 1990; 108(1-2):201-6.
1519. Prasad AS. Zinc deficiency in women, infants and children. *J Am Coll Nutr* 1996; 15(2):113-20.
1520. Cordova A, Alvarez-Mon M. Behaviour of zinc in physical exercise: a special reference to immunity and fatigue. *Neurosci Biobehav Rev* 1995; 19(3):439-45.
1521. Kieffer F. Trace elements: their importance for health and physical performance. *Dtsch Z Sportmed* 1986; 37(4):118-123.
1522. Oteiza PI, Olin KL, Fraga CG, Keen CL. Zinc deficiency causes oxidative damage to proteins, lipids and DNA in rat testes. *J Nutr* 1995; 125(4):823-9.
1523. Hsu JM. Zinc deficiency and alterations of free amino acid levels in plasma, urine and skin extract. *Prog Clin Biol Res* 1977; 14:73-86.
1524. Dorup I, Flyvbjerg A, Everts ME, Clausen T. Role of insulin-like growth factor-1 and growth hormone in growth inhibition induced by magnesium and zinc deficiencies. *Br J Nutr* 1991; 66(3):505-21.
1525. Ghavami-Maibodi SZ, Collipp PJ, Castro-Magana M, Stewart C, Chen SY. Effect of oral zinc supplements on growth, hormonal levels and zinc in healthy short children. *Ann Nutr Metab* 1983; 273:214-219.
1526. Hartoma TR, Nahoul K, Netter A. Zinc, plasma androgens and male sterility. *Lancet* 1977; 2:1125-1126.
1527. Hunt CD, Johnson PE, Herbel J, Mullen LK. Effects of dietary zinc depletion on seminal volume of zinc loss, serum testosterone concentrations and sperm morphology in young men. *Am J Clin Nutr* 1992; 56(1):148-157.
1527a. Ehara Y, Yamaguchi M. Zinc stimulates protein synthesis in the femoral-metaphyseal tissues of normal and skeletally unloaded rats. *Res Exp Med* 1997; 196(6):363-372.
1527b. Singh A, Failla ML, Deuster PA. Exercise-induced changes in immune function: effects of zinc supplementation. *J. Appl. Physiol.* 1994; 76(6):2298-303.
1528. Brilla LR, Haley TF. Effect of magnesium supplementation on strength training in humans. *J Am Coll Nutr* 1992; 11(3):326-9.
1529. Lefebvre PJ, Scheen AJ. Improving the action of insulin. Clinical & Investigative Medicine — *Med Clin Exp* 1995; 18(4):340-7.

1530. Richardson JH, Palmerton T, Chenan M. Effect of calcium on muscle fatigue. *J Sports Med Phys Fitness* 1980; 20(2):149-151.
1531. Anderson RA, Polansky MM, Bryden NA, et al. Effect of exercise (running) on serum glucose, insulin, glucagon, and chromium excretion. *Diabetes* 1982; 31(3):212-216.
1532. Lefavi RG, Anderson RA, Keith RE, et al. Efficacy of chromium supplementation in athletes: emphasis on anabolism. *Int J Sport Nutr* 1992; 2(2):111-22.
1533. Anderson RA. Chromium metabolism and its role in disease processes in man. *Clin Physiol Biochem* 1986; 4(1):31-41.
1534. McKenna MJ. The roles of ionic processes in muscular fatigue during intense exercise. *Sports Med* 1992; 13(2):134-45.
1535. Nassar-Gentina V, Passonneau JV, Rapoport SI. Fatigue and metabolism of frog muscle fibers during stimulation and in response to caffeine. *Am J Physiol* 1981; 241(3):C160-6.
1536. Kossler F, Lange F, Caffier G, Kuchler G. External potassium and action potential propagation in rat fast and slow twitch muscles. *Gen Physiol Biophys* 1991; 10(5):485-98.
1537. Renaud JM, Light P. Effects of K^+ on the twitch and tetanic contraction in the sartorius muscle of the frog, Rana pipiens. Implication for fatigue in vivo. *Can J Physiol Pharmacol* 1992; 70(9):1236-46.
1538. Flyvbjerg A, Dorup I, Everts ME, Orskov H. Evidence that potassium deficiency induces growth retardation through reduced circulating levels of growth hormone and insulin-like growth factor-1. *Metab Clin Exp* 1991; 40(8):769-75.
1539. Dorup I, Clausen T. Effects of potassium deficiency on growth and protein synthesis in skeletal muscle and the heart of rats. *Br J Nutr* 1989; 62(2):269-284.
1540. Schmidt GR. Therapeutics Of Fish Oil. Abstract of Meeting Presentation. ASHP Annual Meeting 1989; 46:1-33.
1541. Kremer JM, Bigauoette J, Michalek AV, et al. Effects of manipulation of dietary fatty acids on clinical manifestations of rheumatoid arthritis. *Lancet* 1985; 1:184-187.
1542. Herold PM, Kinsella JE. Fish oil consumption and decreased risk of cardiovascular disease: a comparison of findings from animal and human feeding trials. *Am J Clin Nutr* 1986; 43:566-598.
1543. Kelley VE, Ferretti A, Izui S, Strom TB. A fish oil diet rich in eicosapentaenoic acid reduces cyclo oxygenase metabolites and suppresses lupus in MRL-lpr mice. *J Immunol* 1985; 134:1914-1919.
1544. Hodgson JM, Wahlqvist ML, Boxall JA, Balazs ND. Can linoleic acid contribute to coronary artery disease?. *Am J Clin Nutr* 1993; 58(2):228-234.
1545. Smith RS. The cytokine theory of headache. *Med Hypotheses* 1992; 39(2):168-174.
1546. Alexander JW, Saito H, Trocki O, Ogle CK. The importance of lipid type in the diet after burn injury. *Ann Surg* 1986; 204:1-8.
1547. Trocki O, Heyd TJ, Waymack JP, Alexander JW. Effects of fish oil on postburn metabolism and immunity. *J Parenteral Enteral Nutr* 1987; 11:521-528.
1548. Baracos V, Rodemann HP, Dinarello CA, Goldberg AL. Stimulation of muscle protein degradation and prostaglandin E sub 2 release by leukocytic pyrogen (interleukin-1). A mechanism for the increased degradation of muscle proteins during fever. *N Engl J Med* 1983; 308:553-558.
1549. Goodnight SH, Harris WS, Connor WE, Illingworth DR. Polyunsaturated fatty acids, hyperlipidemia and thrombosis. *Arteriosclerosis* 1982; 2:87-111.
1550. Needleman P, Raz M, Minkes MS, et al. Triene prostaglandins: prostaglandin and thromboxane biosynthesis and unique biologic properties. *Proc Natl Acad Sci U.S.A.* 1979; 76:944-948.
1551. Endres S, Ghorbani R, Kelley VE, et al. The effect of dietary supplementation with n-3 polyunsaturated fatty acids on the synthesis of interleukin-1 and tumor necrosis factor by mononuclear cells. *N Engl J Med* 1989; 320:265-71.
1552. Dray F, Kouznetzova B, Harris D, Brazeau P. Role of prostaglandins on growth hormone secretion: PGE2 a physiological stimulator. *Adv Prostaglandin Thromboxane Res* 1980; 8:1321-8.
1553. Ip C, Singh M, Thompson HJ, Scimeca JA. Conjugated linoleic acid suppresses mammary carcinogenesis and proliferative activity of the mammary gland in the rat. *Cancer Res* 1994; 54(5):1212-5.
1554. Ip C, Scimeca JA, Thompson HJ. Conjugated linoleic acid. A powerful anticarcinogen from animal fat sources. [Review] *Cancer* 1994; 74(3 Suppl):1050-4.
1555. Pariza MW, Ha YL, Benjamin H, et al. Formation and action of anticarcinogenic fatty acids. *Adv Exp Med Biol* 1991; 289:269-72.
1556. Shultz TD, Chew BP, Seaman WR, Luedecke LO. Inhibitory effect of conjugated dienoic derivatives of linoleic acid and beta-carotene on the in vitro growth of human cancer cells. *Cancer Lett* 1992; 63(2):125-33.
1557. Cook ME, Miller CC, Park Y, Pariza M. Immune modulation by altered nutrient metabolism: nutritional control of immune-induced growth depression. *Poult Sci* 1993; 72(7):1301-5.
1558. Miller CC, Park Y, Pariza MW, Cook ME. Feeding conjugated linoleic acid to animals partially overcomes catabolic responses due to endotoxin injection. *Biochem Biophys Res Commun* 1994; 198(3):1107-12.
1559. Jahoor F, Peters EJ, Wolfe RR. The relationship between gluconeogenic substrate supply and glucose production in humans. *Am J Physiol* 1990; 258(2 Pt 1):E288-96.

1560. Gleeson M, Maughan RJ, and Greenhaff PL. Comparison of the effects of pre-exercise feeding of glucose, glycerol and placebo on endurance and fuel homeostasis in man. *Eur J Appl Physiol* 1986; 55:645-52.
1561. Zanoboni A, Schwarz D, Zanoboni-Muciaccia W. Glycerol metabolism. *Lancet* 1973; 2:628-633.
1562. Lyons TP, Riedesel ML, Meuli LE, Chick TW. Effects of glycerol-induced hyperhydration prior to exercise in the heat on sweating and core temperature. *Med Sci Sports Exerc* 1990; 22(4):477-83.
1563. Stanko RT, Sekas G, Isaacson IA, et al. Pyruvate inhibits clofibrate-induced hepatic peroxisomal proliferation and free radical production in rats. *Metab Clin Exp* 1995; 44(2):166-71.
1564. Borle AB, Stanko RT. Pyruvate reduces anoxic injury and free radical formation in perfused rat hepatocytes. *Am J Physiol* 1996; 270(3 Pt 1):G535-40.
1565. Stanko RT, Robertson RJ, Galbreath RW, et al. Enhanced leg exercise endurance with a high-carbohydrate diet and dihydroxyacetone and pyruvate. *J Appl Physiol* 1990; 69(5):1651-6.
1566. Stanko RT, Robertson RJ, Spina RJ, Reilly JJ Jr. Greenawalt KD. Goss FL. Enhancement of arm exercise endurance capacity with dihydroxyacetone and pyruvate. *J Appl Physiol* 1990; 68(1):119-24.
1567. Stanko RT, Diven WF, Robertson RJ, et al. Amino acid arterial concentration and muscle exchange during submaximal arm and leg exercise: the effect of dihydroxyacetone and pyruvate. *J Sports Sci* 1993; 11(1):17-23.
1568. Stanko RT, Tietze DL, Arch JE. Body composition, energy utilization, and nitrogen metabolism with a 4.25-MJ/d low-energy diet supplemented with pyruvate. *Am J Clin Nutr* 1992; 56(4):630-5.
1569. Stanko RT, Reynolds HR, Hoyson R, Janosky JE, Wolf R. Pyruvate supplementation of a low-cholesterol, low-fat diet: effects on plasma lipid concentrations and body composition in hyperlipidemic patients. *Am J Clin Nutr* 1994; 59(2):423-7.
1570. United States Patent numbers 4,158,057; 4,645,764; 4,874,790; 5,480,909; 5,134,162; 5,294,641; 5,283,260.
1571. McNaughton LR. The influence of caffeine ingestion on incremental treadmill running. *Br J Sports Med* 1986; 20(3):109-112.
1572. Williams JH. Caffeine, neuromuscular function and high-intensity exercise performance. J *Sports Med Phys Fitness* 1991; 31(3):481-489.
1573. Jacobson BH, Weber MD, Claypool L, Hunt LE. Effect of caffeine on maximal strength and power in elite male athletes. *Br J Sports Med* 1992; 26(4):276-280.
1574. Dodd SL, Herb RA, Powers SK. Caffeine and exercise performance. An update. *Sports Med* 1993; 15(1):14-23.
1575. Dulloo AG, Miller DS. Ephedrine, caffeine and aspirin: "over-the-counter" drugs that interact to stimulate thermogenesis in the obese. *Nutrition* 1989; 5(1):7-9.
1576. Horton TJ, Geissler CA. Post-prandial thermogenesis with ephedrine, caffeine, and aspirin in lean, pre-disposed obese and obese women. *Int J Obesity* 1996; 20:91-97.
1577. Daly PA, Krieger DR, Dulloo AG et al. Ephedrine, caffeine, and aspirin: safety and efficacy for treatment of human obesity. *Int J Obesity* 1993; 17:S73-S78.
1578. Sinha MK, Ohannesian JP, Heiman ML, et al. Nocturnal rise of leptin in lean, obese, and non-insulin-dependent diabetes mellitus subjects. *J Clin Invest* 1996; 97(5):1344-1347.
1579. Conley MS, Stone MH. Carbohydrate ingestion/supplementation or resistance exercise and training. *Sports Med* 1996; 21(1):7-17.
1580. Blommaart PJ, Charles R, Meijer AJ, Lamers WH. Changes in hepatic nitrogen balance in plasma concentrations of amino acids and hormones and in cell volume after overnight fasting in perinatal and adult rat. *Pediatr Res* 1995; 38(6):1018-25.
1581. Di Pasquale, MG. Vanadyl sulfate. *Anabolic Res Rev* 1996; 1(4):11-13.
1582. Diamond F Jr, Ringenberg L, MacDonald D, et al. Effects of drug and alcohol abuse upon pituitary-testicular function in adolescent males. *Adolesc Health Care* 1986; 7(1):28- 33.
1583. Barnett G, Chiang CW, Licko V J Effects of marijuana on testosterone in male subjects. Theor Biol 1983, 104 (4) p685-92.
1584. Mendelson JH, Meyer RE, Ellingboe J, et al. Effects of heroin and methadone on plasma cortisol and testosterone J Pharmacol Exp Ther 1975; 195(2):296-302.
1585. Cicero TJ, Meyer ER, Bell RD, Koch GA. Effects of morphine and methadone on serum testosterone and luteinizing hormone levels and on the secondary sex organs of the male rat. Endocrinology 1976; 98(2):367-372.
1586. Mendelson JH, Mello NK, Teoh SK, Ellingboe J, Cochin J. Cocaine effects on pulsatile secretion of anterior pituitary, gonadal, and adrenal hormones. J Clin Endocrinol Metab 1989; 69(6):1256-1260.
1587. Berul CI, Harclerode JE. Effects of cocaine hydrochloride on the male reproductive system. Life Sci 1989; 45(1):91- 5.
1588. Sarnyai Z, Mello NK, Mendelson JH, Eros-Sarnyai M, Mercer G. Effects of cocaine on pulsatile activity of hypothalamic-pituitary-adrenal axis in male rhesus monkeys: neuroendocrine and behavioral correlates. J Pharmacol Exp Ther 1996; 277(1):225-234.

1589. Budziszewska B, Jaworska-Feil L, Lason W. The effect of repeated amphetamine and cocaine administration on adrenal, gonadal and thyroid hormone levels in the rat plasma. *Exper. Clin. Endocrinol. Diabetes* 1996; 104(4):334-8.
1590. Zgliczynski W, Nowakowski J, Roslonowska E, et al. Alcohol decreases the alpha subunit, LH and testosterone secretion in response to LH-RH]. *Endokrynologia Polska* 1992; 43(3):257-62.
1591. Heikkonen E, Ylikahri R, Roine R, Valimaki M, Harkonen M, Salaspuro M. The combined effect of alcohol and physical exercise on serum testosterone, luteinizing hormone, and cortisol in males. *Alcohol Clin Exp Res* 1996; 20(4):711- 716.
1592. Karila T, Kosunen V, Leinonen A, Tahtela R, Seppala T. High doses of alcohol increase urinary testosterone-to- epitestosterone ratio in females 2E *J Chromatogr B Biomed Appl* 1996; 687(1):109-116.
1593. Cigolini M, Targher G, Bergamo Andreis IA, Tonoli M, Filippi F, Muggeo M, De Sandre G. Moderate alcohol consumption and its relation to visceral fat and plasma androgens in healthy women. *Int J Obes Relat Metab Disord* 1996; 20(3):206-212.
1594. American College of Sports Medicine. The use of alcohol in sports. *Med Sci Sports Exerc* 1982; 14: 481-2.
1595. Yardimci S, Atan A, Delibasi T, Sunguroglu K, Guven MC. Long-term effects of cigarette-smoke exposure on plasma testosterone, luteinizing hormone and follicle- stimulating hormone levels in male rats. *Br. J. Urol.* 1997; 79(1):66-9.
1596. Green KG, Heady A, Oliver MF. Blood pressure, cigarette smoking and heart attack in the WHO cooperative trial of clofibrate. *Int J Epidemiol* 1989; 18:355-360.
1597. Attia AM, el-Dakhly MR, Halawa FA, Ragab NF, Mossa MM. Cigarette smoking and male reproduction. *Arch Androl* 1989; 23(1):45-49.
1598. Meikle AW, Bishop DT, Stringham JD, Ford MH. Relationship between body mass index, cigarette smoking, and plasma sex steroids in normal male twins. *Genet Epidemiol* 1989; 6(3):399-412.
1599. Patterson TR, Stringham JD, Meikle AW. Nicotine and cotinine inhibit steroidogenesis in mouse Leydig cells. *Life Sci* 1990; 46(4):265-272.
1600. Yeh J, Barbieri RL, Friedman AJ. Nicotine and cotinine inhibit rat testis androgen biosynthesis in vitro. *J Steroid Biochem* 1989; 33(4A):627-630.
1601. Segarra AC, Strand FL. Perinatal administration of nicotine alters subsequent sexual behavior and testosterone levels of male rats. *Brain Res* 1989; 480(1- 2):151-159.
1602. Favaretto AL. Valenca MM. Picanco-Diniz DL. Antunes- Rodrigues JA. Inhibitory role of cholinergic agonists on testosterone secretion by purified rat Leydig cells. Archives Internationales de Physiologie, de Biochimie et de Biophysique. 101(6):333-5, 1993 Nov-Dec.
1603. Sellini M, Sartori MP, Baccarini S, Bassi R, Dimitriadis E. [ACTH and cortisol after cigarette smoke exposure during the dexamethasone suppression test in smokers and non-smokers]. *Boll Soc Ital Biol Sper* 1989; 65(4)
1604. Sellini M, Sartori MP, Letizia C, Dimitriadis E, Bassi R, Baccarini S. [Changes in the levels of ACTH and cortisol after passive exposure to cigarette smoke in smokers and non-smokers]. *Boll Soc Ital Biol Sper* 1989; 65(4):365- 369.
1605. Field AE, Colditz GA, Willett WC, Longcope C, McKinlay JB. The relation of smoking, age, relative weight, and dietary intake to serum adrenal steroids, sex hormones, and sex hormone-binding globulin in middle-aged men. *J. Clin. Endocrinol. Metab.* 1994; 79(5):1310-6.
1606. Eriksen WB, Brage S. Bruusgaard D. Does smoking aggravate musculoskeletal pain?. *Scand. J. Rheumatol.* 1997; 26(1):49-54.
1607. Nair KS; Woolf PD; Welle SL; Matthews DE. Leucine, glucose, and energy metabolism after 3 days of fasting in healthy human subjects. *Am J Clin Nutr* 1987; 46(4):557-62.
1608. Forbes GB; Brown MR; Welle SL; Underwood LE. Hormonal response to overfeeding. *Am J Clin Nutr* Apr 1989, 49 (4) p608-11.
1609. Kelley DE, Slasky BS, Janosky J. Skeletal muscle density: effects of obesity and non-insulin-dependent diabetes mellitus. Am. J. Clin. Nutr. 1991; 54(3):509-15.
1610. Marks BL, Ward A, Morris DH, Castellani J, Rippe JM. Fat-free mass is maintained in women following a moderate diet and exercise program. *Med Sci Sports Exerc* 1995; 27(9):1243-1251.
1611. Marks BL, Ward A, Morris DH, Castellani J, Rippe JM. Fat-free mass is maintained in women following a moderate diet and exercise program. *Med Sci Sports Exerc* 1995; 27(9):1243-1251.
1612. Marks BL, Rippe JM. The importance of fat free mass maintenance in weight loss programmes. *Sports Medicine* 1996; 22(5):273-81.
1613. Bouchard C, Perusse L, Deriaz O, Despres JP, Tremblay A. Genetic influences on energy expenditure in humans. [Review] [23 refs] Crit. Rev. Food Sci. Nutr. 1993; 33(4-5):345-50.
1614. Oppert JM, Nadeau A, Tremblay A, et al. Plasma glucose, insulin, and glucagon before and after long-term overfeeding in identical twins. *Metabolism: Clinical & Experimental* 1995; 44(1):96-105.
1615. Horton TJ, Drougas H, Brachey A, Reed GW, Peters JC, Hill JO. Fat and carbohydrate overfeeding in humans: different effects on energy storage. *Am. J. Clin. Nutr.* 1995; 62(1):19-29.
1616. Flatt JP. Use and storage of carbohydrate and fat. [Review] *Am. J. Clin. Nutr.* 1995; 61(4 Suppl):952S-959S.

1617. *The Anabolic Diet.* By Mauro Di Pasquale, M.D. Published by OTS. 1995.
1618. Hill JO, DiGirolamo M. Preferential loss of body fat during starvation in dietary obese rats. *Life Sci* 1991; 49(25):1907-1914.
1619. Sidery MB, Gallen IW, Macdonald IA. The initial physiological responses to glucose ingestion in normal subjects are modified by a 3 day high-fat diet. *Br J Nutr* 1990; 64(3):705-13.
1620. Bhathena SJ, Berlin E, Judd JT, et al. Dietary fat and menstrual-cycle effects on the erythrocyte ghost insulin receptor in premenopausal women. *Am J Clin Nutr* 1989; 50(3):460-4.
1621. Fawcett JP, Farquhar SJ, Walker RJ, et al. The effect of oral vanadyl sulfate on body composition and performance in weight-training athletes. *Int J Sport Nutr* 1996; 6(4):382-390.
1622. Gil J, Miralpeix M, Carreras J, Bartrons R. Insulin-like effects of vanadate on glucokinase activity andfructose 2,6-bisphosphate levels in the liver of diabetic rats. *J Biol Chem* 1988; 263:1868-71. 14
1623. Tsiani E, Abdullah N, Fantus IG. Insulin-mimetic agents vanadate and pervanadate stimulate glucose but inhibit amino acid uptake. *Am J Physiol* 1997; 272(1 Pt 1):C156-C162.

REFERENCE BOOKS AND NEWLETTERS

The following books and newsletters have been written by Mauro Di Pasquale, M.D.

Drug Use and Detection in Amateur Sports, five updates, published 1984-1989.
Beyond Anabolic Steroids, published 1990.
Drugs in Sports, newsletters published 1991-1995.
Anabolic Research Review, newsletter by Mauro Di Pasquale. Published 1995–1996 by Iron Man Publishing, Oxnard, CA.
Bodybuilding Supplement Review, by Mauro Di Pasquale. OTS, Visalia, CA, 1995.
Anabolic Diet, by Mauro Di Pasquale. OTS, Visalia, CA, 1995.

The following books have been published by CRC Press Inc., Boca Raton, FL.

Adaptation in Sports Training, by Atko Viru. Published 1995.
Advanced Nutrition: Macronutrients, by Carolyn D. Berdainier. Published 1995.
Amino Acid Metabolism and Therapy in Health and Nutritional Disease, edited by L.A. Cynober. Published 1995.
Foods and Nutrition Encyclopedia, Volumes I and II, 2nd edition, edited by A.H. Ensminger, M.E. Ensminger, J.E. Konlande, and J.R.K. Robson. Published in 1994.
Handbook of Dairy Foods and Nutrition, edited by G.D. Miller, J.K. Jarvis, and L.D. McBean. Published 1995.
Hormones in Muscular Activity, Volumes I and II by Atko Viru. Published 1985.
Nitrogen Metabolism and Excretion, edited by P.J. Walsh and P. Wright. Published 1995.
Nutrition in Exercise and Sport, 2nd edition, edited by I. Wolinsky and J.F. Hickson, Jr. Published 1994.
Nutritional Ergogenic Aids For Sports and Exercise, by Luke R. Bucci. Published 1993.

The following books have been published by other publishers.

Exercise Metabolism, edited by M. Hargreaves. Published by Human Kinetics, Champaign, IL, 1995.
Exercise Physiology, 3rd edition, edited by W.D. McArdle, I.F. Katch, and V.L. Katch. Published by Lea & Febiger, Philadelphia, 1991.
Periodization of Strength, by T. O. Bompa. Published by Veritas Publishing, Toronto, Ontario, Canada, 1993.
Textbook of Medical Physiology, 9th edition, edited by A.C. Guyton and J.E. Hall. Published by W.B. Saunders, Philadelphia, 1996.
The World of the Cell, 2nd edition, edited by W.M. Becker and D.W. Deamer. Published by Benjamin/Cummings, Redwood City, CA, 1991.

INDEX

A

B

C

H

I

J

K

L

R

T

U

V

W

Y

Z